LANGUAGE PRODUCTION

Volume 2

Development, Writing and Other Language Processes

Edited by

B. Butterworth

Department of Psychology,
University College London,
England

1983

ACADEMIC PRESS

A Subsidiary of Harcourt Brace Jovanovich, Publishers

London   New York
Paris   San Diego   San Francisco
São Paolo   Sydney   Tokyo   Toronto

ACADEMIC PRESS INC. (LONDON) LTD
24/28 Oval Road,
London NW1 7DX

United States Edition published by
ACADEMIC PRESS INC.
111 Fifth Avenue,
New York, New York 10003

British Library Cataloguing in Publication Data
Language production
    Vol. 2
    1. Psycholinguistics
    I. Butterworth, B.
    418   P37
    ISBN 0-12-147502-6

Typeset by Oxford Verbatim Limited
Printed in Great Britain by
St. Edmundsbury Press,
Bury St. Edmunds

Contributors

Dr B. BUTTERWORTH, Department of Psychology, University College London, Gower Street, London WC1E 6BT, UK

Dr W. E. COOPER, Department of Psychology, 1204 William James Hall, Harvard University, 33 Kirkland Street, Cambridge, Massachusetts 02138, USA

Dr J. DOCKRELL, Department of Psychology, University of Stirling, Stirling, FK9 9LA, UK

Dr N. HARVEY, Department of Psychology, University College London, Gower Street, London WC1E 6BT, UK

Dr W. H. N. HOTOPF, Psychology Department, London School of Economics, Houghton Street, London WC2A 2AE, UK

Dr P. HOWELL, Department of Psychology, University College London, Gower Street, London WC1E 6BT, UK

Dr J. MCSHANE, Department of Psychology, London School of Economics, Houghton Street, London WC2A 2AE, UK

Dr L. MENN, Aphasia Research Center, Boston V. A., Medical Center, 150 S. Huntington Avenue, Boston, Massachusetts, USA

Dr G. TERZUOLO, Department of Physiology, Medical School, University of Minnesota, 6-255 Millard Hall, 435 Delaware Street S.E., Minneapolis, Monnesota 55455, USA

Dr P. VIVIANI, Istituto di Fisiologia dei Centri Nervosi-CNR, 9 via Mario Bianco, Milan 20131, Italy

Dr E. ZURIF, Aphasia Research Center, Boston V.A. Medical Center, 150 S. Huntington Avenue, Boston, Massachusetts 02130, USA

Preface

In this volume, we complete our survey of language production, by focusing on the relation between speaking and other language abilities. Each chapter is intended as a detailed review of an aspect of this relation.

In the first section, the development of speech in children comes under scrutiny. *Lise Menn* describes the emergence of articulatory skills in the context of the development of wider phonological abilities, abilities which underlie understanding as well as speaking. *John McShane and Julie Dockrell* discuss the child's growing control of vocabulary and syntactic constructions in speech against a background of conversational interaction with adult language-users, and general demands of cognitive processing and cognitive growth.

In the second section, we turn to language production in a non-speech modality – writing, and we ask what special motoric and cognitive constraints shape our ability to produce language in this way. *Paolo Viviani and Carlo Terzuolo* examine the organization of control of writing movements, and also typing, in relation to more general issues of motor control on the one hand, and to linguistic units on the other. *Norman Hotopf* compares errors of writing – "slips of the hand" – with errors in speech, to tease out the structural homologies and the processing connexions between the two.

In the third section, we examine more generally the relations among speech and the other language modalities. *Peter Howell and Nigel Harvey* explore the different and often competing demands of articulation and of hearing on the structure of linguistic units. *William Cooper and Edgar Zurif* review evidence from language breakdown to assess the extent of structures and processes common to production and comprehension. In the final chapter, I look at how words are stored in memory, and whether speakers need separate lexical representations for speaking, hearing, reading and writing.

Since Volume 1 was published, a contributor to that volume and one of the pioneers of psycholinguistic research, Frieda Goldman-Eisler, has died. Volume 2 is dedicated to her memory.

London, July 1982   Brian Butterworth

Contents

Preface vi

Section I. Development of speaking skills 1

1. Development of articulatory, phonetic, and phonological
   capabilities 3
   L. MENN
   I. Introduction 3
      A. Background
      B. Plan of exposition
   II. The transition from babbling to speech 5
   III. Constructing a model of early phonological knowledge 8
      A. The input lexicon: representation of the adult word
      B. Segments, phones, and phonemic contrasts
      C. Strategies for dealing with words and sounds
   IV. Rule creation 21
      A. Extending the notion of "ease of articulation"
         One key to a new theory
      B. "Natural processes"
      C. Non-natural rules
      D. Rule origin and growth
      E. Overgeneralization
   V. Towards a psychological model of phonological
      development 28
      A. The theoretical importance of lexical exceptions and
         overgeneralizations
      B. Phonological idioms
      C. Canonical forms
      D. Motor programming: a psycholinguistic account of
         output constraints and canonical forms
      E. The articulatory program and the general model
   VI. Saying what one hears: task variables 36
      A. Imitation, self-monitoring and spontaneous speech
      B. The word as means to an end
   VII. The acquisition of allophones and allomorphs 41
   VIII. Summary and conclusion 43

2. Lexical and grammatical development 51
   J. McSHANE and J. DOCKRELL
   I. Developmental considerations for a model of
      production 52

II. Lexical development 54
    A. What develops in a lexicon?
    B. Overextension of names
    C. Production and comprehension of names
    D. "Nouns", "verbs", and other objects of wonder
    E. Input for lexical development
III. Grammatical development 70
    A. What develops in a grammar?
    B. Early studies of two-word combinations
    C. Semantic models of two-word combinations
    D. Beyond two-word combinations
    E. Inducing syntactic rules
    F. Input for grammatical development
IV. Conclusion 90

Section II. Production of language in non-speech modalities 101

3. The organization of movement in handwriting and typing 103
   P. VIVIANI and C. TERZUOLO
    I. Introduction 103
   II. Biomechanical and control aspects 105
    A. Handwriting
    B. Typing
  III. Linguistic factors in typing 124
    A. Words are the basic units of motor action
    B. Evidence of higher order contextual imprints in
      the motor prosody
  IV. Conclusions 138

4. Lexical slips of the pen and tongue: what they tell us about
   language production 147
   W. H. N. HOTOPF
    I. Introduction 147
   II. Summary with elaborations of previous position 149
    A. Description of the samples and types of slip at
      lexical level
    B. Categories of lexical slip
    C. Basis of distributional differences between slips
      in speech and writing
    D. Distributional differences between speech and
      writing at the phoneme/letter level
  III. Is input to writing at the lexical level exclusively
    phonological or not? 165
    A. Procedure for identifying structural slips by
      phonemes or by letters

IV. Causes of structural slips of the pen 169
    A. How language is produced in speech and writing
    B. Slips in verbal thinking and in the phonological and
       graphological programs
    C. Deterioration in short-term memory
    D. Misspelling
    E. Access malapropisms
    F. Contextual causes of structural slips
    G. Misinterpreting visual feedback
    H. Summing up

**Section III. Commonalities and differences between production
and perception** 201

5. Perceptual equivalence and motor equivalence in speech 203
   P. HOWELL and N. HARVEY
    I. Introduction 203
    II. Problems of equivalence 204
      A. Production of the same signal in different ways
      B. Articulators in the same position with the signal
        varying
      C. Variation in both articulator positioning and the
        signal
    III. Proposed solutions to problems of equivalence 209
      A. Perception and production as independent processes
      B. Non-independence of perception and production
    IV. The state of play: summary and assessment 219

6. Aphasia: Information-processing in language production and
   reception 225
   W. E. COOPER and E. B. ZURIF
    I. Introduction 225
    II. Some clinical phenomena 226
    III. Comprehension deficits and their relation to production
      deficits in Broca's aphasia 228
      A. Parallels between comprehension and production
      B. Processing accounts of the grammatical limitation
      C. Relations between comprehension and production
        reconsidered
    IV. Comprehension deficits and their relation to production
      deficits in the fluent aphasias 233
      A. Wernicke's aphasia
      B. Anomic aphasia
    V. Speech prosody in aphasia 238
    VI. Broca's aphasia 241

    VII. Wernicke's aphasia 246
   VIII. Conclusion 250

7. Lexical representation 257
  B. BUTTERWORTH
     I. Introduction 257
    II. The full listing hypothesis 261
      A. FLH: evidence from speech production
      B. FLH: evidence from speech perception
      C. FLH: evidence from reading
   III. Unit type 273
      A. Unit type candidates
      B. Evidence from speech production
      C. Evidence from reading
      D. Evidence from writing
      E. Conclusions on unit type
   IV. Modality-specific lexical representations 280
      A. Evidence from the comparison of modalities
      B. Modality-specific language breakdown
    V. Organization of lexical representations 286
      A. Frequency organization
      B. Are content words and function words listed separately?
      C. Are compound forms listed under their bases?
   VI. Conclusions 289

AUTHOR INDEX 295

SUBJECT INDEX 303

I

Development of Speaking Skills

1

Development of Articulatory, Phonetic, and Phonological Capabilities

L. Menn   *Boston University School of Medicine*

I. Introduction

A. Background

A rather large body of information about the early stages of the acquisition of phonology of English and some other languages (Spanish, Mandarin, Thai) has become available over the last decade or so, and the theory of acquisition of phonology has not only grown, but has changed its nature considerably. Since about 1974, we have moved away from a model in which phonological development was considered to resemble the differentiation of an embryo. In its place we have evolved a notion of the young child as a creature of some intelligence who is trying to solve a problem: the problem of sounding like her companions when communicating with them. This shift of model took place as more diary and small-group studies were published, and in the context of Slobin's similar approach to the acquisition of morphology and syntax (Slobin, 1966; 1973).

In recent years, the study of child phonology has also become distinctly more psychological in the explanatory concepts that it employs. This is largely because the richer data base has made it possible to see a considerable range of individual differences among children. Faced with such diversity, we have had to look below the surface for an underlying unity; and in doing so, we have begun to invoke notions of processing and storage of information in addition to the linguistic notions of articulatory control and phonemic contrast.

In this chapter, I will review the strategies that children are presently believed to use in acquiring phonology, and I will give an account of the psycholinguistic model of early phonology which I think is presently the

LANGUAGE PRODUCTION VOL. 2
ISBN 0-12-147502-6

most adequate. For more extensive discussion, in addition to the references which will be cited, the reader should see the many important papers collected in Yeni-Komshian *et al.* (1980).

B. Plan of Exposition

We will begin this summary of the acquisition of phonology by looking at the transition from babble to speech in Section II. This is necessary so that we can understand the problems of defining which early vocalizations a theory of child phonology attempts to account for.

Then we shall undertake the construction of a model of child phonology that will allow us to deal separately with three different kinds of information that the child is acquiring: (1) knowledge of how words sound, (2) knowledge of how to pronounce them, and (3) knowledge of allomorphy or abstract phonology, manifested as the relationships among words or morphs that sound somewhat different but are the same in meaning.

In Section III.A, we shall discuss the child's perceptual knowledge of the sounds of language; in Section III.B, we will pause to discuss problems with the notion of "phoneme" in early stages of phonological development. In Section III.C, we will turn to the traditional subject matter of child phonology: the ways in which children pronounce the words of the adult language (Section III.C.2). We will see, however, that modifying the pronunciation of a word is only one type of reaction to the complexities of adult phonotactics; the other type of reaction is the avoidance of particular sound patterns (Section III.C.1). These behaviours can be unified, at least in the early stages of acquisition, by the formal descriptive device of saying that children obey phonological output constraints (Section III.C.3), and data from variety of children are presented which support this description.

In Section IV, we consider how a child may go about inventing rules to derive her output forms from the forms spoken by adults; Section IV.A extends the idea of "ease of articulation" by including skill already acquired at a point in time as a factor affecting the "ease" of a new sound. In Section IV.B, the notion of "naturalness" in child phonology is discussed, and we consider how it can be related to our account of rule-creation. In Section IV.C, we note the non-natural rules that children can also create, including those which appear to stem from a dim awareness of the fact that allomorphy exists in the adult language. Section IV.D describes data on rule origin and growth, and Section IV.E concerns rule overgeneralization.

Section V presents the notion that early phonological development should be viewed as the development of skill in the ability to program and execute complex motor sequences. It begins by noting the theoretical importance of the two irregular phenomena that are most difficult for conventional approaches to deal with: overgeneralizations of rules of child phonology (Section V.A) and phonological idioms (Section V.B). Then the regular pattern of the arrangement of children's early words into families of canonical forms is recalled in Section V.C. Section V.D attempts to account for these three fundamental types of data within a unified two-stage model of articulatory motor programming.

In Section V.E, we see how this model can be fitted into the overall picture of child phonology that was set up in Section III.A; we flex its explanatory muscles in dealing with rules and rule changes, and we consider some of its conceptual limitations in subsection V.E.3 entitled "Caution: The Limitations of the Programming Metaphor".

In Section VI, we deal with some difficult logical and methodological topics: the relation of imitated to "spontaneous" productions and the nature of children's metalinguistic ability to focus on pronunciation as a task (Section VI.A). These are related to the perennial problem of why some sounds may appear in babble but not in speech (Section VI.B). (Section VI may be considered logically prior to most of the rest of the chapter).

Section VII, "The Acquisition of Allophones and Allomorphs", turns to the other major branch of developmental phonology, and gives a brief outline of this topic, especially as it relates to questions of psychological reality. The reader is referred to MacWhinney's (1978) monograph on this topic, since including a full account of it would double the length of the chapter.

Finally, Section VIII, lists the major findings of the past decade of research in developmental phonology, recalls the motor programming model for the beginning stages of acquisition of phonology which was proposed in Section V, and briefly contrasts the working assumptions of the current approach with those of the preceding "Jakobsonian" era.

Note: Some longitudinal studies will be cited repeatedly in this chapter. For convenience, unless otherwise noted, references to "Hildegard" are from Moskowitz 1970b (originally, of course, from Leopold 1939), to "Daniel" from Menn (1971), to "Si" from Macken (1979); to "Jacob" from Menn (1976a,b); and to "Amahl" from Smith (1973).

II. The Transition from Babbling to Speech

We can usually assume that phonology deals with sound patterns of words, but even in adult languages we must decide whether the phonology that we write should attempt to include certain marginal items, for example onomatopoeic representations of animal cries and noises. In studying early child phonology, this problem, marginal in dealing with most adult languages, becomes central. There is no ready-made solution to it; in this section, I will just attempt to show the nature of the difficulty.

There seem to be three definable types of utterances found during the transition period that we call "the onset of speech": sound-play, proto-words, and modulated babble. Modulated babble refers to the use of strings of sounds which appear to carry meaning only by their intonation contour.

This is also called "jargon" and it can be very eloquent and effective vocal communication. Since our concern is with the development of articulation, we will not discuss modulated babble further here; the reader is referred to von Raffler-Engel (1973) and Menn (1976a,b).

Sound-play, which may include word-practice, is not communicative behaviour; in other words, when we classify an utterance as sound-play, we do so because there is no indication of any association between recurrent context and recurrent sound-play patterns. One can of course say that sound-play is expressive of a cheerful mood, but in that weak sense, any evidence of mood is communicative. Joint sound-play is another matter; it is certainly communicative action, but it seems to be absent or rare in adult–child pairs in our culture when the child appears mature enough to be on the threshhold of speech, although it is certainly found with young infants (see Sterne *et al.*, 1975; Snow 1977).

Proto-words are articulated meaningful utterances; some of them are directed to others (one can tell because the child gets annoyed if no-one responds), and some are solo performances. These are our objects of study, for only here can we be certain that the child is trying to say a word – that is, trying to match a desired perceived target. And again, we judge that they are meaningful because of a recurrent association between sound and situation, (although obviously if what appears to be a clear token of an adult word is uttered just once in a context for which it is strikingly appropriate, it is usually included as a meaningful utterance).

A child may have all of these utterance types for a period of several months. Some utterances, furthermore, may contain elements that belong to more than one class: for example, a child may start playing sound-games with a "real" word (Weir 1962; Menn 1976a), or he may address one with an utterance that has a real word or two embedded in modulated babble (Jones, 1967). And of course, in practice, some utterances are hard to classify, since classification depends in part on surmising the child's intent.

The important point here is that clear cases can easily be found, and that a child may have one, two, or all three of these utterance types for a period of many months. The "silent period", despite the emphasis given to it in the older literature, is a rare phenomenon.

There is a fourth type of utterance that we should mention. Some children's early attack on language proceeds by global approximation to long phrases rather than by attempts at single words or short phrases. Their early efforts at speech are characterized by variable and often "loose" articulation which is extremely hard to transcribe; Ann Peters (1977) dubbed these children "mush-mouth kids". In this chapter, we shall consider only children who take the more segmental word-by-word approach to phonology; the reader who is interested in the "global" approach should see the Peters article and also Branigan (1979).

Proto-words now need to be defined more carefully. They are vocables (articulated utterances) which recur in definable contexts. One might fear that this notion of recurrent definable contexts would be very difficult to use, but it generally is not, because a one-year-old's activities tend to fall into identifiable behavioural routines, some solo and some partnered. These include favourite manipulations on objects (putting things into things), games (peekaboo), directing an adult's attention (pointing), obtaining things (requesting/demanding), offering things, greetings, farewells, and so on. Halliday (1975) describes such pairs of vocalization and behavioural routine in elegant detail; see also Menn (1976a), Clumeck (1977). The meaning of a proto-word is originally very limited, and is best characterized as "what you say when you do X". Proto-words may thus usefully be considered as one type of vocal signal; they are not yet symbols, because each of them is bound to the performance of its routine; it cannot be used freely in new contexts. At some point, however, first singly and then more rapidly, some of the proto-words start to be used in more situations, and thus they begin to acquire the symbolic autonomy of the true word. For example, a "woof-woof" vocable may be initially used only when a child is pointing to a picture of a dog; then it may be generalized rapidly to pointing to real and toy dogs, and yet it may take months to become usable in requesting a toy dog. Incidentally, proto-words do not have to have adult words as models (Halliday, 1975), and some without adult models may even make the transition to becoming true symbols (Menn, 1976a, Menn and Haselkorn, 1977).

Proto-words are, by definition, the first units for which a child is trying to produce a particular articulated sound-pattern for communication (always excepting the whole-phrase efforts of the "mush-mouth kids"). If we wish to make generalizations about the child's first phones, or to evaluate the applicability of terms such as "phoneme" to the onset of speech, we must look into the period when proto-words are first being produced. Sometimes what we see is a handful of nicely-defined CV(CV) shapes, as tradition would have it: [papa], [mama], [dada]. A good example is given in Ferguson, Weeks, and Peizer (1973). But more often, apparently, the early picture shows quite a mixture of forms: some vowelless items, perhaps, such as [m::], or Hildegard's [ʃ::]; some "traditional" CV(CV) shapes and/or some (C)VC and VCV shapes; perhaps an isolated word with a consonant cluster (Hildegard, again); and some wildly fluctuating forms that seem to originate from rather complex adult target words (e.g. Jacob's renditions of "thank-you", which showed an endless variation including [deigʌ], [geigu], [gigo], [giːdo], [dejo], [dido], [dætʌ], [ɣitʌ]).

Summarizing this section: the transition from babbling to speech is typically gradual, and may involve any combination of four types of utterances: sound-play, modulated babble (using meaningful or possibly meaningful intonation contour), whole-phrase efforts, and proto-words. Proto-words are meaningful utterances with phonetically definable targets; however, the phonetic definition may be quite loose by the standards of adult phonetic target-matching and the meaning may be very limited and situation-bound. We will take child phonology as beginning with proto-words, and, in Section III.B we will examine the problem of applying adult-based phonological concepts to these "first words".

III. Constructing a Model of Early Phonological Knowledge

In this section, we will undertake the description of some aspects of "early phonological knowledge". This includes what children, in the first months of speaking, seem to know about the sounds of words in adult language (perceptual knowledge), about the relations among those sounds (phonological knowledge, including knowledge of segmentation and phonemic contrasts), and about how to pronounce words.

The most striking fact about early child words has always been how simplified most of them are compared to their adult models. What has made child phonology an object for study has been three realizations about these "simplified forms": that there are generally systematic relations among a given child's words, that there are generally systematic relations between the child's word and the adult model word, and that it is possible, by comparing children who have very different ways of dealing with adult words, to come up with a general theory of why and how these "generally systematic" relations exist. These three realizations will be developed in this section and in the two which follow.

Note: Beginning in this section, I will occasionally draw small flow-chart diagrams in order to keep track of the various capacities for processing and storage that we postulate in order to account for the child's language behaviour. It is important to keep in mind that the entities and processes represented by these boxes and arrows are only hypothetical constructs, and that even the best guesses among them must be grossly oversimplified compared to whatever it is that we have in our heads.

A. The Input Lexicon: Representation of the Adult Word

"Lexicon" is a word whose precise meaning varies from user to user, but it at least denotes a collection of stored, accessible, memorized bits of information about the sounds and meanings of words and/or their component meaningful parts. We must grant that something which should be called a lexicon exists in the human individual; that is, there must be some form of long-term storage containing at least a sketchy encoding of the sound-pattern and meaning which is accessible when we recognize and understand a word.

In order to say a word spontaneously and meaningfully, one must also have access to stored information about how it sounds and what it means; a standing controversy is whether this knowledge is best represented by postulating a separate "output lexicon" or whether both recognition and production information are best conceived of as being in a single lexicon. [See Chapters 6 and 7.]

To advocate a single lexicon in a psycholinguistic model of child phonology is to hypothesize that the rules which create the child's output form from her input form operate in real time; to advocate a two-lexicon model is to claim that a form "closer" to the output form is also stored and that this second form is used as a basis for production. Much of the data that we will consider can be handled more gracefully in a two-lexicon model than in a one-lexicon model; I think the two-lexicon model is likely to be a better approximation to what we really utilize in speaking, and so I will use it in this chapter. It is by no means universally accepted as the superior model (cf. N. V. Smith, 1978), however, and formally all the data that it handles can be managed in a one-lexicon system, by the use of markings on each lexical entry specifying which rules apply to it in the event of competing rules applying to the same domain.

We shall say, then, that two forms may be stored for each word: a recognition form and a production form. The collection of words (form-meaning pairs) that a speaker can recognize and understand is called the "input lexicon"; it could equally well be called the "recognition lexicon" or the "passive lexicon". The collection of words that a speaker can use (that is, the information necessary to use them meaningfully and to pronounce them) is referred to as the "output lexicon", but could also be thought of as the "active lexicon". (This active/passive dichotomy is usually thought of as a matter of knowledge of word meaning rather than pronunciation, but the extension of it to include knowledge of pronunciation seems to capture the right distinction.) So far, then, we have the rudimentary diagram shown in Fig. 1.

[Collection of percepts/understandings]
↓
[Input lexicon]
↓
[Output lexicon]

FIG. 1

Let us explore the properties that can be ascribed to the input lexicon. We know that speech perception is an active process: the hearer filters and structures the incoming sound. Several researchers, including Waterson (1970, 1972), Ingram (1974), Hawkins (1973), Macken (1979) and Wilbur (1980), have called attention to the possibility that a child may not succeed at first in getting a complete picture of a word he has begun to learn. Therefore, we may be more accurate in particular cases if we represent the child's knowledge of some part of the word's sound pattern by "noise" (Ingram, 1974) or by underspecified phonemes (archiphonemes, macrophonemes). These are useful notational devices whenever we have reason to believe that, for example, a child has not figured out what sounds are present in the unstressed syllable of a word or has been unable to tell which of several fricatives a word ends with. To be more explicit, these devices are useful notations whenever the child apparently cannot distinguish perceptually among particular sets of similar words.

Note that we cannot rely on the child's pronunciation to let us know what perceptual distinctions she is making, for children can in fact frequently tell the difference between two words while they are still unable to pronounce either one of them. (Wilbur points out in personal communication that in adults, cross-dialect phenomena continue to give examples of perception outstripping production: American Midwesterners who do not distinguish among /ɛ,æ,e/ before /r/ in their speech nevertheless can reliably distinguish "merry", "marry", and "Mary" in the speech of those who do make the distinction.)

To give two simple examples of the use of these notations for incomplete phonetic input information: suppose that a certain child appears unable to distinguish between two words which differ only in the shape of a pretonic syllable, such as "along" and "belong", but that she can distinguish them from "long". Then "noise" marker would be appropriate to represent the first syllable of iambic words in the input lexicon.

Now suppose that we have a child who cannot distinguish /bæs, bæθ, bæf/ from one another at an above-chance level in an appropriate test situation, but who can tell them from /bæt, bæv/. Here, the child has some knowledge of the final sound of, say, "bath", so we would not use a noise-marker. Instead, we would say that "bath" is entered as /bæ (unvoiced fricative)/ in the child's input lexicon.

So, what we have been saying is that the child's ability to use acoustic features to discriminate meaningful words is typically well ahead of her ability to control those features for making contrasts in production, but may well be inferior to the linguistic discrimination ability of the adult. Some discrimination which the child appears to make may in fact be carried out partly on the basis of extra-linguistic information and linguistic context. For, like all of us, a child's ability to "hear" is conditioned by her expectations of what she is about to hear. This factor is important to emphasize for two reasons. One will be discussed in Section VI. where we will explore some implications of Barton's (1976) work which shows that unfamiliar words in minimal-pair tests of discrimination ability tend to be misheard as familiar ones. This biases the tests and increases the difficulty of ascertaining what the child's input lexical representation of a word "really is".

The other reason for bringing up the notion of the child's expectations is the following phenomenon: Macken (1979) and Platt and MacWhinney (1983) have argued that we sometimes have good evidence for the following sequence of events. First, a child learns to recognize the sounds of a word adequately but cannot produce it very well: we say that the input representation is good, but not the output representation. Usually, the child will then slowly bring the production into line with the target, but in certain cases, expected improvements fail to occur in particular words or sets of words. The child maintains his old pronunciation in such a way that it seems that he is no longer even trying to match the adult model. Instead, it seems that he has replaced his original input representation with a new one which is based on his own output. For example, Macken (1979) gives this analysis for certain events reported by Smith (1973). Amahl, his subject, produced the word "take" as [Geik] at an early stage, using a general velar assimilation rule (a type of rule which we will shortly be discussing in some detail). The rule stopped operating for all other words by Smith's "stage 14", but Amahl retained a velar-harmonized form for "take" until "stage 22", and even created a participle [kukən] for "taken" at "stage 18".

Now, if a child maintains his own form when he is capable of improving it, it must mean that he has temporarily stopped monitoring, stopped really listening to himself and/or to the adult model. He expects that he is correct, and does not bother to check up. Indeed, many of us have adult acquaintances who have an idiosyncratic pronunciation of some word, and who seem quite unaware that they are not speaking as other people do. Many irregularities in children's phonological behaviour thus seem to be explainable in terms of the biasing of perception by expectation.

B. Segments, Phones, and Phonemic Contrasts

Now we will consider the early stages of the production of proto-words and words. Early child speech is often called pre-phonemic (Nakazima, 1972; Menyuk, 1977). There are very good reasons for this. One is that phonemic contrast and phonetic control do not develop in synchrony. One example of this sort of uneven development can occur when a child honours a contrast without being able to handle the relevant phonetics at all. So we may find a child who renders the voicing contrast in word-final position by deleting voiced final stops and producing the unvoiced stops as a glottal stop. In such a case, for example, the pair "bead, beat" would be rendered as the pair [bi, bi?]. This hypothetical child has preserved a phonemic contrast without being able to produce either adult phone involved.

The converse case can occur as well: phonetic control can develop ahead of phonemic contrast. It is very common for all initial stops, regardless of target, to be produced by a child learning English as "voiced" (more precisely, to have voicing onset time between 0 and 20 msec; see Macken and Barton, 1980). In such a case, the phonetics of voiced (short-lag VOT) initial stops could be under control, but not the phonetics of unvoiced (long-lag) initial stops. One could correctly say that the child at this stage had acquired the *phones* [b,d,g], but it would be quite wrong to say that she had acquired the *phonemes* /b,d,g/ since she does not have the contrast between them and /p,t,k/. (For further discussion with examples, see Moskowitz, 1975).

The second reason why the concept of phoneme is difficult to apply in the early stages of language development is that for many children, minimal pairs (pairs of words differing only by the contrast in question) are so rare as to make statements about the presence or absence of contrast impossible (see Itkonen, 1977).

And the third good reason for calling early speech pre-phonemic is even more linguistically unsettling. At least we can speak of phones in the first case above, and nothing prevents us from doing so in the second case. That is, we appear to have phonetic targets which are comparable to one another, independent of the lexical items – the particular words – in which they are located. In adult language, we expect that any difference between, say, an /a/ in one word and an /a/ in another will be completely due to the sounds surrounding them, the stress pattern, and possibly to some kinds of morpho-syntactic factors (e.g. being used as a clitic) or more social factors (formality, rate). We are not prepared to see arbitrary variation in phonetic targeting between one lexical item and the next. Yet it does happen; it even occurs in adult language in special marginal cases.

Let us first consider a special case in adult English where a segment fails to satisfy the criteria for being a phone. The "o" of "no" is subject to a huge amount of variation in realization because of the expressive roles it plays; it can occupy almost all positions in the English vowel space "below" a diagonal from [æ] to [o], including for example [ɔ, a, æ], and [ə] as well as the citation form [o]. We must therefore record as a lexical fact about the word "no" the colours its vowel would take – in other words, we cannot describe the vowel in "no" as the phone [o], and if we insist on saying (for good reasons outside the scope of this paper) that it is still the phoneme /o/, we must have a special marking in the lexicon preventing this /o/ from having its usual phonetic spelling-out as [o] in certain usages.

The child phonology case to be cited here, from Jacob, parallels the adult one; the problem is caused by inconsistencies in the amount of variation found for what should be two instances of the same phone. Jacob produced many tokens of the targets "down" and "round", both favourite action words. The vowels of the two words differed in output: the renditions for "down" were much more variable than those for "round". But there was no reasonable way to ascribe this difference to phonetic conditioning or to any of the other factors just cited as causing variation. Thus, these two segments could not be considered tokens of the same phone.

Similar problems in the definition of consonant phones were noted by Ferguson and Farwell (1975), and contribute to Ferguson's repeated sugges-tions that the earliest productive stage of language acquisition should be considered a lexical acquisition period rather than a period of acquisition of primitive phonemes. In this chapter we will be working towards a com-promise model that allows for both the idiosyncratic properties of segments in particular words and the general properties of those segments which do seem to be comparable from one word to the next.

C. Strategies for Dealing with Words and Sounds

There seem to be a number of strategies that children may draw on as they try to render adult words within their limited articulatory abilities. Two types of strategies have been clearly identified in the literature to date. The first type induces little distortion in the model word, while strategies of the second type tend to modify it considerably. Most children probably draw on all of these strategies to varying degrees. However, some of them rely quite heavily on those which do little violence to the model word, while other children show no compunction about making gross changes in a fair number of the words that they attempt. (It has often been speculated that this is a matter of cautious v. bold temperament on the child's part, but to date there has been no systematic attempt to compare phonological behavior with any aspect of personality, or even with the strategies chosen for acquiring any other aspect of language.)

1. *Non-distorting strategies: avoidance and exploitation*
The non-distorting strategies, which may also be termed "selection strategies", are (a) avoidance and (b) exploitation of favourite sounds.

(a) Avoidance. By avoidance we mean that the child does not even attempt to say words containing certain adult sounds. The confirmation that this phenomenon can exist in normal children as young as 15 months old, and not merely in the older child who has required articulation therapy, is a matter of major importance on both linguistic and psychological grounds. Linguistically, it is important because it lies entirely outside the range of behaviour considered by Jakobson and requires the construction of additional acquisition theory (see Ferguson and Macken, to appear). Furthermore, it provides one of the clearest demonstrations of the fact that perceptual discrimination can precede production by many months; if there are two similar sounds and one is avoided while the other is attempted, the child must be able to discriminate between the two sounds while being able to make only one of them. Psychologically, avoidance is a stunning phenomenon because it implies considerable metalinguistic awareness on the part of a child who has only recently begun to speak. After all, avoidance must be the result of a kind of decision.

Consider a child who imitates and uses a set of words beginning with, say, /d/, but who will not attempt any with /b/ even though he has demonstrated comprehension of b-initial words like "ball", "block", "box", and so on. At the very least, such a child must have the feeling that there is something special the matter with b-initial words, some reason why he does not want to say them. Ferguson and Farwell (1975) suggested that this might be happening in some of their subjects; Menn (1976a) was able to demonstrate the b/d case just cited for Jacob, including showing that the child knew the meanings of a good number of b-initial words; and Schwartz and Leonard (1982) showed that avoidance could be demonstrated experimentally in children near the onset of speech (having less than 50 words), although not in somewhat older ones (Leonard, Schwartz, Folger, and Wilcox 1978).

(b) Exploitation of favourite sounds. Some children early in their speaking-lives seem to seek out adult words that contain particular sounds and add

these words preferentially to their output, although they learn other words as well. Farwell (1976) is the first study to document this strategy; her case, from the collection of the Stanford Child Phonology Project, was a little girl who apparently especially liked fricatives and affricates, for her output was loaded with words like "juice", "choo-choo", "shoes".

It is clear that both avoidance and exploitation are strategies that we should expect to find if a child is, in fact, treating the mastery of pronunciation as a problem to be solved, and is capable of avoiding perceived areas of difficulty and of capitalizing on perceived areas of success.

2. *Modification strategies: rule use*

Now let us consider modification strategies, those which result in changes to the shape of the word. One case has become familiar: the case of rule-use. Here, the child has a systematic method of dealing with adult words, one that can be described by a set of rules for substitution, omission, and occasional metathesis of the sounds of the adult word. First we will consider some typical examples of this well-studied type of modification strategy, and then, in Section IV.4.C, we will study some more unruly modifications.

Child-phonology rules represent the child's modifications of the adult model word in a segment-by-segment fashion. They are usually written as direct maps from the adult sound to the child's sound. When the rules are written this way, of course, a step is left out: the psychologically intermediate but inaccessible step of the child's internal recognition encoding of the adult model word which we just discussed in Section III.A. For the present, we will write rules without that intermediate step; when we discuss the construction of a psychological model for child phonology in Section V., we will put it back in again, and also hypothesize some other intermediate processing levels.

To begin with, let us consider a hypothetical child near the beginning of speech who has the following list of words:

$$\text{hat [æ']; boy [bɔj]; cat [kæ]}$$
$$\text{nice [naj]; house [æw]; dog [da]}$$
$$\text{please [pi]; blue [bu]; clock [ka]}$$
$$\text{drum [dʌ]; up [ʌ]; down [dæw]}$$

This "child" would appear to substitute glottal stop for final /t/ and to delete other final consonants. Initial /h/ is also deleted. Liquids are dropped from consonant clusters. These statements may be translated into formal terms like this:

$t \rightarrow ?$ / __   (/t/ becomes glottal stop and then

$C \rightarrow ø$ /   all other consonants are deleted word-finally)

$\begin{bmatrix} +\text{cons} \\ +\text{voc} \end{bmatrix}$ (liquids are deleted from initial clusters)
$\rightarrow ø / \#C\_V$

$/h/ \rightarrow ø / \#\_\_$ (h is deleted word-finally)

The reader may have noted that these four rules are not the only ones that can be devised to describe the observed behaviour. It is important to understand that in most cases we do not get enough different words from a young child to determine her set of rules fully. Rules are always to be regarded as the analyst's tentative hypotheses about the child's mental operations. And it is also important to remember that a rule is no more than a description of a hypothesized regularity of behaviour. It is not an explanation of anything to say that a child "has" a deletion rule or a substitution rule, just as it is no explanation to say that an apple falls because of gravity.

Now let us examine in more detail two of the best-known rule types of child phonology: assimilation and voicing/devoicing. Towards the end of this section we shall also see that there are other strategies that children use which produce the same effects that these rules do.

(a) Assimilation and consonant harmony: assimilation rules. We often notice that young children have rules which change the consonants in a word to make them more similar to one another. As in general phonology, these are called consonant assimilation rules. For example, a child who can say "daddy" with a good initial [d] and "egg" with a good final [g] may yet say [gɔg] for "dog". Such a child usually also says [gʌk] for "duck" and "truck", etc. These rules may be so strict for a time that all the consonants in any given output word must be homorganic – that is, made with the same position of the articulators. "Boat", for example, would have to be produced as either [bowp] or [dowt].

Assimilation involving the feature [nasal] is common, too, in child phonology: "dance" may become [næns], with the /d/ assimilating in nasality to match the following nasal; or "meat" may become [dit], with the /m/ losing both its nasality and its labial position as it assimilates to the final /t/. (Both of these forms are from Daniel, Menn 1971).

Sometimes a child may produce some non-harmonic sequences and yet apparently require harmony in other words: he may say "gate" correctly, but produce [gɪg] for "big" and [gejk] for "take". In this case, the assimilation of labials or dentals to velars occured only if the velar was word-final; if it was word-initial, both stops were produced correctly. Relative position of the consonants in a word is often a factor when some sort of asymmetry of consonant harmony is found (Ingram 1974). Vihman's (1978) survey suggests that sounds at the beginning of a word are somewhat more likely to be the ones which are changed when there is an assimilation rule, but this is merely a tendency.

Assimilation rules can be found in great numbers in adult language as well, but there is an important difference. In adult language, the usual type of consonant assimilation is contact assimilation: a segment changes and becomes more like one that is next to it. Although many adult languages have vowel harmony, which occurs even when consonants lie between the vowels, very few adult languages have consonant assimilation at a distance; Vihman finds it in only three of the 88 languages in the Stanford Phonology

Archive (not including some cases in which the intervening vowel is "coloured" by nasalization in nasal harmony, or by pharyngealization in pharyngeal harmony; these cases are called "prosodies" by Vihman). Something special is taking place in child phonology.

When we find deletion rules, as in our initial examples for this section, or contact assimilations like the change of "ask" to [æst], we usually feel that mechanical "ease of articulation" should account for them. But when we contemplate distance assimilation, we find our intuitive notion of simplicity challenged. Why should a child who can say "dad" and "egg" find [gɔg] easier than [dɔg]? Is this to be explained in "natural" terms? In a sense, yes – but in terms of a different kind than we have previously considered, terms which are very important to the construction of a theory of child phonology.

In trying to understand distance assimilation, we can get some help from considering general motor behaviour. Under what circumstances is an ABA pattern of behaviour "easier" than an ABC pattern (assuming that A and C are equally easy to carry out in themselves and as sequels to B)? The only way that doing A again can be "easier" is if the sequence is to some extent pre-assembled or preprogrammed, for in a memoryless series of events it would not matter whether an element is one that has recently been used. In other words, doing A the second time is easier than doing "C" only if we know that we are going to do "A" again and can make use of that information. So the argument goes as follows: young children often use distance assimilation. We take as a working assumption that this must make words easier for them. It cannot make words easier for them unless there is a stage of production at which a word is programmed or assembled before it is spoken. Therefore, I think that a model of how words are produced by young children must have such a stage in it. Later on, we will come back to this point and try to deduce more about the properties of this stage from the data that we have available.

(b) Other strategies: consonant harmony as a goal. Assimilation rules are not the only way that children deal with disharmonic sequences. Some children omit one of the offending consonants: Daniel, who used assimilation on "dog", "boat", and a good many other words, said [gej] for "gate", rather than [gejk] or [dejt]. Other children use a glottal stop in place of one of the adult sounds. Such patterns of rule use linked by similar input and similar output strongly suggest that we should take a functional approach to child phonology rules; that is, they make more sense if we think of them as means to some end. And in fact, we have been doing just that: we have been assuming that these rules are somehow designed to eliminate disharmonic sequences.

3. *Output constraints and conspiracies: first mention*
At this point it will help to develop some terms for dealing with sets of rules which appear to serve some common function. Suppose none of the forms produced by a child contain consonant clusters, for example, or that none

have final stops, or that none have disharmonic sequences. A statement that a particular sound-pattern does not appear in a corpus and is not expected to appear if we get a larger sample is a statement of an output constraint. Adult languages have output constraints as well; consonant clusters are absent from many languages, and every language has restrictions on how many and what kind of consonants form a pronounceable cluster (Bell, 1971). Vowel harmony, present in quite a number of languages, is also describable as an output constraint.

Following Kisseberth (1970), when we have a set of rules that all contribute to eliminating sound patterns which would violate a particular output constraint, we say that those rules form a conspiracy. In the example from Daniel, assimilation rules and a (limited) deletion rule were part of the conspiracy to eliminate disharmonic sequences.

Conspiracies of rules are not the only devices that children use to maintain output constraints, however. Selection strategies may also contribute – children may avoid adult words which violate a constraint. Sometimes, this may be a very minor strategy for a particular child (Daniel probably avoided the word "cup"), but sometimes it is a major contributor to the maintenance of an output constraint.

Let us now look at some cases involving another very common output constraint in young children. This one actually involves a pair of phenomena collectively referred to by Ingram (1976) as "voicing": the constraint that initial stops be voiced and final stops be unvoiced. A child may have only one of these or neither, but the pair is very common for English-learning children.

At the acoustic-phonetic level, the statement is slightly different: initial stops tend to be voiceless-unaspirated (short-lag VOT) and final stops to be partially devoiced (see again Macken and Barton, 1980; N. V. Smith, 1973; B. Smith 1979). This difference in statement is not important within English phonology, but it becomes very important cross-linguisically, since voiceless unaspirated stops count as "voiced" in English phonology, but as "unvoiced" in Spanish, French, and many other languages. An explanation for this pair of phenomena should be in terms of the regulation of glottal air-flow – for discussion see Flege and Massey (1980) and Westbury and Keating (1980). If there is any rule which deserves to be called a "natural process", surely it is the rule of final devoicing: it is not only found in child language, but is one of the most frequent rules in adult language, appearing in many forms from a low-level tendency (as in American English) to the familiar German and Russian final devoicing rule and Turkish syllable-final devoicing.

So, many children use the natural-process rule of devoicing final stops, and many also use the natural-process rule of voicing initial stops; Joan Velten is undoubtedly the best-known example. She said [bat] for "pocket", [ba] for "pie", [bat] for "bad", [ap] for "up" and [zas] for "sauce", to choose from a long list (pp. 86–87 in Velten 1941). There are no examples involving velar stops in output, for at this age (23 months) Joan changed all adult velars to coronals (except for [bup], "book"). Other children who have the same voicing constraint may use a selection strategy: words beginning with /p,t,k/ or words ending with /b,d,g/ may be avoided, and words which begin and end with the preferred sounds may be selected.

Now let us look at a more complicated case, one in which all the three principal stop positions of English were being produced by the child. Here the voicing constraint is in full force in final position: final [p,t,k] have been mastered, while the final voiced stops /b,d/ are avoided, and final /g/ is modified by being devoiced or deleted.

The constraint has been overcome in initial position: the contrast between initial /d/ and /t/ has been mastered and initial [k] has been acquired. Initial /p/ is avoided, but so is initial /g/. (Ferguson (1975) has commented on similar asymmetries of consonant distributions in child phonology and across adult languages.) These statements are summarized in tabular form (Table I). Another important point is exemplified by these data; notice that the voicing contrast has been mastered for initial dentals, but not for initial velars or labials, and that in this case we cannot even say that one value of the feature is present for all three initial stops. A feature that has been mastered (in either the control sense or the contrast sense) in one phoneme may or may not spread to other phonemes in the same word-position. We presently do not know whether it is possible to explain the difference between the cases in which a feature generalizes and the cases in which it remains "bound" to a particular phone.

TABLE I
Jacob's consonants

	Initial				Final		
p	absent	b	mastered	p	mastered	b	absent
t	mastered	d	mastered	t	mastered	d	absent
k	mastered	g	absent	k	mastered	g	devoiced deleted

Other rule strategies besides the use of voicing or devoicing rules can be found in children obeying the voicing constraint. We have just mentioned Jacob's occasional deletion of final /g/, but there are much more interesting cases to be found. These are the children who add extra segments in order to render a voicing contrast. It has been claimed that some children add a vowel to the end of a word with a final voiced stop; this brings the sound into the interior of the word where it could be managed. "Bag" might be produced as [bægə] or [bægæ].

Also, two cases are now reported in which children added nasals rather than vowels in their apparent efforts to preserve the voicing contrast in final position. Fey and Gandour (1979) presented a study of a child who found that he could preserve the voicing of adult final stops by adding a final homorganic nasal: "bag" became [bægŋ]. (Phonetically this is rather less exotic than it looks written out; the effect is just produced by releasing the velar closure before releasing the stop articulation. However, this cannot well be considered a natural process; there is no evidence that there is a general tendency for speakers attempting to maintain voicing through a final closure to fail with this result.) Bowerman (pers. commun.) reports a different use of added nasal segments: one of her daughters added a homorganic nasal before final voiced stops, so that for example "Bob" became [bamp]. The stops themselves were still devoiced, but contrast was maintained (and the insertion of the nasal should have helped to maintain the vowel-lengthening which precedes final voiced stops in English and which in fact serves to carry the final voicing contrast in some dialects).

Now that we have seen how the notion of output constraint can serve to bring together several rules and/or strategies under the observation that they all "serve to maintain the same output constraint", it is time to take a critical look at the notion itself. So far, all we have is description, not explanation. To say that a rule "serves an output constraint" or "is part of a conspiracy" is only organization of data. But once we organize the data in this way, a plausible explanation jumps out at us: the child is modifying unfamiliar sound patterns to make them like the ones he has already mastered. *And that means that the child has to learn sound patterns, not just sounds.* Again, output contraints are only descriptive devices; what they describe are those sound patterns which a child has mastered v. those that he has not. That is why words which do not fit the constraints are almost all avoided or modified. This is the central thesis of this chapter; we shall explore its empirical support and its implications in many of the remaining sections.

4. *Another modification strategy: template matching*

Now let us consider another type of modification strategy, one evidenced primarily in work done by Vihman (1976, 1981), Macken (1979), and Priestly (1977). These cases involve fairly violent rearrangements of sounds of adult words to match "templates" of preferred sound patterns. The simpler cases can just as well be considered cases of rule use, and usually are described in terms of metathesis (place-exchanging) rules. The more complex cases, however, cannot be described by rules without a lot of artificial special-case magic, for what makes them so complex is the fact that the child's attack on the adult word is not fully systematic.

A good simple case to begin with is Vihman (1976). A child learning Estonian as her first language seemed to have learned to say words containing two different vowel sounds only if the first vowel was lower than the second. The Estonian words for mother, /ema/, and for father, /isa/, do not happen to follow this pattern. For a little while, the child said just [sa] for "father"; then for four months she failed to attempt either word, although "both father and mother made earnest attempts to elicit the words /ema/ and /isa/". At fifteen and one-half months, the child began to rearrange those words to conform to her output constraint: "/ema/ emerged as [ami] or [ani]

. . . at which time /isa/ also reappeared, now pronounced [asi], and the word /liha/, 'meat', was reproduced, following the same rule, as [ati]".

An example of a case where the child was less systematic about the map from the adult word to output is given in Priestly (1977) (also discussed in Ingram, 1979). Priestly's son Christopher treated virtually all stop-final adult two-syllable words and a fair number of vowel/sonorant-final two-syllable words according to the following patterns: Consonant selection:

$$C_1 - C_2 \rightarrow C_1 - j - C_2$$

examples: pillow [pijal]; Brenda [bajan]; tiger [tajak]

or

$$C_1 - C_x - C_2 \rightarrow C_1 - j - C_2$$

examples: rabbit [rajat]; melon [majan]

with a few cases of idiosyncratic rearrangements, such as "streamer" being produced as [mijat]. There was also a choice of vowel treatments; sometimes Christopher was able to match two vowels of the target, but at other times he replaced one or both by [a] In addition to the cases already listed, consider the apparent metathesis of vowel features involved in his rendition of "woman" as [wajum]!

Other two-syllable words which ended in a vowel or sonorants were treated without these special medial-[j] rearrangements: examples are "bacon", produced almost correctly as [bejkan], "kitchen', where the medial affricate apparently caused the only problem, rendered [kɪkɪn, kɪtɪn], and 'scissors", [sɪzɪz].

While it is possible to discern some tendencies in Christopher's assignments of particular adult forms to particular outputs, Priestly makes it clear that there is considerable arbitrary variation from word to word. This fact of lexical variation is further emphasized by Christopher's variation across tokens of the same word: "monster" was recorded as [majos] in weeks 4 and 6 of the study, but as [mejan] in week 5; "dragon" was given as both [dajan] (week 3) and as [dajak] (week 4).

In Priestly's case, then, the child had a favourite output shape to fill, but only a few constraints on which consonants and vowels he picked to fill it with. Macken's 1979 subject Si, acquiring Spanish, shows us a much more constrained output template – that is, one which allowed a very limited set of consonants – and a much greater abandon in her treatment of the model word. (The latter fact probably also reflects the much greater proportion of polysyllabic words among her targets.)

Si could produce disharmonic sequences in a word only if one target consonant was labial and another was dental. Adult words which met this criterion were produced so that the labial preceded the dental; much deletion and occasional metathesis occurred.

examples: manzana [mana]   pelota [patda]
zapato   [patda] elefante [batte]
Fernando [wanno] sopa   [pwæta]

In Si's case, the details of what is deleted and what is selected defy organized statement in terms of rewrite rules. As Macken says, this is goal-directed behaviour: the child is looking for consonants that she can fit into her output template and ignoring the rest.

IV. Rule Creation

A. Extending the Notion of "Ease of Articulation"
One Key to a New Theory

When a child's production of a word fails to match the adult model, we cannot help assuming that there must be some sense in which what he does produce is easier than what he has failed to produce. But what sense is this? How can [bada] be easier for Macken's Si than [daba]? Why will some children use [1] for /y/ and others use [j] for /l/? Why do some children exploit fricatives while others delete them, avoid them, or replace them with stops? Clearly, if we stick to our common-sense starting assumption, then it must be the case that what is easier for one child can be harder for another. Perhaps a little of the variation is due to anatomical differences, but we simply do not have the means to investigate that hypothesis. A much more fruitful approach is to assume that a great deal of "ease" and "difficulty" is not a matter of physiology at all – or, to put it another way, that phsyiological causes are only one factor in determining "ease of articulation" for the individual child. The other factor, and I propose that it is the major factor, is the state of a child's knowledge at a given time.

Let me give an example. A child may, as we have said, discover "how to say [l]" before "how to say [j]", or the reverse may be true. Suppose a particular child has discovered [l] first, by chance. We notate this discovery as the invention of a rule taking /l/ into [1]. Now this child may slip into her [l] while trying to say [j], either accidentally or on purpose. If she finds the approximation good enough, she will continue to use it: she will have thus discovered or invented a modification rule. Again, in this case, [l] is "easier" than [j] only because this child happens to have found out how to make an [l] first.

I suggest, in short, that a two-stage discovery process is probably involved in a child's establishment of a new articulatory gesture as her way-of-saying a particular target sound. The first stage is a matter of trial-and-error attempts to match the sound sequence; the second stage is one of deliberate or accidental overgeneralization of the success of that articulatory gesture – that is, the use of it to render similar adult targets.

Let us consider the hypothesized scenario here in more detail, for it is the heart of this chapter's proposal for dealing with one of the fundamental problems of child phonology, namely, how can there be so much individual variation and yet such strong general tendencies? We suppose, then, that variability across children originates with each child making trial-and-error starts at matching adult sound patterns. For each given sound or pattern, some children will succeed and some will fail. "External" factors, such as the frequency and salience of the sound in the speech of others, may contribute to the likelihood of success; so will "internal" factors: the probability of accidentally hitting on an acceptable way to produce it and the salience of the sound in one's own speech.

We frankly do not know why some sounds are more probable than others; Stevens' (1972) notion that favoured phones are those which are acoustically stable (i.e. permit a certain sloppiness in articulation without showing appreciable acoustic change) is certainly an attractive idea, but we cannot yet simulate the child's vocal tract accurately enough to test this idea with acoustic modelling. (However, progress has recently been made in this area – see Goldstein, 1980). The accidental aspect of learning to produce target sounds is a principal source of individual variation, but it is also a principal source of the probablistic universals of order of acquisition; roughly and with all due caveats, stops usually are acquired before fricatives, labials usually before velars, nasals usually early, liquids usually late. (See Sander, 1972, both for data on English and for methodological considerations.) If the reader will permit me some licence in the statement of probabilities, we might say that a [b] is a low pair, [k] is jacks or better, [l] is a flush, [θ] is a straight flush, and the fricative [r̝] which Jakobson dwelt on as the latest-acquired Czech phoneme is a royal flush in spades: some kid somewhere in Czechoslovakia is going to get it phonetically right in her first ten words, but don't bet on her being in your data sample.

We should stress one more thing about this proposed initial trial-and-error stage of discovery: a child may accept her rendition of a sound even when it is quite inaccurate. Some rules that give inaccurate renditions of adult targets therefore arise at this first stage. But many more may arise in the second stage, as the child makes use of her initial accomplishment.

B. "Natural Processes"

It is quite reasonable to say that both /l/→[j] and /j/→ [l] are "natural phonetic processes", in that articulatory factors make it quite likely that a clumsy attempt at either of them will produce the other, rather than, say, a [t] or a [b]. Put another way, a child with a certain amount of experience at making speech sounds with his mouth is likely to get some of the properties of, say, [l], correct (in a word that does not present a host of other problems): perhaps the voicing, the continuancy, the central tongue place-ment, or the lack of rounding. [l] and [j] share all of these properties, so a child who is doing well at approximating one of these two phones is quite likely to end up with the other as his approximation to it.

Informal observation suggests that [l] and [j] are roughly equally likely to be found substituting for one another ([w] or a similar sound is also found frequently for "dark L" [ɫ], of course). In other cases, there is a heavy bias in favour of one of a pair of phones. For example, in word-initial position, stops are much more likely to be discovered before fricatives and then to be used to substitute for them. Similarly, voiced stops are likely to be used for unvoiced stops in initial position, as we have already seen. We certainly have enough reason to say that "stopping" (use of stop for fricative) and "voicing" are natural in initial position; that is, we have reason to believe that there is a high, physiologically-governed probability that the child making a first attempt at an initial fricative will produce an initial stop, and that the child first attempting an initial unvoiced stop will produce a voiced stop instead. This, I think, is the only coherent interpretation of the notion "natural process", although other views certainly appear to be held (see Stampe, 1969; Ingram, 1976, but also Ingram, 1979).

In summary, I propose that "natural processes" are really descriptions of those pitfalls of learning to articulate which are commoner and more heavily determined by physiology. To build a rigorous theory of the acquisition of phonology, one must also be able to explain why children fall into those particular pits.

And that step would still be only a beginning, for physiology only dictates what articulatory goals are likely to be surrounded with what traps. To explain how children succeed in avoiding or climbing out of them, we need a problem-solving theory, a cognitive theory. The essence of such a theory for the acquisition of phonology, again, is the trial-and-error discovery followed by application of the discovered skill to new cases – a model which will be very unsurprising to any developmental psychologist.

C. Non-natural Rules

There remain some kinds of rules that are at a considerable remove from the solution of particular articulatory problems.

A very important kind of non-natural rule arises as the child begins to attend to the fact that what appears to be the same morpheme is not always produced in the same way by adults. Sometimes that child is correct in interpreting her observations this way – that is, sometimes she has indeed run into a case of allomorphy or of stylistic variation. However, sometimes she is incorrect; what appears to be variation in the shape of a single morpheme is in fact a case in which the adult is sometimes using one morpheme and sometimes using two which the child has failed to segment. For example, if a child notices the "Z"-morpheme of the English possessive and plural appearing on certain nouns but does not yet understand that the final sibilant has one or both of those meanings, he may develop his own phonological "hypothesis" about where those final sibilants are supposed to appear. Daniel (Menn, 1971) created a rule adding [s] to the end of all English words ending in /r/, apparently because there was an accidental abundance of plurals and possessives on names and objects in /r/ in his environment. He may have figured that the sibilant-final forms which he heard were the full and correct forms of the words which he also heard with final /r/ – that is, he took "pears" as the full form of "pear", "Peter's" as the full form of "Peter", etc.

It is also the case that rules which once had an articulatory base, after they have been invented, seem to acquire considerable autonomy and may generalize without any further articulatory motivation. A child may apply a rule for one segment or (sequence of segments) to a similar one *even though he could have produced the latter correctly*. This seems to be the case for several rules used by Amahl (see Smith, 1978). Rules are much more than articulatory habits, then; they are transduction habits, habits of rendering perceived targets in particular ways. Illustrations and further discussion will be presented in Section IV.E., "Overgeneralization'.

It is too early to make strong generalizations about the ages at which transduction rules of different kinds can be found, but roughly, it seems that the very youngest children's rules are mostly those which lend themselves to explanations in terms of seeking solutions to articulatory problems; as these problems are overcome, we begin to see more instances of rules that arise from overgeneralizations of other rules, and more rules which reflect the child's guesses about the reasons for variation in words of the adult language.

D. Rule Origin and Growth

We have already found ourselves considering the topic of rule origin; let us now do so in more generality and depth. We have characterized transduction rules as systematic correspondences between adult and child sound-patterns, ranging from correct renditions (/d/ → [d]), omissions, and natural substitutions (/ð/→[d]) to the idiosyncratic rule inserting [s] after word-final /r/ that we have just discussed. There is also a range in how systematic a rule is. Some are exceptionless; most have a few lexical exceptions which typically consist of forms that were learned before the child invented the rule in question, or of forms which are the forerunners of a new rule. And some rules have so many exceptions that they reach the point where we are better off abandoning the attempt to write them; the Priestly case was one example of such a state of affairs.

The evidence for the nature of rule-change is somewhat sketchy, because rule-changes can take place in a short time, sometimes within a few hours. Fine-grained longitudinal study is needed to give a picture of Before, During, and After in such cases. This is emphatically not to say that all rule-change is rapid. Replacement of one well-established rule by another may take place over a period of weeks (and fossil forms created by the old rule may survive indefinitely).

1. *Rule origin*
We have already discussed trial-and-error experimentation as a source for correct transduction rules (/d/→[d]) and for natural transduction rules. But

it should be noted that a child's trial-and-error sessions do not always lead to the formation of a rule. Even if the child manages a perfect rendition of some sound pattern, she may be unable to capture the trick of doing it at will. For example, Daniel (Menn, 1971) made dozens of attempts at the word "peach" during the period when his consonants were subject to assimilation.

If he had been able to make the beginning of the word affricate to match the end, he presumably would have had no problem. But he had not learned to produce any initial affricates, and his versions of the word included [dits, citʃ, nits, its, pipʃ] and [pitʃ] itself at various times. He settled on none of them.

Yet sometimes a rule actually emerged within hours: Daniel tried [φαφs] and [dæts] for "box" at 10:16, and later the same day his assimilation rule made its first true appearance, with "dog" as [gVg], a form it kept stably for months (as far as the consonants were concerned).

The other case of rule origin in the literature has been called consolidation (Menn, 1976a). This term is used to describe the situation in which two similar adult target sound patterns are involved in very similar trial-and-error sequences, and end up being handled in the same way. Correct versions of both of the patterns may be produced in the course of the trials. Jacob varied between [ei] and [i] for the vowel of both "tea" and "table" for some weeks before settling on [i] for both. The mutual influence of similar sound patterns is clearly demonstrated in such cases. Template matching can also originate in this fashion – see Vihman (1981).

2. *Rule generalization*

Rule origin can occur through rule generalization, for of course dividing a rule from its predecessor is often difficult or arbitrary – there is often no sense to the question "is this a new rule or a generalized version of an old one?" Rule generalization basically means the extension of a rule to new cases, and this covers two different kinds of events. To discuss them, we need the concept of the domain of a rule. The domain of a rule is simply the set of cases to which it is actually applied. For example, the domain of a rule that applies to all English voiced obstruent is just the set of all instances of /bdgvðzʒdʒ/.

Formally, if we have an exceptionless rule, its domain is specified in its structural description. In the example given, the structural description could be written [+ obstruent, + voice].

If a rule has lexical exceptions, sounds in the excepted words are not in its domain even if they meet its structural description. Thus, if the word "bad" were simply listed as a lexical exception to a rule otherwise applying to all voiced obstruents, the /b/ and /d/ in it would be outside the domain of the rule. If, at a later time, "bad" ceased to be an exception, it would by definition have been brought into the domain of the rule and thus, the rule would have become more general without any change in its structural description at all. We might term this type of rule generalization "lexical smoothing". Lexical smoothing is important in child phonology because lexical exceptions to rules are so frequent. Yet it is not really a change in the rule; it is only a change in the set of exceptions to it.

The other type of rule generalization is formally expressible as a relaxation of the structural description, allowing additional phonologically-defined sets of words to be operated on by the rule. For example, a rule which at some point applies only to final /b/ might at a later time apply to all final labials, or to all final obstruents, or to all instances of /b/. Any of those changes would bring new sets of sounds into the domain of the rule, thus generalizing it. A relatively technical note: in child phonology, we often have trouble determining the domain of a rule for various reasons. Here is one interesting problem: Consider the data from Joan Velten given above (Section III.C.3). She had no velars in her output; she had initial voicing and final devoicing of other stop consonants. Should velars be considered to be in the domain of the voicing and devoicing rules? It is easy to write the rules either way (with voicing and devoicing rules applying directly to all stops before the conversion of velars to dentals, or with "fronting" preceding voicing and devoicing). Only in the latter order can the voicing rules be written excluding velars and still give us the observed distribution of forms. Now the fact is that when velars show up, they may not be subject to either of the rules obeyed by the other stops, so it is preferable to write the rules the second way, and thus to make no vacuous claims about the velars. If the velars do show up obeying the voicing and/or devoicing rules, that would then count as a generalization of the two rules.

E. Overgeneralization

Just as in the acquisition of morphology or syntax, rule generalization can create incorrect forms, and thus, from the adult point of view, be overgeneralization. The term is used loosely; typically it is used when a rule produces some "good" results and some "bad" ones. If a rule always produces modified forms ("bad results"), we do not bother to call extensions of it "overgeneralizations" except when they make a child's approximations worse than they were before the rule affected them. Let us consider some examples.

Daniel (Menn, 1971) had the two words "down" and "stone" rendered as [dæɔn] and [don] from the time of his first attempts at them. Then he developed a rule of nasal harmony – he made all of the stops in a word nasal if the final stop was nasal. "Down" and "stone" remained lexical exceptions to this rule; that is, after he had been saying [næns] for "dance" and [ŋein] for "train" for two weeks, he still maintained the two older words in their unassimilated form. Eventually, however, there was a period of time in which he varied between [næɔn] and [dæɔn] for "down", and between [non] and [don] for "stone". Finally, the assimilated forms for these two words took over completely and they were no longer lexical exceptions to the rule.

From the adult point of view, these two words were poorer approximations to the adult model after the rule had applied to them than before (indeed, "down" had been perfect). Therefore, the generalization involved in extending the domain of the assimilation rule to include "down" and "stone" (a case of lexical smoothing, to use the term introduced above) is an overgeneralization of the assimilation rule.

A change in the structural description of a rule can also produce over-generalization ("recidivism" in N. V. Smith's terminology). Here is his example from Amahl (1973, pp. 152–53): "At stage 1, /s/ and /l/ were normally neutralised as [d], together with all the other coronal consonants . . ." (I omit his description of exceptions to this rule, which generally made coronals into [d].) Then "/l/ began to appear in A's speech befor any coronal consonant" – for example, "lady" was rendered either [de:di] or [le:di] So /l/ was optionally excepted from the general treatment of coronals in certain environments. "Then at stage 5 /s/ (and shortly thereafter /ʃ/ became [1] before any coronal consonant . . .: sausage [lɔdid]; shade [le:t] . . ."

Here, the new rule for realizing /l/ as [1] in some environments had added /s/ and /ʃ/ to its domain. So it had generalized by a change in the structural description: the input to the rule had originally been /l/, but later included /l,s,ʃ/. What makes this an overgeneralization? Smith says: "Now originally two words such as "side" and "light" were both [dait], but after the appearance of /l/ before any coronal consonant they became distinct as [dait] and [lait] respectively. However, once /s/ was "liquidised" the two words fell together again – perfectly regularly, as [lait]."

What is lost when this /l/-realization rule is generalized, then, is the contrast between /l/ and the sibilants /s,ʃ/. (Of course there is a compensating gain in this case, because there is contrast of /s,ʃ/ with /d/ only after the /l/→[1] rule generalizes.)

Reviewing this section: we have seen that rule creation can take place through probable or natural failures, such as the production of a stop for an initial fricative, or through the consolidation of similar forms. It is not to be forgotten that the discovery of a correct articulation for an adult sound is also a rule in the sense of a connection between what is heard and what is produced. The child's existing repertoire has a great deal to do with what form new rules may take.

Non-natural rules can arise when a child misapprehends an allomorphic variation and treats it as a purely phonetic rule without semantic significance, or when a child performs major alterations to get a target to fit a canonical form.

Rules can grow and generalize in two ways: by overcoming lexical exceptions (lexical smoothing) or by generalizing the class of sound patterns to which they apply; overgeneralizations can occur as a result of either of these kinds of rule growth.

V. Towards a Psychological Model of Phonological Development

A. The Theoretical Importance of Lexical Exceptions and Overgeneralizations

Lexical exceptions and overgeneralizations are important data for developing a psycholinguistic theory of language acquisition. To begin with, overgeneralizations are inexplicable if one holds the view that the child makes word-by-word progress towards correct productions; that is obvious.

Lexical exceptions are also inexplicable on the neo-Jakobsonian view that the acquisition of phonology is purely a matter of acquiring distinctive features (Menn, 1981). After all, Daniel was able to make the distinction between nasal and non-nasal dentals in production before, during, and after the time his nasal assimilation rule applied: he had no problem producing "daddy" with initial [d] and "no" with initial [n] during the time that he said [næns] for "dance" and so on. So the fact that these words were originally exceptions to the nasal assimilation rule cannot be described in terms of distinctive features. Overgeneralizations cannot be accounted for in terms of acquisition of distinctive features either. "Lexical smoothing" – e.g. the overgeneralization of the nasal assimilation rule to "down" and "stone" is certainly not a matter of learning to make a new distinction, and neither is the loosening of structural descriptions. If we re-examine Smith's "recidivism" case, we see that it only involves a shift in mapping input distinctions onto output ones, not the introduction of new output features. (Amahl mapped /l/ onto [l] in certain environments and all other coronals onto [d]; the overgeneralization which then took place resulted in his also mapping two other coronal continuant consonants, [s] and [ʃ], onto [l] in those environments.)

Similarly, one cannot explain lexical exceptions or lexical smoothing (although one can handle recidivism) within a theory which says that the acquisition of phonology is purely a matter of overcoming natural processes. Consider: if nasal harmony is not a natural process, then the natural process approach is not able to deal with one of the commoner rules of child phonology. On the other hand, if it is a natural process, one has to explain why it did not apply to "down" and "stone" (i.e. why it was "suppressed", in Stampe's terms, for these two words) initially, and then began to show up on other words and eventually on these two themselves.

Finally, one cannot explain lexical exceptions or overgeneralizations within a theory which might claim that the acquisition of phonology is purely a matter of overcoming output constraints, as I might have tempted you to think in Section III.C.3, "Output Constraints and Conspiracies". Such a theory would be subject to exactly the same inadequacies as Jakobson's in these cases – for example, it could not deal with the existence of lexical exceptions to rules.

Summarizing, if we want a functional, explanatory theory of the acquisition of phonology – a theory that does more than say "children have rules, but the rules sometimes have exceptions", we need a theory which is more complicated.

B. Phonological Idioms

One thing that we have just seen is that articulatory success on particular sound patterns sometimes cannot be extended to new instances of very similar patterns. The ability to say "down" and "stone" without nasal harmony apparently was not generalizable to "dance" (let alone to "prune" or to "jump").

The most spectacular cases of non-generalizable articulatory accomplishments were analysed by Moskowitz (1970b); she aptly named them "progressive) phonological idioms". By this she meant words which are pronounced quite well, sometimes perfectly, and, crucially, much better than words of similar adult sound pattern. These are, in short, words which are exceptions to the child's modification rules and/or output constraints. The classic example is Hildegard Leopold's "pretty". She produced this word quite accurately as one of her first words at about 9 months of age. However, then and for many months thereafter, she produced no other consonant clusters and only one other word violating consonant harmony, "tick-tock". Finally, at a point after she had learned to break the consonant harmony constraint in general, "pretty" was changed to roughly [bidi], thus becoming part of the system in effect at that time. (See also Moskowitz, 1970a.)

A good many of the children studied have a few progressive phonological idioms among their early words. These phenomena as well as the less spectacular lexical exceptions discussed in the preceding section are clearly material which must be explained. Note that such lumpy pattern-and-exception landscapes are characteristic of the most closely related psychological areas that we know of: adult language is full of idioms, and cognitive development is full of instances in which the mastery of special cases long precedes the mastery of general skills. It seems that child phonology is more complicated than was once thought, but it still appears to be no more complex than adult syntax or cognitive development. (This rather silly-sounding remark is provoked by those who complain that if one introduces all these complexities, there is no elegant theory left any more. I believe it is one of the corollaries to Murphy's law, however, that nothing is as simple as it originally appears to be.)

C. Canonical forms

Ingram (1974) and Waterson (1971, 1972) have both shown that a young child's output forms can be sorted into sets of canonical forms (Ingram) or prosodies (Waterson). Prosody is here used in the Firthian sense of a sequence of several archiphonemes (partially specified phonemes), and is exactly equivalent to the notion of canonical form. The members of such a set of forms have some strong syllable-structure restrictions in common: a set will be, say, just CV words, or just CVC and VC words, etc. What makes them interesting, indeed surprising, is that these sets are also restricted as to what phones can appear in them.

For example, taking Waterson's data, one set consists of forms for "fly", "barrow", and "flower"; these are all realized by forms consisting of an open syllable with voiced, continuant, labial onset: [wæ], [bβæ]. Another set consisted of "fish", "fetch", "vest", "brush", and "dish"; these were rendered as [(C)Vʃ], with the vowel always mid-high as it is in the targets. A third set was made up of CVCV forms in which the C's were stops and the second syllable was an exact reduplication of the first; the targets mapped into this canonical form included "Bobby", "biscuit", "kitty". Another set, which allowed the vowels to differ, was of the form [ɲVɲV], used for "Randall", "finger", "window", and "another".

Such sets may be maintained by any of the strategies that we have discussed: by selection of adult words that "fit" a form, by use of a rules, or by template-matching. We can thus see in phonological development a gradual weakening of restrictions on the co-occurrence of phones and the realization of more combinations of syllable structure with phonetic content, until we can no longer sort the child's output into these neat sets. In this progression, phonological idioms represent the most primitive level in the sense that they are the forms with the tightest relationship between phonetic content and syllable shape. A little set of lexical exceptions to a rule like "down" and "stone" represent a slight weakening in that relationship – they were produced, remember, as [dæɵn] and [don], two forms differing only in the vowel.

D. Motor Programming: A Psycholinguistic Account of Output Constraints and Canonical Forms

In the preceding section, we implied an interpretation of early output constraints and their gradual relaxation: it is as though the beginning speaker cannot vary some feature values in the course of a single word even though he can make the different sounds in separate words. To take a familiar example, a child with a consonant harmony constraint may be able to make consonants at two or more positions of articulation, e.g. be able to say "toy" and "boy", yet be able to say only [bʌb] for "tub". As Waterson says (1972, p. 13), there is "difficulty in the planning and production of rapid changes of articulation in a short space of time". There is a sense in which the whole word, for a child such as this, can be thought of as bearing a single specification for place of articulation. (This idea has antecedents in several theories of vowel harmony in adult language, e.g. Wellmers and Harris

1942, Waterson 1956/1970.) For a child like Waterson's P, an output word must conform to one of the given canonical forms, and within that restriction, only few degrees of freedom are left for the individual word.

We can tie all of these phenomena together and understand how they fit into an acquisition process if we make an analogy with computer programming. Suppose that learning to pronounce a sequence of sounds is like creating a program that the articulators and the larynx execute. A phonological idiom would then be like an invariant program, one which has no variable parameters that the user is free to set. A canonical form would be like a program in which some parameters are fixed, but others are settable. Let us consider some examples using this metaphor. Assume a child has CV(CV) as the canonical form subsuming, say, "bye-bye" and "baby" as [baba], "ball" as [bɔ], "doggie" as [dʌdʌ], and "there" as [de]. In this hypothetical case, the "program" can either stop after one CV cycle or produce a second CV. The only stops are [b] and [d], which means that there are two choices for consonant position: labial or dental; this choice is made once for the whole word. It also means that there is no choice for voicing or nasality within this program (which means that the canonical form should in fact have been written out as C[+voice, −nasal] V (CV)). Note that there is considerable freedom of choice for the vowels, but that the vowel is also specified once for the whole word.

This child might also have another canonical form, say (C)Vʃ, like Waterson's child. This form is like a program that allows some leeway for specifications of the initial consonant and the vowel, but always finishes the word with an [ʃ]. Such forms have always been puzzling before – it is easy to imagine why assimilated forms are simpler than non-assimilated forms, but what good are canonical forms like CVʃ?

If the "programming" metaphor is roughly accurate, we now have an answer to that question. Even though a form like CVʃ requires a change in the articulatory position for the production of "bush" or "fish", it has very few variable parameters. Therefore, once it has been learned, it can be highly automatic to "run". The program is called up, the initial consonant is chosen, the vowel is chosen, and it runs with no more attention than would have been necessary to produce an open syllable. Waterson (1972, p. 17) noted: "each word appeared to be learned as an individual item . . . at first there were only one or two examples of a particular pattern and then there would be quite a sudden increase."

So now, we can describe phonological development by saying that the child gradually learns to improve in three areas of production control: (1) she learns to increase the number of parameters that can be freely assigned values in a given word; the consequence of this is that more of the segments in a word can vary (2) she learns to increase the number of values that each parameter can take on; this increase means that there is a wider range of possible phones that can be put into each segmental position in a word (3) she learns to link up short programs to make longer ones which can generate polysyllabic words.

In summary, the patterns of language behaviour that we have surveyed suggest that the child must initially discover (by trial and error) how to make sequences of sounds, not merely how to make segments in isolation. Some of these sequences she learns to vary systematically in one or two respects; these we see as groups of similar words, that is, as sets of words belonging to canonical forms. Other sequences she does not learn the trick of varying for a long time, possibly because they were among the most complicated to begin with; these remain phonological idioms. Some canonical forms run into developmental dead ends: Daniel learned only to vary the vowel in his [dVn] canonical form, producing only "down" and "stone" ([non]) with it. But apparently he could not go on from there to learn to vary the place of articulation of the consonants; he had to abandon his temporary conquest of nasal disharmony and make a fresh start.

E. The Articulatory Program and the General Model

1. *The Output Lexicon*
We have described many typical rules of child phonology, we have considered what might be difficult about certain sound sequences that children seem to avoid producing, and we have seen that many rules may be explained as devices which children invent to get around those difficulties. We have found rules that get rid of consonant clusters, of consonant disharmony, and of particular sounds in particular environments. We have also seen that there are some rules and looser strategies that cannot be explained in terms of articulatory simplification, at least not in the usual sense. Instead, we have had to invoke the idea that getting a word out involves the assembly of some sort of articulatory program.

Let us now go back to another aspect of psycholinguistic modelling. There is another important property of children's output that we have mentioned but not really discussed: the fact that some rule changes are carried out gradually. Sometimes this can be explained, following Macken (as we did earlier), by postulating that the child has misheard some word to begin with or has replaced an originally correct encoding of the word by an erroneous version based on his own output. In either case, the result can be that when a new rule comes in which should apply to the word, it will fail to do so because the word has the wrong stored form. Recall that in Macken's example, taken from N. V. Smith, the child had apparently stored "take" as [geik], because when all other velar-final words had broken free of the consonant-harmony rule, that word remained harmonized as an exception.

But often enough, there is quite a delay in applying a new rule to a word that is already established in the output vocabulary, and this can happen even when it is quite unlikely that there has been any miscoding of the word. For example, we mentioned that it took about two weeks for the nasal assimilation rule to begin to affect Daniel's "down" and "stone", and several more before the new forms replaced them entirely. What accounts for the persistence of these forms? The most straightforward account, I think, is given by the two-lexicon model. What we can say with this model is that ways-to-say words are stored, too, in an output lexicon; application of a new rule to a word that is already in a child's active vocabulary involves the ouster of the old form which was stored in the output lexicon and its replacement by the new form. In this model, rules are the links from the input lexicon to the output lexicon. To show this our original figure is relabelled in Fig. 2.

[Collection of percepts]
↓
[Input lexicon]
Rules ↓
[Output lexicon]

FIG. 2

Lags in the adoption of a rule, in this model, simply are cases in which a child has formed the habit of saying a certain word a certain way and maintains that habit instead of "updating" it.

Now we need to fit the notion of articulatory programming, which we developed in the previous section, into the two-lexicon model. This proves to be very easy to do. What we did in that section was to factor the stored information about how to pronounce a word into two parts: (1) information as to which canonical form it belongs to, and (2) information on how the variable parameters in that canonical form should be chosen in order to produce the word. For example, suppose that the child has an accurate rendition of "dish" as part of a $C[+voice]V[-tense][ʃ]$ canonical form. We view its entry in the output lexicon as consisting of the information that (1) it belongs to the canonical form just mentioned and (2) the variable consonant parameters should be set at $[+dental, -continuant]$, giving [d] since the voicing parameter has been fixed at $[+voice]$; meanwhile the variable vowel parameters should be set at $[+front, +high]$, giving [ɪ] since there is already a fixed vowel parameter of $[-tense]$.

The actual production of a word that belongs to a canonical form thus takes place in two stages. The first is recall of the canonical form and the stored variable-parameter values from the output lexicon, and the second stage is plugging the values into the articulatory program specified by the canonical form. Figure 3 shows this elaboration of the two-lexicon model.

Phonological idioms remain as output lexical entries that cannot be factored – that is, as entries in which there are no variable parameters to be set. This means that in our model, the output lexicon contains only the specification of the program; when it is called up, there is no plugging in of settings to be done – the articulatory program (alias the canonical form) has been stored fully specified.

|collection of percepts|
↓
|Input lexicon|
Rules |
↓
|Output lexicon: entry for each word consists of specification of canonical form plus specification for each variable parameter|
↓
|Articulatory instructions|

FIG. 3

2. Rules in the Two-lexicon Model

We have occasionally used the cover term "transduction" to mean all the steps from hearing to speaking a word. As we have analysed this process in terms of perception, storage, and production, we have steadily been breaking it down into finer steps. We have said that one of those steps is the connection between the input lexicon and the output lexicon, and that step is mediated by rules. But we have really only talked about rules in the usual informal mode of relating the adult model word to the child's output word. We need to go back and see what we can deduce about the nature of the rules that would fit into our model.

These rules must account for the difference between what the child knows about the sound of a word as stored in the input lexicon and what is stored as canonical form membership plus variable parameter settings in the output lexicon. In the immature speaker, there is generally a loss of information at this step – that is, kids do not make in production all the distinctions that they can make in perception. The major function of the rules, then, is the selection of which pieces of information about the adult word will be preserved in the output lexicon and which will be abandoned; for this reason, we will refer to the rules in our model which link the input lexicon with the output lexicon as "selection rules".

Let us first consider how selection rules should look for a child who has developed beyond the stage of having obvious canonical forms. For such a child we gain very little by introducing the theoretical complexity of the factored output lexicon, and we make our work easier if we go back to the older model in which the output lexical entry for a word contains all the information needed to say it (see Fig. 2 again).

The notion of selection rule is especially convenient in discussing different children's treatment of consonant clusters, so we will use that topic as an example. The commonest pattern of initial cluster reduction for children acquiring English seems to be the one used in baby talk: stops and nasals are retained, liquids and fricatives lost; /sl/ and /sw/ clusters seem to be indeterminate. (Incidentally, parents tend to perceive their children as adhering to this stereotypic pattern even when the child actually uses a different one; see Menn, 1977; Menn and Berko Gleason, forthcoming.)

Some children find ways of breaking clusters apart, inserting [ə] or moving one of the segments to another part of the word (e.g. saying [nos] for "snow" (Hamp, 1974; also Waterson, 1971). In this discussion, however, we need to focus on those children who do reduce an adult initial consonant cluster to one segment, but who do not do it just by omitting one of the segments. For /sp, st, sk/ we can find some children who use the roughly corresponding fricatives [φ or f, s, x or s] to represent the cluster (also [fw] for /skw/); for /sm, sn, sl/ some children use the devoiced counterparts [m̥, n̥, l̥]. It is easy to describe what is happening here: the child is mapping the cluster into one segment by selecting some of the features belonging to the first adult segment and some to the second one. This is usually done with considerable regularity; that is, a given child will preserve either the fricative character or the stop character of all s + stop clusters. (The treatment of s + nasal clusters may differ from the treatment of s + stop clusters, however.)

Selection rules which produce effects such as these can be considered as selecting features from a particular portion of a word in the input lexicon and then putting them in a designated slot in the output lexical entry. Here, certain position and manner features from initial consonant clusters are taken and "put into a slot" so that they will designate the initial consonant of the output word.

Now let us consider briefly the character of the selection rules that would have to be written to characterize the behaviour of a child who is still operating with strict canonical forms. These rules must map the input lexical entry onto the two-part output lexical entry which we constructed in Section V.D. Therefore, they must be able to take each word in the input lexicon and specify both the canonical form (which articulatory routine will be used) and how any variable parameters are to be set.

A great deal of the variation from one child to the next is reflected right here. Take the word "snow"; for some young children, this will be treated as a CV word and most likely be produced as [no], [do] or [n̥o]. Other children may put any target word containing a sibilant into a (C)Vs class, and so produce "snow" as [nos] or [dos]. A child who tries to break up the cluster with an inserted vowel, giving [səno'] would probably have a CVCV canonical form to map it onto (but this raises problems of stress, which is clearly fixed for some polysyllabic canonical forms). A syllabic [s] for the first syllable is another possibility.

It is by no means clear how a child goes about picking what canonical form to assign an adult word to. She may be quite systematic about it – say assigning all two-syllable words with initial consonants to CVCV and all fricative-final monosyllables to CVs. But her assignments may seem rather more haphazard, especially for words which could fit equally well into either of two forms and for words that do not fit well into any form.

When we consider children whose transduction patterns are less regular and more like template matching, it is no longer possible to write selection rules; we must be content with guidelines. Note, however, that it is possible for there to be a fairly reliable rule for the choice of canonical form coupled with some roughness in the way that variable parameter values appear to be selected (Macken's Si; Priestly's child – both discussed in Section III.C.4). I do not know if any case has been analysed as having irregularity in the choice of canonical forms coupled with regular rules for setting the variable parameters once the form has been chosen.

3. *Caution: the limitations of the programming metaphor*

We set up all this apparatus because it does a nice job of rationalizing the transduction patterns that we seem to find, although there are some data that do not fit as easily as one would like. This model is valid only to the extent that producing a word is like running off some fairly simple sort of speech synthesis program. I enjoin the reader to consider how the theory presented in this chapter might be modified so that it simulates the behaviour of real children better than it presently can.

VI. Saying What One Hears: Task Variables

A. Imitation, Self-monitoring, and Spontaneous Speech

We have been using the term "transduction" occasionally as a cover term for the whole process of hearing and then saying a word (regardless of the time delay between those events). One of the major phenomena of child phonology is the great variability that can be found in the accuracy of a single child's transductions, and the apparent relation of that accuracy to the conditions under which the word was produced. There are three reasons why we must be able to deal with this variability: first, obviously, since it exists we must be able to incorporate it in our theories; second, we must take it into account in data collection so as to get a proper sample of a child's performance, and third, in the assessment of phonological development for clinical purposes, we face the same sampling problem as in research data collection but with much greater urgency because of the need for efficient use of time and because of the consequences for the child.

In this section, we shall review some of the factors that are believed to be involved in the observed variations. It is well-known that imitated productions of words may be much better than spontaneous ones; it is also known that they may be just the same (Korte and Bond, 1979) or simply different (Moskowitz, 1975); and under some conditions, imitations can be worse than spontaneous productions. This means that the factor of being imitated cannot be the only one which produces variations in accuracy of transduction; other factors must be interacting with it if the relation of spontaneous to imitated production is unstable. We shall see that one of these factors is whether the target is already in the child's output vocabulary. However, when this is taken into account there is still a large residue of variation which does not seem to be a matter of the choice of test words and tasks at all. Perhaps it is truly random, but there is some evidence to suggest that another possible factor is the child's own moment-to-moment appraisal of what task she is really being asked to do.

Let us first consider why imitation, so often used as a research or assessment tool, is expected to improve a child's performance, and then why it may fail to do so. Recall that "spontaneous" is actually used to describe utterances elicited from the child by any (humane) means, as long as no-one says the target word itself within several minutes prior to the child's attempt at saying it. The intended essence of this distinction between "spontaneous" and imitated speech is that spontaneous utterances require retrieval of some encoding of the sound pattern of a word from long-term memory, while imitation is supposed to rely on short-term auditory memory. Thus imitation should be able to reflect the child's perceptual and articulatory capacity unencumbered by incorrect stored information.

But careful consideration of this supposition and of the data that we actually have about perception and about imitated production shows that it is, in general, false, especially for very young children. One always relies to some extent on old knowledge in both perception and production, and no imitation task can be assumed to escape this reliance. Perhaps it is minimized when the subject succeeds in categorizing and imitating novel sounds, as in Kent's task of imitating foreign vowel sounds (1978). But in general, imitation does not mean listening and reproducing without the interference of old habits; and if imitation relies entirely on old knowledge, as it may when the child is asked to repeat a familiar word, then imitated and spontaneous tokens of a word should be identical.

Now let us see how imitated tokens might be worse than spontaneous tokens. Barton's extensive work (1976, 1980), shows that children aged two years or under have a strong tendency to mis-hear unfamiliar words, re-interpreting them as familiar words which are phonetically similar. Barton attempted to do minimal-pair word-discrimination tasks with very young subjects, and often they had to be taught one of the words – for example, a twenty-month-old might know "coat" but not "goat". Such a child could learn to choose pictures correctly when one picture was a goat and the other was a bull, but given the minimal pair "coat – goat" to discriminate, the child tended to pick "coat" regardless of whether he heard "coat" or "goat". (The bias depended only on this familiarity factor, not on any phonemic factors.)

The implication of Barton's comprehension study for our consideration of imitation should be clear: he was running into a perceptual bias, and the same bias should be present in imitation tasks, unless they use words which are firmly in the child's passive vocabulary. Even tasks using all nonsense syllables may be affected, since any of them may be misperceived as a familiar word. (It is worth remembering that this bias for hearing the novel as the familiar remains throughout life, as anyone who has an uncommon name that resembles a common one can testify.)

Another variable which is involved in transduction is self-monitoring. Conscious monitoring is likely to improve the quality of one's output, and in adults such self-monitoring seems to be maximal when other cognitive loads are reduced; we assume that the same is true for children. Waterson (1978) has certainly shown that for one child's spontaneous speech, phonetic quality declined as the length of the phrase produced increased; this is suggestive, but the "cognitive load" variation producing the phonological variation was a very highly linguistic one, namely the length of the utterance the word was embedded in, so one must be cautious about generalizing from it.

At any rate, children do indeed go off and quietly practice new sounds (Weir, 1962, is the classic reference). Some children are also observed to whisper new words and sounds (Leopold, 1939). As an aside, we might reflect that the observations of children practising, whispering, and showing off new sounds make the problem-solving theory of child phonology more credible (though they in no way make the old embryonic development theory less credible). It would be difficult to make sense of the claim that the acquisition of the ability to pronounce is a matter of problem-solving, if children never acted as though they were trying to solve a problem.

However, a large part of self-monitoring must also take place below the level of consciousness, for the amount of feedback that must be involved in the achievement of the fine control of the native speaker's accent is immense.

Returning to the main topic, now we must ask whether self-monitoring is improved during imitation. It could be; during imitation, a child has an opportunity to compare her short-term phonetic memory of a word with her production of it and/or with her long-term stored memory of how it should sound. Sometimes such comparisons are made, sometimes they obviously are not. There are plenty of recorded instances in which a child imitates an adult, produces a deviant pronunciation ([ote] for "okay", [fɪs] for "fish"), shows no signs of dismay, and denies hotly that what she has said differs from what the adult has said. Why the failure to spot such major discrepancies? In a good many of these cases, we are sure that it is cannot be ascribed to perceptual difficulty, for if the adult goes on to imitate the child's faulty pronunciation, the child also hotly rejects the adult's parody. The child can tell the difference. True, sometimes the adult produces a very crude parody; in such cases one can argue that the child would have accepted an accurate one. But in many cases, this dodge is not available; the child would have been capable of distinguishing her version from the correct version, if only she were paying attention. An unpublished observation of Daniel will illustrate this point. During the period in which all initial dental and labial stops were assimilated to following velar stops, Daniel was requested to get his toy duck; the toy was out of sight, and the adult simultaneously pointed in the direction in which it lay. Daniel echoed the word as [dʌk], went and looked in the indicated place, said [gʌk], and toddled away with no further interest. I suggest the following interpretation for this sequence of events: in the absense of non-verbal supporting context, Daniel failed to comprehend the word "duck". He repeated it correctly under this condition, clearly demonstrating that he had no perceptual problem with the adult word whatever. Then he went and found it, and repeated his familiar form for it.

It must be the child's self-monitoring that is at fault when he is at this level of discriminatory ability and still fails to recognize that there is a difference between his output and the adult's. I suggest that there are two factors contributing to this lack of attention. One has been mentioned above; if the child has somehow arrived at the opinion of his word is adequate, he is likely to believe that he always does it right. (See Zwicky, 1982 on classical malapropisms.)

The other factor is a problem which also besets many Piagetian-style interviews of children: the problem of making sure that the adult and the child are actually directing their attention to the same phenomenon. Suppose that we consider an adult correcting a child's production of "fish" (to take a frequently-used example). The child says [fɪs], the adult says "No, say [fɪʃ::]", and the child indignantly responds "But I did say [fɪs::]." The adult wants the child to attend to the pronunciation, but how is this desire to communicated to the child? Language is usually used, not contemplated; children expect to listen for meaning, not for sound. The child is more often disposed to understand the request to "say fish" as "say the sound pattern that designates the object with fins and scales that swims" than as "pronounce the word 'fish' accurately".

At the beginning of this section, we said that these transduction variables are of theoretical, methodological, and practical importance. By now these claims are obvious. First, as for theory, what we have seen is that the variables of attention and task orientation need to be incorporated into any model of child phonology. We have developed the outlines of a model of child phonology without taking account of these variables. We will not discuss in any detail how it can be modified to allow for them, but for example some more boxes and arrows need to be introduced into Fig. 3 to represent the following statement: spontaneous productions come from storage in the output lexicon, but imitated ones, to the extent that they are better than spontaneous ones, bypass the output lexicon and draw on less-automatic production mechanisms (Menn, 1979). Second, if we want to assess a child's ability to pronounce, whether our goals are research or remediation, we want to know whether the child is using her "best" pronunciation or an old familiar one. Recognizing that we have no control over this variable, we need to think of tasks that would make attention to pronunciation instead of meaning more or less likely.

Some speech pathologists and researchers attempt to test a child's best articulatory capacities by asking her to imitate nonsense words. This is intended to reduce the child's reliance on her habitual ways-of-saying known words; it is a very reasonable procedure, but we have seen that a child may assimilate a nonsense word to a known word in perception.

Her target word would then be different from the one that the examiner said, and thus there would be two sources of error: the misperception of the target and the effects, if any, of drawing on established articulatory habits. A very useful discussion of these and other task variables in assessment is Menyuk (1980).

B. The Word as Means to an End

We have introduced the problem of task variables in the context of observing and testing the child who has begun to talk. We should also consider the role of task variables during the transition from babbling to speech.

One of the perennial puzzles of child phonology is the phenomenon that got exaggerated into the legend of the universal "silent period": frequently a child will be able to produce a sound in babbling even though she cannot put it into any words. How can this come about? Like any other voluntary motor performance, the production of a sound or sound-sequence is easier in some contexts of action than others. Consider producing a given sequence of sounds under each of the following conditions:

(i) having just made the sound(s) by accident (the context for "circular" babble);
(ii) having just heard someone else make the sound(s) (the context for imitation);
(iii) having decided to make the sound for its own sake or to execute the motor sequence that will produce the sound(s) (the context for sound-play);
(iv) having decided to obtain a goal which requires the use of the sound(s) as a subgoal (the context for meaningful utterances).

Observation tells us that (i) is the earliest, and therefore the easiest of these four conditions, while (iv) is the hardest. It is not clear whether (ii) is easier than (iii), however. But the important point is that (iv) requires the ability to carry out (ii) or (iii) plus attention to the goal of the act of speaking. We might hypothesize that the means–ends gap found here is the reason why sounds can appear in babble before being used in speech, drawing on general principles of cognitive development.

But there may be some other factors involved in this delay. For example, a child might fail to realize that a sound made in play is just the one needed for certain words. This might happen because the recall memory for the sounds in those words is not strong enough to bring them to mind without supportive contexts, even though the child can recognize them when others say them. Second-language learners will certainly recognize this kind of recognition/recall disparity.

In conclusion, we cannot say with certainty why a child is unable to use in words a sound that he can produce in play, but there are many possible cognitive reasons why this might happen, so there is no point to invoking some mystery of the "language faculty" until it is shown that none of these possible reasons is plausible.

Note: It is important to make one's analogies carefully when comparing language with other cognitive abilities. There is possible confusion about my use of the terms "means" and "end". Children can indeed learn to produce words for various social and personal ends well before they show the innovative means–ends behaviour that is called for on Piagetian developmental scales. But the kind of means–ends behaviour required for the onset of meaningful speech is of the most primitive variety; early words are acquired by plenty of practice and are deployed in familiar situations for familiar purposes.)

VII. The Acquisition of Allophones and Allomorphs

So far, we have concentrated on the development of the child's ability to go from a shallow phonemic input representation of the adult's word to some tolerable output approximation of it. But this, of course, is only the surface of the acquisition of phonology. How do children begin to dig below the phonetic surface?

This is a major topic, and in this section we will only discuss some theoretical issues and cite some of the recent studies in this area. To begin with, there are terminological problems that I would like to avoid, so I will specify the terms I will use in this section. A morphophonological or morphophonemic rule is one which requires morphological information for its operation, e.g. a rule which applies to verb stems, to plural morphemes, to members of a declensional class. An allophonic rule is one which requires only phonological information: the identity of neighbouring sounds, boundaries, assigned stresses, etc. (Boundary and trace markers are essentially devices for recasting morphophonological rules as allophonic rules.)

A productive rule is one which would apply to new words coming into a language and which can therefore be tested on nonsense words of properly chosen shapes. The effects of non-productive allophonic rules may persist for a long time in redundancy rules, which specify possible output shapes of morphemes without giving directions as to how aberrant morphemes are to be rearranged.

A rule of any type, morphophonological or allophonic, productive or not, may produce allomorphy: the appearance of a given morpheme in two or more shapes that would be written distinctly in phonetic transcription. (Examples will be supplied in the text as needed, rather than being given here.)

The distinction between superficial and cognitive aspects of acquisition has been kept in clear focus – in fact, has been the focus of debate – in studies of the acquisition of morphophonology. Berko Gleason's "wug test" (Here is a wug. Now there are two of them; there are two . . .) (Berko, 1958/1971) contrasted the child's ability to produce forms which might have been memorized (one glass, two glasses) with non-word forms which could not have been heard before (tass, tasses; gutch, gutches). Here, the pattern of $/-s, -z, -\partial z/$ allomorphy is productive in the adult language, and the test distinguishes between the child who can produce the correct allomorphs only on familiar words and the more advanced child who can supply them for novel words and therefore must know the underlying pattern.

When a pattern does not reach productivity in the adult language, as is the case with many of the alternations in the late-acquired "learnéd" vocabulary in English, it is more difficult to assess the degree to which a speaker has acquired a pattern rather than a list of surface forms. As McCawley (ms) has pointed out, when a pattern is non-productive, it is probably not necessary to go beyond memorization of a short list of words to be a competent user of the language.

However, some techniques show that a degree of awareness of such patterns does develop in many speakers. It should be noted that the cognitive demands of the acquisition of the common non-productive rules of English (tri-syllabic laxing, various stress-shift rules, velar softening) are no greater than the demands of the acquisition of the complex productive morphophonemics of German or Russian. (Review of the acquisition of complex morphophonologies is beyond the scope of this chapter; the reader should consult MacWhinney 1978.)

Several techniques have been developed for studying knowledge of non-productive morphophonemic rules. There are the memory-reversion technique of Myerson (1975), the meaning-guessing technique of Wilbur and Menn, and the concept-forming technique most recently used by Jaeger. The Wilbur and Menn (1974, 1975) technique is the simplest: here subjects were given pseudo-words created from Latin or English morphemes according to regular non-productive patterns, and asked to pick among three possible meanings – for example, for "chibble" the choices were (a) light rain, (b) a kind of smooth cloth, (c) coarse sawdust. Responses of experimental subjects showed that attenuated sound–meaning correspondences were indeed available to the subjects for most of the obsolete allomorphic patterns: for "chibble", 65% of the subjects chose "coarse sawdust", 22% chose "light rain", and only 12% chose "smooth cloth"; for the test word "abducive", 72% chose "distracting", 10% "conserving", and 18% "informing".

But as Linell (1979) correctly warns, one cannot infer awareness of particular rules (e.g. the rules postulated by SPE) just by showing awareness of the allomorphy that those rules describe. Much more work is required in this area, and Jaeger's, which is too complex to discuss here, is a good start.

So far we have been discussing allomorphic relations that clearly go across phoneme boundaries: equivalences of /s,z, əz/; or of /p/ and /b/ (chip, chibble). How do we study the acquisition of strictly allophonic rules, that is, rules which have purely phonological conditioning? Some of these also go across phoneme boundaries (i.e. produce neutralization) and some do not. For example, final devoicing of consonants in a language with a voice–voiceless distinction produces neutralization (e.g. "Hund", /hɔnt/; "Hunde" /hɔnd /, where the underlying /d/ in the singular cannot be distinguished from an underlying /t/ unless one looks at the plural or another inflected form). On the other hand, the lengthening of vowels before voiced segments in English does not cause neutralization – there is no problem reconstructing an underlying segment different from the surface form.

Allophonic rules are easy enough to study if their context can be manipulated – if the segment can be made to appear both in the conditioning context and out of it. Vogel (1975) studied nasal assimilation to following stops in Spanish and Drachman and Malikouti-Drachman (1973) studied the same phenomenon in Greek. The overall impression from such studies is that stages of acquisition can be understood only from the perspective that the child is trying to work his way "back" from the surface to account for the patterns he observes; intermediate stages of rule acquisition need not look like simplified versions of the rules written for adult phonology.

These two nasal assimilation rules, incidentally, both function in two kinds of contexts: across morpheme boundaries, where they are easy to study by manipulation of context, and within morphemes, where their productivity is much harder to demonstrate. The techniques for appropriate tasks now exist, however, such as repetition of synthetic stimuli which violate the rules, and we can expect considerable progress on this front. In the meantime, some studies are available on the achievement of adult-like control of the surface manifestations of these rules: for example, Hawkins (1973, 1979a) on the acquisition of proper stop duration within consonant clusters in English, and Naeser (1970) on the duration of children's vowels before voiced and unvoiced stops in English.

VIII. Summary and Conclusion

It would be pleasant to say: these are the facts about the acquisition of phonology. However, we must hedge, this being a human science, and say instead: these are the major conclusions about the early stages of the acquisition of phonology that appear to be justified at the present time.

(1) Some children take a very "holistic" approach to the acquisition of phonology; their speech is so hard to transcribe and describe that we can say little about them in existing theoretical frameworks (Peters, 1977). Even the more analytical children sometimes resort to holistic approaches to varying degrees.

(2) The child's early acquisition of phonology has two aspects: the acquisition of phonetic control and the acquisition of phonemic contrast. Later, the same dichotomy extends to the acquisition of the surface forms of words v. the acquisition of the patterns that they are instances of.

(3) For most of the children whose approach we currently can handle, we find a rough division into an early period of very slow growth of the output lexicon, and then a period of more rapid growth. However, some children never show such a marked point of acceleration.

(4) Most of the words of the early period will have alternating vowels and consonants. Some words will probably be very well controlled and be more complex in structure (progressive phonological idioms); others may be extremely vague and variable in their output token forms.

(5) During the early period and for a while thereafter, most words will fall into groups. The words in such a group will be similar in both syllable structure and phonetic content; they will be describable as instances of a canonical form.

(6) The acquisition of phonemic oppositions can be studied only in terms of syllable structures: the typical picture is for a child to have a particular feature contrast in one position (initial, intervocalic, preconsonantal, final . . .) well before it appears in others. Within a given position, phonemic contrast may be evidenced indirectly before the child achieves good control of the pair of adult phonetic features involved in the contrast, but on the other hand there may be good phonetic control of one value of a feature without the presence of a contrasting phone.

(7) The mismatches between adult model and child word are the results of the child's trial and error attempts; they are shaped by the child's articulatory and auditory endowments (and thus to that extent are "natural") and by the child's previous successes at sound production. All rules of child phonology are learned in the sense that the child must discover for herself each correspondence between the sounds that she hears and what she does with her vocal tract in an attempt to produce those sounds.

(8) Knowledge gained by articulatory success on a particular sound or sound-pattern does not always generalize to cases which we phonologists feel to be similar: a feature or a phone or a string mastered may remain an isolated success for a long time.

(9) Regular mapping patterns (rules) grow, generalize, and often overgeneralize, even to the point of diminishing the child's accuracy of production of some words.

(10) Whole-word mapping strategies are used to varying degrees and are a major type of irregular mapping. Even in later stages of acquisition, such strategies can be found on the more difficult polysyllables.

(11) Instead of modifying adult words which are not within her capacity to produce accurately, a child may use selection strategies, avoiding problematic sounds and sound sequences and/or exploiting favourites.

(12) As implied by the phrasing of all these statements, individual variation among children is considerable. A deterministic theory would therefore have to be so weak as to be meaningless. Yet typical patterns emerge. The prevailing theories allow for individual variation by considering the child to be experimenting with solutions to the problem of how to say words. As we look across children, trying to discover what tends to be earlier, and therefore presumably easier, and what tends to be later, and therefore presumably harder, we find three articulatory sources of difficulty for the young speaker: the articulation of certain phones (e.g. [ɹ, θ]), the sequencing of dissimilar consonantal targets, and departures from CVCV . . alternations. Difficulties also arise from perceptual sources, including a tendency to perceive unfamiliar forms as similar familiar ones, and (probably) an inability to take in all the information about a relatively long word until its most salient sounds have already been well-learned.

Finally, unexpected hindrances and aids may arise from the child's current array of strategies: a sequence which "should" be easy may be difficult for a particular child because it does not fit into the rules or prosodic strategies that she happens to have developed up to that time.

(13) This chapter presents the view that the child's mastery of production mechanisms can be described as learning to (a) control the accuracy of articulatory movements, (b) specify more contrasting articulatory targets in a given sequence position, (c) produce more different sequence types, and (d) concatenate sequence types.

Let us conclude by considering the assertion made in the introduction to this chapter: that evidence from the studies which have become available in the last ten or fifteen years has forced a change in our basic conception of the nature of phonological development. We can no longer sustain the developing-embryo model; we need problem-solving models to make sense of peculiarly skewed output distributions such as we find in children who "avoid" or "exploit" heavily. Just as in the acquisition of morphology and syntax, what has been called the "implicit defining question" of our research has changed. We used to ask: What linguistic theory will explain the order in which the various language behaviours develop? This question assumed that there is such an order, and that it should be explainable by linguistic theory. The new question is roughly: What behavioural predispositions and abilities does the child bring to the task of learning to communicate with language, and how does the individual go about solving the articulatory and phonological problems posed by the language to be learned?

The presuppositions of the second question differ markedly from the first. We now presuppose that there are a variety of "predispositions and abilities" of memory, motor control, perception, etc. – including perhaps some "purely linguistic"predispositions which might have evolved just for handling the special rapid information processing and complex pattern learning involved in the acquisition and use of language. We also presume that the notion of problem solving is the best heuristic for explaining the kind of very rough consensus of developmental order that we find in the data. As for the old assumption that linguistic theory can explain what we find in acquisition, we have seen that the more likely scenario is that linguistic theory and acquisition data will have to come to terms with one another. A theory based only on the performance of the mature skilled user cannot anticipate the temporary learning devices and detours of the unskilled learner.

Note: In this chapter, the feminine form has often been used for the indefinite pronoun. The reader may not realize it, but my female colleagues and I are still receiving professional form correspondence – for example, reprint requests – that address us as "Dear Sir / Sehr geehrter Herr / Cher monsieur". At least until I have evidence that more scientists in this field can conceive of their fellows in two sexes as well as in three languages, I think it well to jog their sense of "markedness" a bit.

Acknowledgements

My grateful thanks to Sarah Hawkins, Paula Menyuk, and Ronnie Wilbur, who spent considerable time and effort working over the first draft of this chapter. At the urging of Charles A. Ferguson, and with the help of Prof. Hawkins, I have attempted to overcome old habits and use IPA consistently throughout it.

References

Barton, D. P. (1976). The role of perception in the acquisition of speech. Doctoral dissertation, University of London. Circulated by Indiana University Linguistics Club.

Barton, D. P. (1980). Phonemic perception in children. In "Child Phonology: Perception and Production" (G. Yeni-Komshian, J. F. Kavanagh and C. A. Ferguson, eds) Vol. 2. Academic Press, New York and London.

Bell, A. (1971). Some patterns of occurrence and formation of syllable structures. In "Working Papers on Linguistic Universals", Linguistics Department, Stanford University, 6, 23–137.

Berko, J. (1958). The child's learning of English morphology. Word 14, 150–157. Reprinted in A. Bar-Adon and W. Leopold, (eds) (1971). "Child Language: A Book of Readings". pp. 153–167.

Branigan, G. (1979). Sequences of words as structured units. Doctoral dissertation, Boston University School of Education.

Clumeck, H. (1977). Studies in the acquisition of Mandarin phonology. Doctoral dissertation, University of California at Berkeley.

Drachman, G. and Malikouti-Drachman, A. (1973). Studies in the acquisition of Greek as a native language. In "Ohio State University Working Papers in Linguistics" 15, 99–114.

Farwell, C. B. (1976). Some strategies in the early production of fricatives. In "Papers and Reports in Child Language Development" (No. 12). Stanford University Linguistics Department.

Ferguson, C. A., Weeks, T. and Peizer, D. B. (1973). Model-and-replica grammar of a child's first words. Lingua 31 (1), 35–65.

Ferguson, C. A. and Farwell, C. B. (1975). Words and sounds in early language acquisition. Language 51, 491–439.

Ferguson, C. A. and Macken, M. A. (To appear). Phonological development in children's play and cognition. In "Children's Language", (Keith E. Nelson ed.), Vol. IV. Gardner Press, New York.

Fey, M. and Gandour, J. (1979). Problem-solving in early phonology acquisition. Paper read at the Annual Meeting of the Linguistic Society of America, Los Angeles, 1979.

Fey, M. and Gandour J. (1982). Rule discovery in early phonology acquisition. Journal of Child Language 9, 71–82.

Flege, J. E. and Massey, K. P. (1980). English prevoicing: random or controlled? Paper read at the Summer Meeting of the Linguistic Society of America, 1980.

Goldstein, U. (1980). An articulatory model for the vocal tracts of growing children. Doctoral dissertation, Electrical Engineering Department, MIT.

Halliday, M. A. K. (1975). "Learning How to Mean: Explorations in the Development of Language". Edward Arnold, London.

Hamp, E. H. (1974). Wortphonologie. *Journal of Child Language* 11, 287–288.

Hawkins, S. (1973). Temporal coordination of consonants in the speech of children: preliminary data. *Journal of Phonetics*, 1, 181–217.

Hawkins, S (1979a). Temporal coordination of consonants in speech of children: further data. *Journal of Phonetics*, 7, 235–267.

Hawkins, S. (1979). The control of timing in children's speech. *Proceedings of the Ninth International Congress of Phonetic Sciences, Copenhagen, 1979.*

Ingram, D. (1974). Phonological rules in young children. *Journal of Child Language* 1, 49–64.

Ingram, D. (1976). "Phonological Disabilities in Children". Elsevier, New York.

Ingram, D (1979). Phonological patterns in the speech of young children. *In* "Language Acquisition" (P. Fletcher and M. Garman, eds). Cambridge University Press, Cambridge.

Itkonen, T. (1977). Notes on the acquisition of phonology. English summary of Huomioita lapsen äänteistön kehityksestä. *Virittäjä*, 279–308.

Jaeger, J. J. (1980). Categorization in phonology: an experimental approach. Doctoral dissertation, University of California/Berkeley.

Jakobson, R. (1968). "Child Language, Aphasia, and Phonological Universals" (Trans. A. Keiler). Mouton, The Hague.

Jones, L. G. (1967). English phonotactic structure and first-language acquisition. *Lingua* 19, 1–59.

Kent, R. D. (1978). Imitation of synthesized vowels by preschool children. *Journal of the Acoustic Society of America*, 63, 1193–1198.

Kisseberth, C. W. (1970). On the functional unity of phonological rules. *Linguistic Inquiry* 1, 291–306.

Korte, S. S., and Bond, Z. S. (1979). Children's spontaneous and imitative speech: An acoustic analysis. Paper read at meeting of American Speech and Hearing Society, November, 1979.

Leonard, L., Schwartz, R., Folger, M. K. and Wilcox, M. J. (1978). Some aspects of children phonology in imitative and spontaneous speech. *Journal of Child Language* 5 (3), 403–416.

Leopold, W. F. (1939–1949). "Speech Development of a Bilingual Child". Vols I–IV. Northwestern University Press, Evanston.

Linell, P. Psychological reality and the concept of phonological rule. *Proceedings of the Ninth International Congress of Phonetic Sciences, Copenhagen, 1979.*

Macken, M. A. and Barton, D. (1980). The acquisition of the voicing contrast in English: a study of voice onset time in word-initial stop consonants. *Journal of Child Language* 7 41–75.

Macken, M. A. The child's lexical representation: evidence from the 'puzzle-puddle-pickle' phenomenon. Stanford University Papers and Reports in Child Language Development (No. 16), 1979; also to appear in Journal of Linguistics.

Macken, M. A. (1979). Developmental reorganization of phonology: a hierarchy of basic units of acquisition. *Lingua* 49 11–49.

MacWhinney, B. (1978). The acquisition of Morphophonology. *Monographs of the Society for Research in Child Development* 43, 1–2.

Menn, L. (1971). Phonotactic rules in beginning speech. *Lingua* 26, 225–241.

Menn, L. (1976a). Pattern, control, and contrast in beginning speech: a case study in the acquisition of word form and function. Doctoral Dissertation, University of Illinois. Circulated by Indiana University Linguistics Club.

Menn, L. (1976b). Semantics of intonation contour in late babble and beginning speech (English). Paper read at the Summer Meeting, Linguistic Society of America, 1976.

Menn, L. (1977). Parental awareness of child phonology. Paper read at the Annual Meeting of the Linguistic Society of America, 1977.

Menn, L. Transition and variation in child phonology: modelling a developing system. *Proceedings of the Ninth International Congress of Phonetic Sciences, Copenhagen, 1979.*

Menn, L. (1981). Review of S. P. Blache, The acquisition of distinctive features. *Language*, **57**, 953–958.

Menn, L. and Haselkorn, S. (1977). Now you see it, now you don't: tracing the development of communicative consciousness. *In* "Procedings of the Seventh Annual Meeting, NorthEast Linguistic Society", (Judy Kegl, ed.) 1977.

Menn, L. and Berko Gleason, J. (to appear). Babytalk as folk phonology: Bias in parents' reports of children's pronunciations. (forthcoming.)

Menyuk, P. (1977). "Language and Maturation". Cambridge, MIT Press, Cambridge, Massachusetts.

Menyuk, P. (1980). The role of context in misarticulations. *In* "Child Phonology", (Yeni-Komshian, G. Kavanagh, J. and Ferguson, C. A., eds) Vol. I. Academic Press, New York and London.

Moskowitz, A. (1970a). The two-year-old stage in the acquisition of English phonology. *Language* **46**, 426–441.

Moskowitz, A. (1970b). The acquisition of phonology. Working paper (No. 34), Language-behavior Research Laboratory, University of California, Berkeley.

Moskowitz, A. (1975). The acquisition of phonetics: a study in phonetics and phonology. *Journal of Phonetics* **3**, 141–150.

Myerson, R. (1975). A developmental study of children's knowledge of complex derived words of English. Doctoral dissertation, Harvard Graduate School of Education.

Naeser, M. A. (1970). The American child's acquisition of differential vowel duration. Technical report No. 144 (in two parts), Wisconsin Research and Development center for Cognitive Learning. University of Wisonsin, Madison.

Nakazima, S. (1972). A comparative study of the speech development of Japanese and American children, part IV. *Studia Phonologica* **VI**, 1–37.

Peters, A. M. (1977). Language learning strategies. *Language* **53**, 560–573.

Platt, C. and MacWhinney, B. (1983). Solving a problem vs. remembering a solution: error assimilation as a strategy in language acquisition. *Journal of Child Language*, **7**, 41–75.

Priestly, T. M. S. (1977). One idiosyncratic strategy in the acquisition of phonology. *Journal of Child Language* **4**, 45–66.

Sander, E. K. (1972). When are speech sounds learned? *Journal of Speech and Hearing Disorders* **37**, 55–63.

Schwartz, R. G. and Leonard, L. B. (1982). Do children pick and choose? An examination of phonological selection and avoidance in early lexical acquisition. *Journal of Child Language*, **9**, 319–336.

Slobin, D. I. (1966). Comments on "Developmental Psycholinguistics". *In* "The Genesis of Language" (F. Smith and G. A. Miller, eds,). MIT Press, Cambridge, Massachusetts.

Slobin, D. I. (1973). Cognitive prerequisites for the development of grammar. *In* "Studies of Child Language Development" (C. A. Ferguson and D. I. Slobin, eds), Holt, Rinehart and Winston, New York.

Smith, B. L. (1979). A phonetic analysis of consonantal devoicing in children's speech. *Journal of Child Language* 6, 19–28.

Smith, N. V. (1973). "The Acquisition of Phonology: A Case Study". Cambridge University Press, Cambridge.

Smith, N. V. (1978). Lexical acquisition and the acquisition of phonology. Summer Forum Lecture, Linguistic Institute of the Linguistic Society of America.

Snow, C. (1977). The development of conversation between mothers and babies. *Journal of Child Language* 4, 1–22.

Stampe, D. (1969). The acquisition of phonemic representation. *Proceedings of the Fifth Regional Meeting of the Chicago Linguistic Society*. 433–444.

Sterne, D., Jaffe, T., Beebe, B. and Bennett, S. L. (1975). Vocalizing in unison and in alternation: two modes of communication in the mother–infant dyad. In "Annals of the New York Academy of Sciences." Vol. 263: Developmental Psycholinguistics and Communication Disorders. (Aaronson, D. and Rieber, R. W. eds).

Stevens, K. N. (1972). The quantal nature of speech: evidence from articulatory-acoustic data. *In* "Human Communication, A Unified View". (Denes, P. B. and David, E. E. eds) McGraw-Hill, New York. pp. 51–66.

Velten, H. V. (1941). The growth of phonemic and lexical pattern in the infant. *Language* 19, 440–444. Reprinted in A. Bar-Adon and W. Leopold (eds.) (1971). "Readings in Child Language". Prentice-Hall, Englewood Cliffs, New Jersey.

Vihman, M. M. (1976). From prespeech to speech: On early phonology. "Papers and Reports on Child Language Development", (No. 12), Stanford University Linguistics Department.

Vihman, M. M. (1981). Phonology and the development of the lexicon: evidence from children's errors. *Journal of Child Language* 8, 239–264.

Vihman, M. M. (to appear). Homonymy and the organization of early vocabulary. Child Phonology Project, Stanford University.

Vihman, M. M. (1978). Consonant harmony – its scope and function in child language. *In* "Universals of Human Language" (J. H. Greenberg, ed.), Vol. III. Stanford University Press, Stanford.

Vogel, I. (1975). Nasals and nasal assimilation patterns in the acquisition of Chicano Spanish. *In* "Papers and Reports on Child Language Development" (No. 10), Stanford University Linguistics Department.

von Raffler-Engel, W. (1973). The development from sound to phoneme in child language. *In* Slobin, (eds.), "Studies of Child Language Development". (Ferguson, C. A. and Slobin, D. I., eds) pp. 9–12. Translated from *Proceedings of the Fifth International Congress of Phonetic Sciences, Munster, 1964*.

Waterson, N. (1970). Some aspects of the phonology of the nominal forms of the Turkish word. *In* "Prosodic Analysis" (F. R. Palmer, ed.) pp. 174–187. Oxford University Press, London.

Waterson, N. (1970). Some speech forms of an English child: a phonological study. *Transactions of the Philological, Society*.

Waterson, N. (1971). Child phonology: a prosodic view. *Journal of Linguistics* 7, 179–221.

Waterson, N. (1972). Perception and production in the acquisition of language. *Proceedings of the International Symposium on First Language Acquisition, Florence, 1972*.

Waterson, N. (1978). Growth of complexity in phonological development. *In* "The Development of Communication". (Waterson N. and Snow, C. E., eds) Wiley, New York.

Weir, R. (1962). "Language in the Crib" Mouton, The Hague.

Wellmers, W. E. and Harris, Z. S. (1942). The phonemes of Fanti. *JAOS* **64** (No. 4), 318–333.

Westbury, J. R. and Keating, P. A. (1980). A model of stop consonant voicing and a theory of markedness. Paper read at the Annual Meeting of the Linguistic Society of America, 1980.

Wilbur, R. B. and Menn, L. (1975). Psychological reality, linguistic theory, and the internal structure of the lexicon. San Jose State University Occasional Papers in Linguistics.

Wilbur, R. B. (1980). Theoretical phonology and child phonology: argumentation and implications. *In* "Phonology in the 1980's". (Goyvaerts, D. ed.) Story-Scientia, Ghent.

Yeni-Komshian, G., Kavanagh, J. and Ferguson, C. A. (eds) (1980). "Child Phonology: Perception and Production". Academic Press, New York and London.

Zwicky, A. M. (1982). Classical malapropisms and the creation of a mental lexicon. *In* "Exceptional Language and Linguistics';, (L. Menn and L. K. Obler, eds), pp. 115–132. Academic Press, New York and London.

2

Lexical and Grammatical Development

J. McShane
J. Dockrell

London School of Economics
University of Stirling

In recent years there has been a tremendous growth in the literature concerned with language development. One difficulty that faces any attempt to
review the relevant literature is the diversity of issues that arise. What role
does the child's environment play in facilitating language development (see,
for example, Gleason and Weintraub, 1978; Snow and Ferguson, 1977)?
Does linguistic communication have precursors in the early vocal and
gestural communications of the young infant (see Bullowa, 1979; Lock,
1978; Schaffer, 1977)? How does the child's production system change over
time? This review will be concerned primarily with this last question. We will
start at a point at which the child has begun to produce recognizable
language and discuss the more influential theories and pieces of empirical
work that have contributed to an understanding of how the child's production system develops.

The realization on the child's part that language is a system in which words
are used symbolically provides the basis for both lexical and grammatical
development (McShane, 1979, 1980). Although the words that a child uses
in structured utterances are obviously words that are in the child's lexicon,
the issues of how the lexicon develops and how grammatical structure
develops can be separated. An example may illustrate one way in which
these issues warrant separate consideration: a child may wrongly believe
that 'duck' denotes all birds, a fact that would be of considerable interest for
theories of lexical development. However, this erroneous belief need not
hinder the child's ability to combine "duck" appropriately with other words
in order to encode such concepts as NONEXISTENCE in *allgone duck*,
RECURRENCE in *more duck*, ACTOR-ACTION in *duck fly* and so on.*

---

* Throughout we use *italics* for utterances, single quotation marks for a lexeme or sentence,
and CAPITALS for conceptual categories. We use double quotation marks for quotation and
for "scare" quotes.

LANGUAGE PRODUCTION VOL. 2
ISBN 0-12-147502-6

The first section of this chapter provides a framework within which the various issues pertinent to lexical and grammatical development can be discussed and the relations among the issues clearly seen. In the second section we will be concerned with issues of lexical development that can be studied independently of grammatical development. The third section will consider how a child learns a system of rules for combining words together. Throughout, our central concern is to address the following question: In following the developmental path he does in learning a language what sorts of inductions, generalizations, and inferences is a child making about how that language is organized?

I. Developmental Considerations for a Model of Production

In General Systems Theory distinctions are drawn among input, state, and output variables. These distinctions will serve as organizing constructs in this review. An adequate theory of language development must explain what the relevant relations are among these variables. Most existing theories only attempt to deal with the functioning of part of the system and there has been little attempt to relate the different partial theories to each other or to construct an overall theory of the system.

Developmental psycholinguistics has been much concerned with the relations between state constructs and output variables. The relative neglect of the input variable is largely due to arguments initially advanced by Chomsky (1957, 1959) that an input–output account of speech was inadequate and that complex state operations had to be postulated to account for the observed complexity of language. Chomsky further argued (1965, 1968) that these state operations could not be derived by children from the input they heard and that one had, therefore, to assume that these operations were innate endowments.

One of Chomsky's main arguments in support of this claim was that the input was so impoverished as to render impossible any inferences by the child about the state operations necessary to reproduce that input. Subsequent research (see Snow and Ferguson, 1977; Vorster, 1975) has shown that the input is not nearly as impoverished as Chomsky had claimed. However, while this literature charts ways in which the speech that children hear differs from adult speech, much of the literature has little to say about the actual effects of adult speech on children learning language. This is a serious neglect and the problem is made more acute by the fact that many of the more obvious hypotheses about input–output relations have not been supported when subjected to test (Newport, Gleitman and Gleitman, 1977).

The state operations which have been the subject of so much theorizing and research (and that will be the main subject of this review) are the rules that are assumed to underlie the utterances that the child produces. The system of rules used is obviously not open to direct inspection. In arriving at a formulation of these rules, inferences must be made from the child's output. To some extent the relations between state operations and output variables can be studied in ignorance of input variables: one can study the output produced, and formulate hypotheses about the structures necessary to account for that output, while remaining neutral about the origins of those structures. However, the independence is, in practice, more illusory than real. The tendency, for example, to postulate powerful innate state variables (e.g. Bloom, 1970; McNeill, 1970) is directly related to beliefs about the relevance of the input. Chomsky's (1965) argument that the input a child receives is so degraded that the necessary production rules could never be inferred was one factor that helped to detach the study of state-output relations from the study of input. Thus, whether or not theorizing about state operations is informed by a knowledge of input variables, it inevitably makes certain assumptions about the nature and relevance of the input.

Output is the behaviour produced by the child. In the case of production this output will usually consist of speech, although other non-verbal behaviours may also constitute relevant output. State and output are inextricably linked in that the inferences made about state operations depend on one's characterization of the output which in turn depend on one's assumptions about state. There are three points that need to be made in relation to this. The first is that it merely emphasizes the fact that research is guided by theories. What aspects of output are chosen for study and the dimensions chosen to describe this output will be dictated by the theoretical issues that are deemed important. The second point is that it is important to preserve, as far as possible, terminological distinctions between state terms and output terms so that the predictive and inferential relations between the two can be tested properly. Output consists of behaviour and so the appropriate description of output is at the level of behavioural events. State consists of inferred rules and categories and so the appropriate description is at the level of hypothetical organizational constructs that determine the structure of the output. Confounding of these levels is common and regretable. For example, there are many descriptions of children's one-word output in terms of nouns, verbs, and adjectives. McShane (1980) has pointed out that such descriptions presume that form-class distinctions are made by the child when there is no warrant whatsoever for such a presumption. As we shall see in Section III below, the origin of form-class distinctions is an issue of considerable complexity. The third point, which emphasizes the importance of the second, is that descriptions of output and inferences about state will be subject to frequent revisions in the light of new theories, new evidence, and re-evaluation of old evidence. For example, it used to be assumed that overextended use of words was unequivocal evidence for feature-by-feature acquisition of word meaning. It is now obvious that the evidence is both much more difficult to interpret than was presumed and does not necessitate a feature-by-feature model of the acquisition of word meaning (see Section II). A similar point can be made in relation to grammatical development. It used to be assumed that the child operated with a small number of powerful general rules for producing structured utterances. It is now more commonly assumed, in the light of Braine's (1976) re-evaluation of the evidence, that the child operates with a more piecemeal system of particular rules of limited scope (see Section III).

II. Lexical Development

A. What Develops in a Lexicon?

The types of questions that are asked about lexical development and, by corollary, the empirical studies that are carried out, depend to a great extent on what is conceived as developing. If lexical development is viewed as development towards standard adult usage then one might examine the various errors or reference that the child makes and attempt to infer the partial intensional criteria that the child uses as a subset of the adult criteria.* If, on the other hand, lexical development is viewed as a process of establishing the relations that exist among words, then one might study the child's errors as indices of greater or lesser degrees of differentiation in a particular semantic field. The difference between the two approaches is the extent to which the meaning of a word is viewed in isolation from the meaning of other words. It must be emphasized that these approaches are not opposite characterizations of lexical development but different perspectives on the issue. However, particular theories have tended to emphasize one perspective and neglect the other. In order to represent the issues clearly it will be necessary to establish an adequate terminology.

Studying lexical development involves studying how the child learns to map relations of meaning between words and the world. This involves tripartite relations among reference, denotation, and sense (Lyons, 1977). Reference describes the relation between a particular expression and an entity referred to on a particular occasion of use. It follows from this that reference is not a property of words *per se* but rather "it is the speaker who refers (by using some appropriate expression): he invests the expression with reference by the act of referring" (Lyons, 1977, p. 177). The entity itself can usually be referred to in a number of ways. In different situations an entity such as a dog might be referred to as *dog, animal, the shaggy one*, and so on. Thus, one issue that confronts theories of lexical development is how contextual and discourse factors determine the selection of a referential expression.

---

* The adult criteria are inferred also, of course. There are considerable problems about establishing the criteria used by adults. Much developmental work asserts that the adult lexicon has such-and-such a structure without producing empirical evidence that this is, in fact, the case. These assertions are frequently derived from formal linguistic theories of the lexicon, which, by now, ought to be regarded as a notoriously unreliable guide to the psychological structure of the lexicon (see Black and Chiat, 1981, for a discussion of formal and psychological models). To the extent that the *terminus ad quem* of the developing system is misconceived, the hypotheses about the processes of development will also be misconceived.

While reference describes the relation between a particular expression and a particular entity, denotation describes a relation that exists between a word and a set of entities – e.g. the word "tree" denotes a particular set of entities (trees) and the individual trees are its denotata. The crucial semantic issue that confronts theories of lexical development is to explain how a child establishes the denotation of a word. Most theories argue that a word's denotation is determined by the set of properties that the denotata have in common. Such a set of properties is generally called the intension of a term.* Thus, the intension of 'cat' is the set of properties that determines what entities are denoted by 'cat' and can therefore be called *cat*†. One common feature of modern theories of lexical development is to relate output and state by using the child's referential errors to infer the set of intensional features that the child uses to determine a word's denotation. A crucial issue in the discussion of intension is whether the properties that determine denotation can be defined as a set of isolated features or whether the contrasts between classes of entities also serve as part of the intension of a word. This latter notion is captured by the term 'sense'.

Sense, as we use it here (following Lyons, 1977), applies to relations existing within the lexicon. There are two important types of sense relations that we wish to focus on: hierarchical sense relations that exist between terms at different levels in a taxonomy, and contrastive sense relations that exist between terms within a semantic field.‡ As an example consider 'cat' and 'dog'. Both terms occur at the same level of a taxonomy and are hierarchically related to the term 'animal'. 'Cat' and 'dog' are thus hyponyms of 'animal' and there are hierarchical sense relations between 'cat' and 'animal' and between 'dog' and 'animal'. 'Cat' and 'dog' have mutually exclusive extensions; an entity cannot be both a cat and a dog. Thus, 'cat' and 'dog' can be contrastively defined; 'cat' implies not-dog and

---

* 'Intension' is usually contrasted with 'extension'. In our terminology 'denotation' and 'extension' are interchangeable terms. We prefer 'denotation' as it admits the convenient 'denotatum' and 'denotata'.

† A number of philosophers have recently claimed that the meaning of many words cannot be determined by intensional criteria (see Schwartz, 1979, for a summary of the argument). The basis of the argument is that many "natural kind" terms do not have a set of intensional criteria that determine their extension. Intensional properties are not necessarily associated with these words but merely empirically associated with them (Kripke, 1972). Putnam (1975) used "gold" to illustrate the argument. It is unlikely that most people could specify the properties that uniquely pick out gold. Further, it is possible for anybody (even experts) to be mistaken about the criteria that identify gold. The same argument can be applied to terms such as 'water' and 'tiger'. From the argument that natural kind terms cannot be defined intensionally it does not follow that intensional criteria do not play a part in the way a child learns the meaning of a term (or even in the way adults use a term). An intension (or a combination of intensions) that is inadequate to specify the true extension of a word may nevertheless function adequately to specify the extension that is relevant to communication and shared understanding. The Kripke/Putnam argument shows that intensions and extensions are imperfectly related. Such imperfections need not hinder socially shared extensions determined by agreed intensions.

‡ For a discussion of semantic fields, see Miller and Johnson-Laird (1976, *inter alia*).

vice versa. That much is uncontroversial. It may also be argued, however, that it is only the contrasts among members of a semantic field that serve to determine a word's denotation and that other criteria are neither relevant nor adequate to the task (see e.g. Barrett, 1978; Harrison, 1972). A more neutral position will be adopted here, which regards denotation as determined both by contrastive and non-contrastive properties.

The three-way distinction of reference, denotation, and sense provides both a working definition of what is involved in knowing the meaning of a word and an instrument with which to examine some of the issues and approaches to lexical development. (We will not, at this stage, be concerned with factors that determine the grammatical privileges that a word has.)

In discussing lexical development some segmentation of the lexicon is necessary. It is convenient to distinguish among words that refer to entities, actions, and properties. The terms 'noun', 'verb', and 'adjective' are frequently used to indicate these distinctions. However, their use in a developmental model of the lexicon is problematic. Describing a child as learning nouns, verbs, and adjectives can carry the implication that a child already understands the grammatical functions of nouns, verbs, and adjectives. This is far from being the case in the initial stages of acquisition and thus the use of these terms can serve to confuse discussion of the state constructs that organize and determine the child's output (see McShane, 1980, for a more detailed discussion).

In general, we will use 'name' for words that refer to entities. Convenient alternatives are not available for 'verb' and 'adjective', so, when the occasion demands we will use these terms within "scare quotes".

The issue that has received most attention in lexical development is the construction of state models to explain the child's output. The referential errors that children make in speech output have been the main source of evidence for these models. Consequently, we will first discuss theories of nominal overextension based on errors of production and then discuss the issue of errors in comprehension and the relation between production and comprehension. We will then extend the discussion to other types of words besides names. Finally, we will discuss the way in which input might be related to the state models discussed. We will not, for reasons of space, discuss the classificatory basis of such prominent early words as *more*, *no*, and *allgone*, although clearly a complete theory of lexical development would have to account for the conceptual categories that underlie the child's use of these words (see McShane, 1980, for some relevant discussion).

B. Overextension of Names

It is apparent, from children's use of language, that words are frequently used to refer to inappropriate referents (see Bloom, 1973; Leopold, 1939–49; Lewis, 1936; see Clark, 1973a for a review). It has often been inferred from this that the overextended words have a different denotation in the child's lexicon than they do in the adult lexicon. While there undoubtedly are words of which this is true, the interpretation of overextension errors is by no means as straightforward as this in general. As we shall see, referential overextension need not imply denotational overextension. Even when it can be argued that this is the case there is still room for theoretical disagreement on how denotational differences between child and adult arise.

The dominant theory of lexical development in the past decade has been Semantic Feature Theory (Clark, 1973a; 1974), which has provided researchers with a framework within which many precise questions can be asked about children's partial understanding of words in many specific lexical domains. Clark's theory is drawn directly from the work of linguists (e.g. Bierwisch, 1970; Katz and Fodor, 1963; Postal, 1966) and anthropologists who view words as a collection of semantic components or features. Semantic components are seen as the basic units of meaning, which combine in different ways to make up the meaning of individual words. Clark (1973a, p. 72) characterizes the process of development as follows:

> The semantic feature hypothesis states that when the child first begins to use identifiable words, he does not know their full (adult) meaning: he only has partial entries for them in his lexicon, such that these partial entries correspond in some way to some of the features or components of meaning that would be present in the entries for the same words in the adults lexicon. Thus the child will begin by identifying the meaning of a word with only one or two 'features' rather than the whole combination of meaning components or features (qua Postal) that are used criterially by the adult. . . . Let us suppose that the child has learnt the word *dog* (or *doggie*); however, he only uses one feature to characterize the meaning of this word, so the set of objects that he will put into the category named *dog* will be larger than the set in the adult category. For instance, he might have characterized the word *dog* as meaning *four-legged*; the set of objects referred to as *dog*, therefore might include cows, sheep, zebras, llamas, dogs and anything else that is four-legged.

Clark assumes, therefore, that the meanings of words are composed of features and that children learn the meanings of words gradually, by adding more features to their lexical entries until the meanings are complete by adult standards. Clark's theory thus implies that there is a quantitative difference between child and adult usage of words in that children have fewer critical features available than adults in deciding on the use of a word.

The Semantic Feature Theory explanation of overextended reference focuses on the denotational differences between child and adult. It has little to say about how sense relations are established among words. Barrett (1978), by contrast, offers an account of lexical development that focuses on sense relations. He argues that the meaning of a word is not learnt by acquiring a set of defining features sufficient to determine the extension of a word but rather by acquiring the features that distinguish the extension of one word from the extensions of closely related words. According to this hypothesis the child abstracts a set of constrastive features that distinguish a referent from other potentially confusable referents. In the case of 'dog', a child will learn "only those contrasts which serve to distinguish dogs from other animals and are needed in order to delimit the extension of *dog*" (Barrett, 1978, p. 209).

The crucial difference between Barrett's views and those of Clark (1973a) is the respective emphasis on sense and intension as *the* key factor in word learning. It is doubtful whether one of these factors should be seen as central to the acquisition process in preference to the other. Both sense and intension are important components of word meaning and it seems reasonable to expect that they would be interdependent in the development of word meaning. To date, little attention has been given to their interdependence. One issue that must be faced in any further theorizing is whether the boundaries of a word's denotation are clear cut (as both accounts would seem to imply) or fuzzy as some theoretical accounts of word classes argue (Labov, 1973).

The views that we have considered up till now regard all members of a category as equally good members and hence all denotata of a word are equally good denotata. This view has been challenged by a variety of writers (Berlin and Kay, 1969; Kay, 1975; Rosch and Mervis, 1975; Rosch *et al.*, 1976) who argue that there are degrees of membership of a category with some members being regarded as more typical exemplars than others. These members are regarded as prototypes and a category is structured around these prototypes. According to one influential view (Rosch and Mervis, 1975) semantic categories consist of prototypes that share a network of overlapping attributes and more peripheral members that have relatively few attributes in common with the prototypical members. On this view one might argue that lexical development begins by learning that an entity, or several entities, can serve as referents for a word. These entities might serve as the prototype for future uses of the word. Bowerman (1978) has advanced such an argument. She also argues that prototypical exemplars are further analysed into salient features. The exemplars will share many features in common but there will not necessarily be any one feature that is common to all. Rather, exemplars will differ in the extent to which they share features with other exemplars.

Let us now consider, with respect to names, to what extent the evidence supports or refutes the various theories. Semantic Feature Theory appears to predict that overextensions will be the dominant pattern in lexical development. However, less than a third of the child's words are actually overextended (Nelson, Rescorla, Gruendel, and Benedict, 1978). Semantic Feature Theory is thus faced with the embarassing difficulty of explaining how the majority of words are used correctly. A theory such as Barrett's (1978) likewise has difficulty in that it predicts that overextensions will occur if a word is learnt in isolation from others in the same semantic field. However, such learning frequently occurs without concomitant overextensions. By contrast, prototype theory has no difficulty in accounting for both the correct use of words, and for overextensions and underextensions. If a word has been learnt with reference to several prototypical exemplars then these exemplars may serve to define the core meaning of the word. If only these exemplars are encountered by the child (or alternatively if other exemplars are encountered but the word is never used except for the prototypical exemplars) then errors of overextension will not occur. Further, the theory predicts that when overextensions do occur the overextensions will not necessarily share any one feature in common. According to the theory a variety of features will be abstracted from the prototypical exemplars and any of these features may be used as criterial in extending a word to cover novel referents. Thomson and Chapman (1977) and Bowerman (1978), both report patterns of overextended use in which no one feature alone is common to all the overextensions of a particular word*.

One major difficulty in interpreting overextensions as evidence for or against particular theories of word meaning is that overextensions do not constitute unequivocal evidence for denotational differences between children and adults. Overextensions occur for a variety of reasons (McShane, 1979). The most obvious case is that in which a child does not know the word for a particular referent (or knows the word but fails to access it) and uses a word with a related sense in order to refer (see Bloom, 1973; Huttenlocher, 1974). It is not always possible, with much of the available evidence, to tell whether a child's overextension has occurred because of a denotational error or because of production difficulties. Many of the observations reported in diary studies do not include a record of the frequency of over-extended use. There is a considerable risk attached to inferences concerning the denotation of a word on the basis of a small number of referential overextensions. In order to distinguish among the different interpretations possible, it is obvious that some other converging source of evidence is needed to indicate which interpretation of the evidence is most plausible. In the case of overextensions, evidence from comprehension studies might be used to establish whether the overextension is due to inadequate denotation or due to lexical impoverishment (i.e. the absence of a suitable alternative term). As we shall see below such evidence indicates that overextension errors occur for various reasons. Before embarking on a discussion of some of the empirical work it is necessary to discuss in more detail the manner in which lexical knowledge is assessed in production and comprehension studies.

C. Production and Comprehension of Names

Very different conclusions can be reached depending on whether the investigator uses production or comprehension data in studies of lexical develop-

---

* Thomson and Chapman (1977) interpret the absence of a single feature common to all overextensions as evidence that the child's concepts are ill-defined in the manner of Vygotsky's (1934) "chain complexes". The presumption is that adult-like well-defined concepts will later replace these ill-defined concepts. However, the errors of overextension reported by Thomson and Chapman can also be interpreted as evidence for the organization of concepts around prototypical exemplars. This view does not assume that the child's concepts are ill-defined (see Bowerman, 1978, for a comparison of the two views).

ment. Diary studies of early lexical development, by their very nature, reflect the productive competence of the young child and tend to capture children's overextensions rather than their underextensions. It is obvious to an observer when a child overextends a word to an inappropriate referent whereas it is less obvious when a word is only used to refer to some subset of the referents to which it has potential reference.

A common view is that comprehension develops in advance of production. Goldin-Meadow, Seligman, and Gelman (1976) conclude that young children initially have receptive vocabularies several times the size of their productive vocabularies. The logic of the comprehension-before-production argument rests on the state assumption that while comprehension involves identifying the entity referred to, production involves both identification and a procedure for selecting a word appropriate to the initial identification and is therefore cognitively more complex. However, Clark *et al.* (1974) argue that production and comprehension are less divergent than is normally assumed. They suggest that there is an association between the child's capacity to comprehend a word and its availability for production – that is, a word that is in the child's productive vocabulary is also more readily perceived and responded to. These authors also emphasize that such factors as redundancy, intonation, and various non-verbal cues facilitates the child in interpreting what has been said to him. Thus, behavioural evidence of comprehension does not necessarily imply sophisticated lexical processes (see Shatz, 1978, for similar arguments in relation to grammatical comprehension).

Clark *et al.*'s suggestion that comprehension of (some) words need not involve semantic knowledge might be taken to imply that production data alone provide a true picture of the child's representation of meaning. However, this implication is acceptable only if it is also accepted that comprehension and production involve differential access to a common lexical store and are thus alternative methods for studying the same phenomenon. If comprehension and production draw on a common lexical store, then we would expect that words over-extended in production would be over-extended in comprehension. The empirical evidence indicates otherwise.

Thomson and Chapman (1977) reported a study of overextensions in production and comprehension. They found that some words were overextended in both production and comprehension and some were overextended in production only.* As we have argued earlier there are various reasons why this might be the case and among the suggestions in the

* Kay and Anglin (1982, p. 96) point out that the method of Thomson and Chapman (1977) virtually guarantees this result. "[The] words chosen for study were ones that according to parents their children overextended . . . Thomson and Chapman (1977) found stimuli that elicited overextensions of those words by the children in production. The test was whether or not the child also would overextend the words to those stimuli in comprehension. Since the stimuli were carefully selected to be ones that elicited overextensions in production, this procedure virtually guaranteed that there would be no case of overextension in comprehension but not production."

literature are the following: children prefer to use a word they know well (Gentner, 1978); retrieval errors occur in labelling a referent (Huttenlocher, 1974); vocabulary limitations force the child to use an incorrect word (Bloom, 1973). However, at least the last of these suggestions could not account for all the errors observed by Thomson and Chapman as there were instances recorded in which the child had an appropriate word in his lexicon but nevertheless used an inappropriate overextension. While the suggestions of Gentner and Huttenlocher might account for these errors, it is difficult to see how these suggestions could ever amount to more than a post-hoc interpretation. A further possibility exists: that it is mistaken to assume a single lexicon for production and comprehension.

Kay and Anglin (1982) have reported a study that questions the presumed relation between production and comprehension. They assessed two-year-old children's production and comprehension of five words and then trained each child to produce one word (in response to a prototypical referent) that had previously been comprehended but not produced. Subsequent to training, the child's comprehension and production was assessed. In addition to the prototype for which he had received training the child was also tested on eight referents and eight nonreferents. Half of the referents had been judged (by adults) to be central referents for the word and half to be peripheral. Half of the nonreferents were "perceptually similar" to the prototype and half were dissimilar. Kay and Anglin found that in both comprehension and production, children made more underextensions to peripheral than to central referents and more overextensions to perceptually similar than to perceptually dissimilar nonreferents. Contrary to previous findings, they found that overextensions occurred more frequently in comprehension than in production and, conversely, underextensions occurred more frequently in production than in comprehension. It seems, from these results, that the relation between comprehension and production in development cannot be simply summarized in terms of differential access to a common lexicon. Further evidence for this conclusion is provided from a study by Campbell, Bowe, and Dockrell (in press). These authors studied children's knowledge of the colour lexicon. Subjects in their study received both an elicitation session and a comprehension session in that order. In the elicitation session children were required to name the colours of 11 wagons of a model train and 22 coloured schematic men who occupied these wagons. Only those colour terms used by the child were included in the subsequent comprehension test in which the child was asked to "Give me all the . . . ones." This question was asked for each colour term previously used by the child. Campbell *et al.* found instances in which the comprehension range was broader than the production range as might be expected but they also found instances in which the pattern was reversed and the production range was broader than the comprehension range. They even found instances in which the production and comprehension ranges were disjoint. They suggest that

> in the early stages of the acquisition of a word there are two lexical representa-
> tions established, one supporting acts of production and the other supporting

acts of comprehension. . . . The wide variety of relations observed to hold between comprehension and production ranges suggested that there was initially no need to suppose that these representations bore any intrinsic semantic connection.

Such conclusions indicate that it can no longer be assumed that there is one central lexical store. Whether this applies to every semantic field, or only to some, is an issue for future research. Such research must, of necessity include data on both production and comprehension. (It must also be borne in mind that evidence of comprehension may not be evidence of semantic knowledge because of other strategies for understanding available to the child.) It is only through a systematic evaluation of these two systems in various contexts and with different word-classes that it will be possible to evaluate the relation between production and comprehension.

D. "Nouns", "Verbs", and Other Objects of Wonder

Names constitute a significant proportion of the child's initial vocabulary (Nelson, 1973). Goldin-Meadow *et al.* (1976) have suggested that there are two stages in the development of the two-year-old's vocabulary: (a) an earlier "receptive" stage in which the child says many fewer names than he understands and says no "verbs" at all, although he understands many and (b) a later "productive" stage in which the child says virtually all the names he understands and also produces some "verbs". However, beyond this early stage the details of further lexical development are extremely sketchy. Children continue to acquire words for many years but, apart from a few well-researched niches of the lexicon, relatively little is known about the later stages of lexical development.

If we consider the acquisition of "verbs", there have been comprehension studies of the relations among 'give', 'take', 'pay', 'trade', 'spend', 'buy', and 'sell' (Gentner, 1975); 'come', 'go', 'bring', and 'take' (Clark and Garnica, 1974; Richards, 1976); 'ask', 'promise', and 'tell' (Chomsky, 1969; Warden, 1981); and 'remember', 'know', and 'guess' (Johnson and Wellman, 1980; Miscione *et al.*, 1978; Wellman and Johnson, 1979). These studies have provided some useful information on the processes by which some semantic distinctions are mastered. However, integration of the information provided by these studies is hampered by the fact that relatively little is known about the more general outlines that concern the acquisition of the semantics of "verbs". The construct "verb" is, in any case, much too global to allow meaningful general comments. Verbs differ. Some denote punctate actions. Some denote enduring actions. Some denote states (either temporary or enduring).* The importance of these distinctions in determining lexical acquisition remains to be explored.

* For a discussion of these issues from a linguistic point-of-view see Comrie (1977) and, from a psycholinguistic point-of-view Miller and Johnson-Laird (1976).

Investigation of other areas of vocabulary development have, for the most part, attempted to test the predictions of Semantic Feature Theory (Clark, 1973a) through comprehension studies. The majority of these studies have investigated children's acquisition of antonymic terms: dimensional adjectives such as 'long'-'short', 'narrow'-'wide' etc. (e.g. Brewer and Stone, 1975; Donaldson and Wales, 1970; Eilers, Oller and Ellington, 1974; Townsend, 1976; Wales and Campbell, 1970); temporal reference such as 'before'-'after', 'first'-'last' (e.g. Amidon and Carey, 1972; Barrie-Blackey, 1973; Clark, 1970, 1971, 1972); locatives such as 'in', 'on' and 'under' (e.g. Clark, 1973b; Grieve, Hoogenraad and Murray, 1977; Hoogenraad, Grieve, Baldwin and Campbell, 1978; Wilcox and Palermo, 1975); comparative adjectives such as 'more'-'less', 'same'-'different' (e.g. Carey, 1978a; Donaldson and Balfour, 1968; Donaldson and Wales, 1970; Glucksberg, Hay and Danks, 1976; Gordon, 1977; Grieve and Stanley, 1980; Palermo, 1973, 1974; Trehub and Abramovitch, 1978); and spatial-relational terms such as 'in front of'-'behind' (e.g. Clark, 1973a; Kuczaj and Maratsos, 1975).

Recently, Richards (1979) has reviewed this literature with the aim of evaluating three of the basic hypotheses of Semantic Feature Theory:

Hypothesis 1 (the top-to-bottom hypothesis). Given the componential nature of word meaning assumed by the theory, it is hypothesized that the more general features will be learnt first and the more specific features gradually added to the lexicon over time.

Hypothesis 2 (the making hypothesis). The linguistically unmarked term will be acquired earlier than the linguistically marked term.*

Hypothesis 3 (the overextension hypothesis). There will be a stage during which the marked term will be treated synonymously with the unmarked term.

Richards (1979) provides a comprehensive review of these hypotheses, which it would be superfluous to repeat. We will summarize his conclusions and cite some illustrative examples, relying for these examples, in large part, on evidence not reviewed by Richards.

The third prediction fares worst of all. It appears that what positive evidence there is can be explained by non-linguistic biases that either originate within the child or are precipitated by the structure of the experiment. These biases lead the child to treat the marked member of a pair as an apparent synonym of the unmarked member. For example, Grieve and Stanley (1980) have shown that children respond to 'less' as 'more' (apparent overextension of 'more') in a context in which a response bias

---

* In this context the unmarked term is the term that applies most neutrally to the dimension in question frames such as 'How – is it?' Thus 'tall' is unmarked and short is 'marked' because 'How short is it?' presupposes that "it" is, in fact, short, whereas 'How tall is it?' does not presuppose that "it" is either tall or short.

operates in favour of an appropriate response to 'more' but they respond to 'less' at random in a context in which there is no such response bias. Carey (1978a) has moreover found that if a nonsense word is inserted into the question frame instead of the marked lexical item the same pattern of response is obtained in both cases. Unless one wants to argue that the child has a partial meaning for a previously unheard nonsense word, there are no grounds for suggesting that marked and unmarked terms are ever treated as synonymous.

Evidence in support of the second hypothesis is likewise equivocal as comprehension has been confounded with the behavioural tendencies of young children in comprehension tasks. Grieve et al. (1977) and Hoogenraad et al. (1978) have studied the child's acquisition of 'in', 'on', and 'under'. They used two boxes, one large and one small, which were designated as different objects in different tests (e.g. a table and chair, a cup and saucer). Even children as young as 2 years made the correct arrangements for 'in' and 'on' (but not 'under') under varying instructions. There was no evidence from these experiments that the understanding of 'in' preceded 'on' (as Semantic Feature Theory predicts). Grieve et al. (1977) make the point that children's responses are determined by how the child views the natural canonical relations of the objects used in the test as well as by the linguistic instructions. When the child fails to understand he construes as appropriate from the context. It may be that the child's own response biases and the contextual constraints provided by particular situations help the child build up meanings for a word. Some contexts will restrict the possible meanings more than others and these restrictions may guide the child's hypotheses concerning the possible meaning of the word. Hence, the child may proceed from being correct in context to a later stage in which he has abstracted the criterial features for acontextual meaning.

The first prediction holds up best, but only in the domain of dimensional adjectives with spatial reference: Terms having more specific dimensions of spatial reference appear to be learnt later than those having fewer specific reference dimensions. Carey (1978b) argues that the main difficulty the child has in learning spatial adjectives is in working out the underlying dimension that is referred to. The child has little initial difficulty in working out that the adjectives refer to spatial extent and little difficulty in discovering the polarity of antonymic terms. However, the exact dimension to which reference is made does present difficulty. Further, Carey found that individual children's error patterns, on tasks that tested the production and comprehension of spatial adjectives, were inconsistent with the notion that children had simply failed to include dimension in their representation. Children did not make errors in a consistent fashion across tasks. Carey argues that the child's representation of the meaning of these words includes general feature information, such as [comparative] and [+pole], and also specific information about typical objects to which the word applies. As an example, Carey (1978b, p. 286) offers the following hypothetical lexical entries for a 3- to 4-year-old:

tall [Adj] [comparative] [+pole] [−building, ground up;
-person, head to toe]
short [Adj] [comparative] [-pole] [-person, head to toe;
-hair, root to end; -distance, direction of motion]

Carey is arguing that the child has learnt a word such as 'tall' exclusively with reference to a limited range of entities – buildings and people in this example. She suggests that the development of a word's meaning will be a reflection of the child's encounters with the word and the world (Carey, 1978b, p. 287):

> suppose the child first learns *deep* and *shallow* as applying to the ends of pools. If he can use the words correctly faced with novel swimming pools, not confusing depth with the length or width of the pool, then certainly he has the concept of depth of swimming pools. But he may not see the similarity between the way that the deep end of a swimming pool is deep and the way that bowls, holes, and puddles are deep. He may not know that *deep* can apply when there is no contrast between two parts of a single object, or that it does not require a liquid medium. Each of these, plus many other irrelevant features, may be part of his unanalyzed conception of the depth of pools.

Such a theory has considerable appeal in that it relates the development of word meaning directly to the child's experience. However, as formulated, the theory is vague in some respects and gratuitously specific in other respects. As it is virtually impossible to know in what contexts a child will have acquired a word it will be impossible to predict patterns of results in advance of a comprehension test. Thus, there is a danger that the theory could become a circular data-driven account of the acquisition of word-meaning. This need not be the case so long as specific predictions can be derived about the relation between particular "adjectives" and entities.

It is not entirely clear what the status is of the "features" that comprise Carey's lexical entries. She does little to justify the more formal features. There is no justification offered for the feature [Adjective] nor any discussion of what the implications of such a feature would be. If, as Carey argues the feature [dimension] has been restricted in scope to some particular entities then there is no reason why the features [comparative] and [+pole] should not be similarly restricted. If this line of enquiry is to be pursued then a good deal more theoretical rigour is necessary in the determination of a word's "features."

E. Input for Lexical Development

Although we have occasionally made reference to input in the preceding sections, we have made little attempt to systematically relate the developments that take place to the input received. This is because the theories reviewed, in general, pay little attention to input variables. It is assumed that a word enters the child's lexicon through casual contact with the environment and is mapped to some concept. If the denotation of that word undergoes change then the task is seen as one of constructing an explanation of state changes to account for denotational changes. Little is said about what causes the state changes to occur. Explanations of change can be couched in state terms or input terms, or a combination of both. Here, we will consider the role that input might play in the explanation of change. We are conscious of the fact that no adequate explanation of change exists. What follows is merely an attempt to review briefly some relevant facts about input that might constitute a part of a more detailed explanation of change.

Several researchers have drawn attention to the way in which the input offered by the child's caretakers could facilitate the initial development of reference. In order for a child to learn a name it is necessary, at minimum, that he hear it spoken in the presence of a relevant entity, while he is attending to that entity. In a naturalistic study of one mother–infant dyad, Ninio and Bruner (1978) found that the mother invariably drew the child's attention to the referent before naming it. Supporting evidence is provided from a laboratory study by Murphy (1978) who also found that a call for attention was a frequent accompaniment to naming by the mother. In Ninio and Bruner's study (1978), 76% of all observed naming occurred when mother and child were looking at picture books; the mother providing the child with an ostensive definition by pointing to the entity and then naming it. Thus the child received regular and repeated pairings of word and object. In a later study of 40 mother–infant dyads, Ninio (1980) found that ostensive definitions were used almost exclusively to name objects; 95% of ostensive definitions referred to the whole object depicted, rather than to its parts, attributes, or actions. When mothers named parts of objects they avoided misunderstanding of the level of reference either by naming the part immediately after naming the whole, or by including a reference to the whole in the definition of the part. However, none of these studies has provided clear evidence of what the relation is between input and output. (Ninio and Bruner do report output measures but a study of one dyad is clearly not sufficient to disentangle causal effects.) Howe (1981) in a naturalistic study of 24 mother–child dyads found differences in naming that were related to the style of conversational interaction between mother and child. Exchanges that frequently began with requests for a name by the mother led to a greater incidence of naming and a greater rate of vocabulary increase than exchanges that simply provided the child with a name. Thus, it is important, and no doubt ultimately more profitable, to study the discourse context of input–output relations than to simply study whether output copies input.

However, it is not entirely clear whether the child's linguistic environment continues to be pedagogically structured in a way that might facilitate the development of specific linguistic skills. Clearly, much more evidence is needed on this and on the relation between input and output. One issue that needs much more thought in input–output studies is whether the measures of frequency correlation commonly employed are appropriately sensitive measure of the relation. It is obviously the case that output derives from input. It is less obviously the case that the state variable between input and output is simply a bucket that is filled by input and emptied by output. However, much of the logic of correlational studies is based on this assumption. It might be more profitable to concentrate on differences in speech-styles in the input from both psycholinguistic and sociolinguistic perspectives and relate these to features of the child's output than to regard frequency as the all-important input variable.

If we conceive of input as encompassing all aspects of the environment that are relevant to lexical organization, then caretaker speech is but one aspect of the input. A second aspect that we wish to discuss is whether there is a preferred level of reference in talking about the environment. Brown (1958) drew attention to the fact that an object can, in principle, be referred to by a variety of different terms. A dog can be called *dog* but can also be called *quadruped* or *animal* at a higher level of generality or *spaniel* at a lower level of generality. Brown argued that when caretakers provide names for children, they provide a name at the level of maximum utility in the child's world. Thus (to use Brown's example), some caretakers may initially call every sort of coin *money*. Brown (1965) elaborated this notion and defined the maximum level of utility as the level at which objects are behaviourally equivalent (i.e. the level at which they share common appropriate behaviours). There is an appealing interdependence of behavioural and linguistic factors in Brown's thesis. Indirect support has been provided by Anglin (1979). He asked adults to rate terms at different levels in a hierarchy for their relative degree of behavioural equivalence for children (e.g. adults were asked whether behavioural equivalence in children was best specified by 'car' or 'Volkswagen'). He found that adult rating of the behavioural equivalence of terms correlated with the order of aquisition of these terms. More direct support is provided in an experimental study by White (1982). He asked mothers to label pairs of items in a category for their children. He found that mothers rarely used a superordinate term to refer to pairs of atypical instances of a category but did so to refer to pairs of typical instances. Thus, while meat and peas were often labelled *food*, candy and ketchup were labelled candy and ketchup rather than food. White argues that atypical items are not usually labelled with a superordinate term because they are associated with different actions on the child's part from the typical items. These experimental findings suggest that the naming practices of parents in the natural environment may provide the child with a very selective input for subordinate–superordinate relations.

There are further issues that might be explored in relation to the issue of the level of lexical specificity chosen by caretakers: To what extent do different caretakers use a similar level of specificity when talking to children? Do children adopt the level of specificity contained in the input or do they have a preferred level of specificity to which terms at a different level are assimilated (in which case some overextension and underextension errors might be the result of the child not being supplied with a word at the appropriate level of reference). In view of the convergence between these issues and the arguments advanced by Rosch and her colleagues (Rosch, 1978; Rosch and Mervis, 1975; Rosch *et al.*, 1976) that taxonomies contain a basic level, which carries more information than other levels, possesses the highest category cue validity, and at which the greatest degree of differentiation can be made, it is surprising that more work has not been carried out on this aspect of lexical development.

The argument that there is a preferred level of reference applies when there is a clear hierarchical arrangement among a group of terms. However, there are many areas of the lexicon (e.g. action and relational terms) in which such a notion may be of little relevance in studying the relation between input and output. Alternative hypotheses are obviously needed for these areas. One such hypothesis mentioned earlier, is that advanced by Carey (1978b) in relation to dimensional adjectives: the child haphazardly hears particular dimensional adjectives used with reference to particular entities and these entities may become criterial for further use of the term (as in 'shallow' being selectively applied to pools). Some further speculation can be entertained also. The salient dimension of an entity (or class) with which an adjective has been paired may dictate an erroneous dimension of generalization to other entities. If, for example, 'big' is regularly heard by a child to describe people whom the child perceives as taller than he is, then that child might judge bigness as extent on the vertical dimension. On this line of speculation, the child's task in eventually arriving at a correct understanding of dimensional adjectives is to disentangle the overlapping and metaphorical uses of these terms in the everyday language he hears.

Further evidence on the relation between input and output is provided by Dockrell (1981). She introduced 4- and 5-year-old children to a novel lexical item and then traced the course of acquisition over a period of five months. In the introducing event children were presented with three building blocks: a red cube, a green sphere, and the test stimulus – a hexagonal prism with silver stripes on a tangerine background. Prior to this it had been established that none of the children had a word for either the shape, the colour, or the pattern of the test stimulus.

The question of interest was how variation in the input would affect acquisition. All children were therefore introduced individually to the same novel word, *gombe*, but under two different conditions of input. Half of the children (the shape group) were asked to *pass me the gombe block, not the round one or the square one, but the gombe one.* The remaining children (the pattern group) were asked to *pass me the gombe block, not the red one or the green one, but the gombe one* (we will explain below why this contrast was used). Over the subsequent five months production and comprehension were periodically assessed. In the final session, a large number of blocks with both known and unknown attributes were presented to the children. If the lexical contrasts in the introducing event provided sufficient information to restrict the denotation of the novel term it would be predicted that children in the shape group would restrict the denotation of the term to hexagons irrespective of their colour or pattern while children in the pattern group would restrict the denotation of the term to a specific pattern irrespective of its shape. By corollary, if lexical contrast provides insufficient information to guide denotation, no generalization, or a variety of random mappings, would be predicted.

In the final session, only one child failed to show any learning. All the remaining children had developed some form of denotation for the term. The children in the shape group had restricted the denotation of 'gombe' to hexagons in both production and comprehension. In a series of questions designed to elicit the children's understanding of shape and colour terms they clearly treated 'gombe' as a shape term. Within the pattern group a variety of mappings was evident. Some children took 'gombe' to denote a striped pattern with specific colours, others any striped shape and yet others either shape or pattern. All of these children had clearly established denotational criteria for 'gombe' but, unlike the children in the shape group, the criteria were not uniform within the group. Why do these differences occur?

The implied contrast in the input for the shape group was shape although the objects were also of visibly different colours. However, as the three objects clearly differed in shape, the most reasonable interpretation (and the one dictated by conversational usage) of the input was that 'gombe' referred to the shape of the third object. The reasonableness of the interpretation would be increased for the child if he actually expected the shape to have a name, even if that name was unknown to him.

The implied contrast in the input for the pattern group is the patterned colour. Here, there are two variables that determine the contrast: pattern and colour. It is evident that both of these variables influenced the denotation of the term. Further, there was evidence that some of the children's productions conflicted with the manner in which they comprehended the term. For example, a child who comprehended the term as denoting only a specific pattern, produced the term in such a way that 'gombe' clearly denoted either pattern or shape. Would the results have been clearer if only one variable had been manipulated? Unfortunately no; at least not with colour as the variable. A previous study (see Dockrell, 1981) had provided evidence that lexical contrast does not work for colour alone in the same way as for shape. When *gombe* was used to refer to a hexagonal block with a colour for which the children did not have a name, children made the inference (as revealed by subsequent testing) that 'gombe' denoted hexagonal shape. When asked to name the colour children simply extended a known colour term to include the new colour. Taken in conjunction these results suggest that the internal structure of the child's lexicon is a crucial determinant of how input is interpreted.

We bring this all too brief section to a close by emphasizing that studying input–output relations is complementary to, rather than a substitute for, studying state–output relations. The solution to one problem may leave the other relatively untouched (although it is debatable whether a reasonable solution to one issue in isolation from the other could ever be arrived at). In all of the approaches discussed there has been an emphasis on some *part* of the acquisition process without any attempt to set this part in the context of the remaining problems. Our point is not that no theory has failed to solve all aspects of the problem (that is evidently the case) but rather that no theory has adequately identified the problem-space within which it is working and recognized that there is a necessary relation between this and other problem-spaces. Given the diversity of meanings among words, it is unlikely that any single consideration, at either input or state level, will explain lexical acquisition. Hence, there is a compelling need to identify the domain of application of different theoretical accounts.

III. Grammatical Development

A. What Develops in a Grammar?

Before considering the theories and the evidence, it is as well to consider, in more detail, what models of grammatical development should and do offer. The first and most obvious thing that a model should offer is a set of rules that describes the child's production system. Here we encounter the first difficulty. The earliest stages of word combination are well documented and there have been many attempts to describe production models for these data. These models are relatively complete in that they encompass most of the utterances actually produced by the children studied. The speech-samples from which these utterances come can also be assumed to be reasonably representative samples in that there is good agreement among different studies on the general outline of the data for consideration. Another reason for having some confidence in the representativeness of these studies is that the child's range of competence is, of necessity, small to begin with, so there is a reduced risk of failing to sample some area of competency. Because the range of competence is small, it is also relatively easy to check the competence assessed by sampling, against caretaker's reports thus offering a further check against failing to observe some area of competence.

However, beyond the initial two-word combinations, language development occurs at an increasingly rapid rate, with many sub-systems of the grammar undergoing simultaneous development. The hope of adequately sampling, much less analysing, a child's range of competence has resulted in a shift in the nature of the evidence available and the nature of the theories offered. Particular investigators concentrate on particular sub-systems. Longitudinal studies, if carried out, selectively gather data on these sub-systems. The intensive study of a few children is, however, more frequently replaced by the experimental study of many children. Experimental studies have the advantage that they focus attention on the particular sub-system being studied, and allow for the controlled collection of a discrete amount of data pertaining to a particular sub-system. They have the disadvantage that the data are more subject to artifact than are naturalistic data. Precautions, of course, are taken to overcome this but nevertheless the lack of convergence of naturalistic and experimental data (Miller, 1977) is not encouraging.

As a consequence of changes in the methods of study adopted, there are many partial production models that deal with linguistic sub-systems but few that attempt any integration across these sub-systems. It may well be that sub-systems develop relatively autonomously but there is little way of knowing whether or not this is the case given the present evidence.

The rules that describe a production system depend on one's view of what the child is learning and so, ultimately, they depend on a broader theoretical orientation. It was Chomsky (1959) who convinced a behaviouristic and cognitively atheoretical psychology that language behaviour had to be described in terms of a speaker's underlying competence to generate a wide variety of novel sentences. The result has been the replacement of input–output models of language (e.g. Skinner, 1957) with (input–) state–output models that attempt to describe the development of production rules. The task facing the psychologist in such an enterprise is two-fold: to describe a production system and to describe a model of acquisition that provides a psychological rationale for the state of the production system at any particular stage in development and for the changes in the system as development proceeds. Psychological theory has, to a large extent, been driven by linguistic theory. As linguistic models changed so did production models. The initial attempts to describe a child's production system in terms of a transformational grammar (e.g. McNeill, 1966) were thus replaced by attempts to describe the production system in terms of a case grammar (e.g. Brown, 1973; Slobin, 1970). Later models have drawn on lexical grammar (e.g. Maratsos, 1978). As conceptions of the production model have changed, so has the psychological grounding of the model. Production models based on transformational grammar tended to argue that the child had innate production rules. The evidence in favour of this claim was never wholly convincing, particularly as there was relatively little attempt to specify what the innate rules were. (For recent discussions see Pinker, 1979; Wexler and Culicover, 1980). Production models based on Case Grammar (Fillmore, 1968; Chafe, 1970) had a stronger psychological grounding in that it was argued that the semantic cases on which production rules operated were the linguistic equivalent of non-linguistic cognitive categories that the child used in understanding and ordering his everyday environment. This view – the cognition hypothesis – left a number of additional, but perhaps more tractable problems:

(a) In what ways are cognitive and semantic categories linked?
(b) Can an adequate developmental account be given of the independent emergence of the cognitive categories from which semantic categories supposedly derive?

The relation between the linguistic rules that characterize a production model and the psychological dynamics of that model have also been affected by a number of other linguistic and psychological developments. Chomsky's insistence on studying generative competence tended to focus attention on the form of the child's utterance to the neglect of their function in the child's activities. There have been many calls for a redress of this balance (e.g. the emphasis on 'communicative competence' by Campbell and Wales, 1970; Hymes, 1971) and a number of attempts to give functional considerations a greater role in models of a production system (e.g. Bruner, 1975a, 1975b; Halliday, 1975; McShane, 1980). Prototype theory has also had some effect on conceptualizations of production rules in that it has been argued that production rules may be learnt selectively for a few core members of a category and only later extended to non-core members (de Villiers, 1980).

Given that various production models posit rules to account for the observed behaviour of children, how are we to decide among competing models? There are no hard and fast criteria but there are a number of guidelines that may prove helpful (see Atkinson, 1982, for a detailed discussion). A model obviously should have developmental plausibility. One way in which this is manifest is the ways, specified or potentially specifiable, in which the production rules can change to account for changes in the child's behaviour. Thus, many arguments that there are innate rules that determine early word combinations lack developmental plausibility in that the rules are too powerful for the behaviour observed – the rules specify a richer output than that which occurs. Bloom (1970) postulates a "reduction transformation" to remove the discrepancy between the production system and the output observed. This involves specifying a more complex production system to account for two-word utterances than would be required to account for three-word utterances. While such a developmental model cannot be ruled out in principle, it needs considerable justification. As the only justification that seems to have motivated such claims was the expediency of preserving the theoretical model we can conclude that such claims lack developmental plausibility.

On grounds of parsimony it can be argued the production rules should be no richer than the data warrant. Thus, *ceteris paribus*, the simpler of two competing accounts is to be preferred. However, the application of this criterion in practice comes less in deciding between systems than in deciding, within a system, what the relative scope of a production rule should be. Thus, if a child appears to have learnt a particular construction with selective application to a small number of words, there is little justification for positing a powerful general rule to account for the child's behaviour. With limited data one always has to tread a route between data as productive examples of a more general competence and data as specific examples of some restricted heuristic. There is no infallible procedure for deciding what is the right level of description but the observed generalization of the rule can be especially useful. If a child learnt a new grammatical construction and employed this construction freely with a wide range of the appropriate terms in his vocabulary then that would constitute good (but not perfect) evidence for the productive use of a general rule. On the other hand, a child might apply a rule to some subclass of the items to which it could appropriately be applied and one might then prefer to posit a rule of "limited scope" (Braine, 1976) rather than a powerful general rule. Ultimately, converging evidence from different methods of data collection could resolve the issue. Experimental evidence on generalization might resolve whether a production rule has general or limited scope. There are other types of evidence that help in the search for the appropriate level of generality. Errors can be particularly informative. The widespread naturalistic observation of the addition of the morpheme -ed, to indicate pastness for both regular and irregular verbs (Brown, 1973; Cazden, 1968; Kuczaj, 1977) is good evidence that the child has acquired a general productive rule for indicating pastness as it is extremely improbable that the child will have heard other speakers utter such forms as *breaked* or *thinked*, and yet these forms are frequently produced at a certain point in development, often replacing the previously correct forms, *broke*, and *thought*. Similarly, the experimental elicitation of errors (e.g. Karmiloff-Smith, 1979) can be informative.

Cross-cultural evidence may also be informative in determining the level of generality at which a rule should be presumed to operate. Assuming that a production rule is not language specific, the same meaning may require different surface constructions in different languages and the way in which these surface constructions are conformed to or overridden across languages can constitute important clues to the underlying production system. (For a review of cross-cultural research see Bowerman, 1981.)

Two further comments can be made in relation to the search for the appropriate level of generality at which to frame a production rule. The first is that the tendency to invoke a general or limited-scope rule will, to some extent, depend on one's general theoretical model. Prototype models of grammatical categories, for example, might readily envisage limited-scope rules as the expected order of things. On the other hand, models that take a more all-or-none approach to grammatical categories might more readily envisage general rules, both because of theoretical predilection and because of the difficulty of accommodating limited-scope rules within the model. There are however, as we shall see, exceptions to these general tendencies. The second comment is that it is easy, in discussing the search for general rules, to lose sight of the fact that although languages obey general rules they are also fraught with irregularities, inconsistencies and idiosyncracies and these must be mastered by a competent speaker. The fact that they are, is testament to the enormous learning capacity of the human organism. It would be a surprise if it were to emerge that language acquisition could be understood as the operation of a few simple principles. In what follows we have necessarily had to be selective in the material surveyed. Our aim has been to illustrate important trends and to point to sources of difficulty that await resolution.

B. Early Studies of Two-word Combinations

Brown and Fraser (1963) and Brown and Bellugi (1964) characterized
children's early word combinations as 'telegraphic'. This description captured the fact that children's utterances contain relatively few function
words (such as articles, prepositions, and auxiliary verbs) and a preponder-
ance of content words. Although grammatically impoverished, such speech
is readily intelligible as the content words establish reference between the
utterance and the situation being talked about. While the term 'telegraphic
speech' neatly encapsulated the essential characteristics of children's early
word combinations it gave no account of the cognitive processes that might
account for such speech. The first attempt to present a model of such
processes was Braine's (1963a) "pivot grammar".

Braine carried out a distributional analysis of the earliest word combinations of three children. He found that most of the initial combinations were
just two words long. The majority of the two-word utterances were characterized by a relatively small number of words occurring in the initial position
and a much larger class of words occurring in the final position. Braine called
these 'pivot' and 'open' respectively. The combination can be represented as
P + O. Braine also found a less frequent O + P combination. The words in
the two O classes seemed to be drawn from the same population but there
was no overlap of the words in the two P classes. Thus, there were two
distinct combination P_1 + O and O + P_2. In addition, words from the O
class seemed to combine freely in O + O combinations.

Braine's model was intended not merely as a model of speech output but
also as a model of the state variables that organize output. The model claims
that a child, in learning to combine words, learns that some words (the
pivots) occupy fixed positions and that other words (the opens) do not
occupy fixed positions. Thus, learning language structure was a matter of
learning the permissible positions of words. The plausibility of this model
was enhanced when Braine (1963b) demonstrated that preschool children
could remember the positions of words in an artificial language.

Bloom (1970) criticized Braine's pivot-grammar because it offered no way
of differentiating among the different meanings the same utterance might
have in different contexts. In her own data Bloom observed the same child,
Kathryn, using the utterance *Mommy sock* on two different occasions: once
when Kathryn picked up her mother's sock and once when the mother was
putting Kathryn's sock on Kathryn. Bloom argued that the two utterances
conveyed different meanings the first of which expresses a POSSESSOR–
POSSESSED relation and the second of which expresses an ACTOR–
ACTION relation. In pivot-grammar both instances of *Mommy sock* would
have the same structural relation: O + O. Bloom therefore argued that
pivot grammar was an inadequate representation of the child's knowledge of
grammar and that there must be a more differentiated organization under-

lying the production of utterances. Bloom's proposed solution was to argue that the utterances had different deep structures.

However, it transpired that Bloom's example of the dilemma that faced pivot-grammar was of more importance than her proposed solution. While semantic considerations had led Bloom to question pivot-grammar, her resolution of the issue had given semantics very little direct role in the production of utterances. Essentially, Bloom (1970) saw semantic analysis as a necessary precursor to the characterization of syntax. However, within linguistics and psychology a number of theorists had begun to argue that semantic considerations had a more direct role to play in a syntactic theory than was envisaged by Transformational Grammar (e.g. Fillmore, 1968; Chafe, 1970; McCawley, 1968; Schlesinger, 1971; Slobin, 1970). This quickly led to a reappraisal of the role semantics might play in a production model.

C. Semantic Models of Two-word Combinations

One of the earliest semantic production models to be worked out in any detail was that presented by Schlesinger (1971). He suggested that speech begins with an intention to communicate and that children convert intentions into utterances by means of realization rules without an intervening deep structure. The content of a child's utterance is determined by innate cognitive capacities, which determine the conceptual categorization of reality. The child begins to communicate with intentions to express certain facts about the world in words and learns a number of specific "realization rules" which determine the structure of the speech output in order to express these intentions. Such is the model in outline. We will now consider it in more detail.

Schlesinger points out that a speaker does not produce just any utterance but an utterance that is appropriate to the particular situation. He argues that utterance production begins with intentions. Not all of a speaker's intentions are realized in speech but some are. These intentions serve as input to the speech production mechanism. This input specifies relations among elements (which elements are determined by the innate cognitive capacity of the child) about which the speaker intends to communicate and the speech production mechanism turns these relations into speech output through "realization rules." Schlesinger argues that there are two kinds of rules that account for primitive utterances: position rules, which determine the ordering of words in utterances and category rules, which determine the grammatical category that is appropriate in a particular position. Schlesinger specifies a variety of position rules for two-word utterances: AGENT + ACTION;   ACTION + DIRECT   OBJECT;   AGENT + DIRECT OBJECT;   MODIFIER + HEAD;   NEGATION + X;   X + DATIVE; INTRODUCER + X; and X + LOCATIVE. Category rules are acquired following these position rules. Category rules restrict position rules to words of certain classes. The justification for this ordering seems to be the "errors" that children sometimes make. Schlesinger cites examples from Braine (1963b) of such errors as *more wet* and *more outside* to indicate that the child has not yet restricted the MODIFIER + HEAD construction to nouns and adjectives respectively. (Schlesinger extends his model to cover more complex utterances by the ordered application of two or more position rules but for our purposes the essential elements of the system are contained in the outline sketched above.)

There are a number of difficulties readily apparent with Schlesinger's model. The difficulties are apparent because the model is relatively exact and it is interesting to pursue them in order to establish possible sources of difficulty that may be less apparent from more vaguely formulated models. Schlesinger does not work out in any detail in what way intentions develop or serve as input to the speech production model. This, he points out (p. 99) would presuppose a psychology of cognition in a more advanced state than the present. He assumes that some part of the speaker's intention serves as input to the speech-producing mechanism. If a speaker has an intention then it must be an intention about something. According to Schlesinger, the content of the child's intentions is determined by an innate cognitive capacity. In speech the child attempts to represent relations between innately determined concepts. It is not entirely clear how concepts themselves are to be treated in Schlesinger's account but, putting that aside, the next stage of the process is for "realization rules" to operate to produce speech output. An obvious difficulty with the realization rules is explaining their origin. Are they innate like the concepts they operate on? If not, how are they learnt?

An acute difficulty with the model is the scope of the realization rules. Let us consider the MODIFIER + HEAD rule. Schlesinger cites such utterances as *pretty boat*, *more nut*, *my stool* and *baby can* as examples of this rule. Do these diverse utterances actually reflect a common underlying organization imposed by the child? Might the category not be more plausibly subdivided to separate recurrence, possession and attribution? And if that course were embarked on why stop there? Why not have a distinct rule for each utterance type? The question at issue is which of many possible distinctions is functional in the child's speech production system? This issue is one that all semantic theories confront and we shall now broaden the discussion to inquire how the issue was treated by different theorists.

There are several issues involved in a discussion of the inferred semantic categories that form the basis of a production model. We can ask, first of all, whether different investigators agree on the nature of the categories. In general there was good, if not perfect, agreement among the categories proposed by the ealiest investigators (Bloom, Lightbown, and Hood, 1975; Brown, 1973; Schlesinger, 1971; Slobin, 1970). The disagreements were of two sorts: the scope of the categories identified (some investigators drew finer distinctions than others) and the assignment of a particular utterance to a particular category. However, the extent of the agreement among early investigators is impressive.

The second issue that arises is the methodology used in inferring semantic categories. There are a number of clues that can be used, often in conjunction. Firstly, the context of the utterance can be an important clue in determining the speaker's intended meaning. It was knowledge of the context of the utterance that enabled Bloom (1970) to argue that *Mommy sock* could be given two different interpretations. Secondly, the response of others to the child can provide information on the child's intended meaning. Caretakers frequently expand the child's utterance and these expansions have often been treated as glosses on the child's meaning. Thus, *doggy ball* might, in a given context, receive the reply *yes, the dog did bite the ball* and the semantic concepts of ACTOR and PATIENT might be inferred. The method is not, however, foolproof. Adults do sometimes misinterpret children's utterances, so expansions cannot be regarded as veridicial readings of the child's intended meaning. Howe (1976) has radically questioned the procedure and argued that adult expansions merely reflect adult modes of conceptualizing the world. The child may conceptualize the world in a completely different way and may therefore intend to express something different from the adult expansion. While such a possibility cannot be ruled out *a priori*, the suggestion should not be accepted without good evidence. Howe does not say what the radically different mode of conceptualizing the world might be. If it were the case that radical differences exist between adult and child conceptualizations this would impose an enormous strain on communication and it would add a new phenomenon to be explained: How does the child make the move from his radically different conceptualization of the world to the conventional adult conceptualization? It is always possible to invoke the type of objection raised by Howe; one can endlessly entertain the possibility that children's concepts are radically different from those of adults. Such entertainment can only be seriously pursued if there is good evidence that such differences exist. Thus, the burden of proof must be with the objector. Howe provides no evidence in support of her proposal. (For further discussion of the issues raised by Howe see Bloom, Capatides, and Tackeff, 1981; and Golinkoff, 1981.) However, this does not mean that all is well with the semantic analyses proposed. A dilemma remains.

The dilemma that researchers face is this: children's initial word combinations seem to express a rich variety of meanings but often lack the grammatical completeness that might allow unambiguous interpretation of these meanings. Thus a child may indicate possession by saying *mommy sock* but not *mommy's sock* or *this is mommy's sock*. In the absence of linguistic evidence* how is such semantic analysis to be justified? The context of the utterance is crucial in determining the child's intended meaning but context provides a means of interpretation, not a justification for that interpretation.

---

* Despite the absence of structural and morphological evidence for the existence of semantic categories, other linguistic factors such as stress and intonation may provide evidence of the intended meaning of an utterance. (see Wieman, 1976).

If semantic categories are, in some sense, intended to be state explanations of the speech output then the output cannot be the sole evidence for these categories without introducing a vicious circularity. It is necessary, at minimum, to provide independent evidence that the child is capable of making the conceptual distinctions attributed to him. Such evidence would not, of itself, establish that speech production is semantically organized. However, it would provide a greater or lesser degree of plausibility for arguing for particular semantic distinctions. Recent research has begun to address these issues. Golinkoff (1981) reviews a variety of nonlinguistic studies that provide good evidence that the 2-year-old child is capable of making many of the conceptual distinctions† implied by the accounts of writers such as Bloom (1970), Brown (1973), Schlesinger (1971) and Slobin (1970). The balance of the evidence at present suggests to us that cognition and semantics are closely linked, at least in the initial stages of word combinations, and that the procedure of using contextual information in conjunction with one's knowledge of the child's current linguistic abilities is the best procedure for making inferences about the organizing categories of a production model. That said, the issue of how to accurately identify categories remains.

Braine (1976) reanalysed the structural patterns of 16 corpora of word combinations that had formed the data base of many of the earlier debates about grammatical development. He points out that in many of the original analyses the inferences from the corpus to the rules of grammar are not spelled out and frequently the inferred rules have not been adequately justified in that they are exemplified, in the corpus, by only a few utterances. Braine's main findings can be summarized as follows:

(1)   Children's word combinations are not based on rules for combining general grammatical categories, whether syntactically or semantically defined, but are based on rules for combining specific words and narrowly-defined categories.

(2)   The rules themselves are rules that order the position of elements in the surface structure. Thus, a child might have a rule that combines *more* and X as *more* + X. The rule thus applies to a single word and a category that remains to be specified (see below for an example). The semantic patterns evident in children's speech are the product of rules for encoding relatively specific and circumscribed meanings.

(3)   There is generality evident in acquisition in that (a) one finds positional rules in all children and (b) the semantic patterns have much the same content in one child as another.

(4)   There is variability in the order of emergence of the patterns suggesting that they are not interdependent but rather there is considerable independence among the patterns acquired.

---

† We say "many of the conceptual distinctions" because the categories offered by various theorists are an odd mix of cognitive, semantic, linguistic, and intuitive distinctions and it is therefore not entirely evident what an agreed list of semantic categories would eventually include.

TABLE I

Patterns identified by Braine (1976) in early word combinations.

Content and/or function of utterance	Typical pattern	Example
Draw attention	*see* + X	*see train*
	here/there + X	*here milk*
Identify	*it/that* + X	*that ball*
Comment on property	*big/little* + X	*big ear*
Possession	X + Y	*Daddy book*
Number	*two* + X	*two spoon*
Recurrence	*more* + X	*more juice*
Disappearance	*allgone* + X	*allgone stick*
Negation	*no* + X	*no water*
Actor–action	X + Y	*Mommy read*
Location	X + *here/there*	*lady there*
Request	*want* + X	*want car*

The main patterns are shown in Table I. Let us consider how Braine arrived at these patterns. The first criterion that Braine used for dividing the speech output into different patterns was whether or not the utterances expressed manifestly different semantic relations. Thus, patterns that draw attention to something can be readily distinguished from patterns that express possession, which can in turn be distinguished from patterns that express recurrence.

But, given this first crude distinction, how can we know that we have identified the correct semantic formulation of the pattern. For example, how is it decided whether there is one general POSSESSION pattern or several specific *my* + X, *your* + X patterns? To resolve questions of this sort Braine used distributional criteria for inferring differences in patterns that expressed the same semantic relation. For example, one child, Andrew, was judged to have a *more* + X pattern and a separate *other* + X pattern rather than a general RECURRENCE pattern on the grounds that in the former the X items comprised both action and object words whereas in the latter the X items were always object words.

While the use of distributional criteria may be relatively easily applied when one member of the pattern has a fixed meaning and determines the semantic relation specified by the pattern, the criterion is more difficult to apply when both members of a pattern may freely vary as in patterns of the X + Y type. The classic example of this type of pattern is the ACTOR–ACTION pattern. How does one determine if there is one ACTOR–ACTION pattern, several more specific patterns, or even a general pattern but not the one captured by the concepts ACTOR and ACTION? If the formula used by the child is a relatively broad one then novel utterances should be common and there should be no obvious restriction on the range of appropriate words appearing in either position. In this context the comparison of data from different subjects may prove instructive. Assuming a common underlying production model among different children one would expect to find wide divergence in the expressions used within say, the ACTOR–ACTION pattern. Evidence of convergence may suggest a more limited formula than that envisaged. Braine's analysis does not include such a comparison which could, in principle, help to resolve issues of the appropriate level of generality for a category. Cross-cultural data provide another possible source of evidence. Slobin (1981) cites evidence collected by Schieffelin (1979) on Kaluli – an ergative language* spoken in Papua New Guinea – that is relevant in this context. In Kaluli there is a grammatical marker that indicates the agent of action for transitive verbs. In Schieffelin's data this ergative marker appears to be initially acquired for nominals used with a selected range of verbs – those that are high in transitivity. (For a consideration of the notion of transitivity see Hopper and Thompson, 1980). The fact that the ergative suffix is limited to nominals in a particular construction and is not used when the same nominals are used in non-transitive constructions (e.g. *Mother is cooking food* v. *Mother is sleeping*) suggests that categories such as ACTOR may be too general a characterization of the Kaluli child's production system (and possibly the English child's also). Slobin suggests that CAUSAL AGENT may be a more appropriate characterization. However, causal agent is not an isolated notion but is part of an entire scene in which the agent is embedded. Slobin argues that such scenes, "prototypical events" as he calls them, provide the basic conceptual framework for grammatical marking. We have previously commented that very little is known about the child's non-linguistic conceptual framework. Slobin's suggestion is an interesting example of how linguistic data can help the formulation of hypotheses about this system. These hypotheses can be tested further by considering the predictions that they make about future development. Whether or not the hypothesis advanced will be supported by future data remains to be seen.

Thus far we have concentrated on the identification of patterns on semantic and distributional criteria. Braine does not advocate pragmatic criteria but these are clearly relevant also. The same semantic pattern may be used to express different pragmatic meanings and the limiting of a pattern to one type of speech act is a further way in which it may be limited in scope. The

---

* An ergative language is one in which the intransitive subject is treated in the same manner as the transitive object, and differently from the transitive subject. In an ergative language the subject of an intransitive clause and the object of a transitive clause share morphological properties (either through case-marking or verb-agreement patterns) while the subject of a transitive clause carries a special ergative marker. Thus, the notion of "subject", which has a unified syntactic and morphological treatment in familiar languages, is divided into two by clause type in ergative languages. (For a discussion of ergativity see Dixon, 1979.)

issue can be highlighted if we choose an example from Braine's analysis. *See* + X is an example of a pattern that draws attention to something. However, the expression could be used to either regulate the attention of another or to describe the child's own experience. Its limitation to one of these uses could suggest (a) that *see* has been learnt as a procedure for regulating attention, but does not yet have other potential uses, or (b) that *see* describes the child's own experiences exclusively but not the experiences of others. Such information could help to integrate our knowledge of the development of the lexicon and the development of grammar. However, the distinction between one speech-act and another is only possible when one possesses adequate contextual information, and the issue of precedence can only be resolved with longitudinal data. Thus, although Braine's reanalysis of speech corpora has made a considerable contribution to our understanding of the child's production model, the analysis is limited by the fact that the semantic differences among patterns are not considered in relation to the pragmatic function of patterns. Further, the analysis does not resolve issues of precedence (and therefore issues of development) in the emergence of related patterns.

The conclusion that emerges from Braine's review is that there is nothing powerfully grammatical about early word-combinations. These combinations seem to be generated by rules that encode semantic relations of limited scope. Braine argues that there are three sorts of semantic patterns. The first sort is a "positional productive pattern", in which the two elements occupy a fixed position; one of the elements is drawn from a small class (in some cases a singleton) and the other is drawn from a much larger class. These are clearly similar to Braine's (1963) original pivot-open classes. Typical examples are expressions of recurrence (*more car*, *more hot*) and of denial (*no car*, *no hot*). The second sort of pattern is a "positional associative pattern", which is like the first pattern in that the elements occupy a fixed position but both classes are now restricted. Either of the examples discussed above could be regarded alternatively as positional associative patterns if the evidence indicated that the formula was not productive but was limited to a specifiable range of items. The third type of combination involves patterns in which there is free word order. This may occur for a variety of reasons: the child may randomly order the elements; the child may have two rules, one for each order or the child may have a rule that word order is free. There are some difficulties in distinguishing these different options. Braine argues that one might distinguish the first pattern from the others if the first pattern is soon to be replaced by a pattern that includes word-order rules. Thus, when an unordered pattern precedes an ordered pattern in the same semantic category it is presumed that the unordered pattern is a random pattern.* A pattern might be said to consist of two rules,

---

* Braine calls such patterns "groping patterns". Further criteria used to identify these patterns are (a) only a small number of combinations occur, (b) the utterances are produced with evidence of uncertainty and effort and (c) the pattern exists for a relatively brief time before being replaced by a positional productive pattern.

one of each order, if it is possible to specify what determines one order as opposed to the other. It is difficult, however, to see how a rule that specifies free word-order could be distinguished from a pattern that is randomly ordered (and thus, presumably, lacks a rule).

An important part of Braine' findings was the fact that the different semantic patterns observed, emerged in different orders across the children. This suggests that children are learning a series of particular rules for the expression of meaning with few interdependencies among the rules. Thus, while there is generality in the semantic concepts expressed in two-word speech there is considerable variability in the order in which particular concepts emerge. This could suggest that there is variability in the order in which the related cognitive concepts emerge but a more likely suggestion is that cognitive development does not automatically lead to related semantic development. Quite what determines the relation between cognitive and semantic development remains to be resolved.

D. Beyond Two-word Combinations

Two-word utterances predominantly consist of content words which are uninflected. Brown (1973) has described the development of function words and of various inflections. He studied 14 "grammatical morphemes" that appeared in the speech of three children between the ages of 2 and 4 years. Averaging the acquisition of each morpheme over the three children Brown found that the earliest morphemes to be acquired were the present progressive -ing, the locatives in and on, and the plural. These were followed by the past irregular, the possessive, the uncontractible copula, the articles the and a, the past regular, the third person regular, the third person irregular, the uncontractible auxiliary, the contractible copula, and the contractible auxiliary. The question arises as to the extent to which these developments can be understood in the same terms as the development of basic semantic relations.

It might be thought that the relatively invariant order of acquisition found by Brown is due to the invariant development of basic cognitive categories of experience. While this is possibly the case, elaboration of the argument is hampered by the fact that there is neither an adequate understanding of the cognitive factors that control the acquisition and use of the morphemes nor an adequate semantic theory to compare among morphemes (see Atkinson, 1982, pp. 120–126, for a more detailed discussion). Further, the notion of what it means to acquire a morpheme requires scrutiny. In Brown's (1973) study a morpheme was judged to be acquired when it appeared in 90% or more of obligatory contexts. While this may seem a stringent criterion it must be borne in mind that the contexts in question are those in which the child expressed a meaning that, in some grammatical sense, required the use of the morpheme in question. Thus, the child's speech controlled the obligatory contexts. The use of this criterion to determine when a morpheme has been acquired thus does not mean that a morpheme is used in the variety of ways it may be used in adult language but merely that it is used when it is obligatory for the meanings that the child attempts to express. The development of the child's comprehension and production of articles (Karmiloff-Smith, 1979) is one example of a process of acquisition that is considerably more complex than the criterion of productivity might suggest. Similar complexities may possibly be evident in the development of the other morphemes. There is some evidence that this, at least, is the case for verb inflections.

Studies such as those of Brown (1973), Cazden (1968), de Villiers and de Villiers (1973) have described correlations between children's use of particular verb inflections and increase in MLU. The implication of these studies is that verb inflections are learnt in a sequence and apply in general to all of a child's verbs. However, a recent study by Bloom, Lifter, and Hafitz (1980) challenges this view. They argue that the different verb inflections emerge at the same time but are distributed selectively with different populations of verbs in ways that depend on the meaning of the verb. Bloom *et al.* claim, in fact, that inflections do not mark tense at first but are redundant aspect markers. They studied the progressive (*-ing*), the regular (*-ed*) and irregular (IRREG) forms of the past tense, and the third person singluar (*-s*) as these emerged in the speech of four children. They claim that the progressive *-ing* was correctly used most often with action verbs that referred to situations that extended over time and had no clear end result. The verbs that occurred with *-ed*/IRREG referred to situations of momentary duration with a clear end result. The most frequent verbs that occurred with *-s* referred to situations that had a clear end result that continued after completion. Although there are serious shortcomings with the method of analysis adopted by Bloom *et al.* (McShane, 1981) it is obvious that there is a complex interaction of semantic and structural factors that needs to be explored in the acquisition of verb inflections.

The elaboration of a production model beyond the two-word-stage is going to be a complicated task in view of findings such as the above. While it is likely that there is a continuing central role for semantics in a production model it is also likely that autonomous syntactic considerations play an increasingly significant role in the further elaboration of the system. Language, as Karmiloff-Smith (1979) has said, becomes a problem-space for the child. We do not envisage that such a development is a stage-like progression but rather, we see the child as a structure-inducing organism with language structure being, of necessity, parasitic on other structures (those of cognition) for its beginning but becoming increasingly independent of those structures. The difficulty that confronts attempts to describe a production model is that the earlier corpora of children's speech are increasingly replaced by detailed studies of specific linguistic sub-systems in isolation from other sub-systems. As many sub-systems are developing simultaneously it is a difficult task to keep track of them all. Rather than discuss particular sub-systems, which would in any case extend this review beyond

manageable proportions, we will consider a model of structural development that has reasonable generality and that offers a fresh challenge to
research on language development: the model advanced by Maratsos (1978)
and Maratsos and Chalkley (1980).

E. Inducing Syntactic Rules

Most of the preceding analysis has concentrated on the child's output and
the rules that might be inferred from this output. Very little has been said
about the environmental origins of the child's output – a point that is
probably of critical importance in the discussion of individual differences
(although this is not to claim that individual differences need or will reduce
to differences in environmental input). None of the models that we have
discussed pays any specific attention to how language is analysed at the input
stage. The model that we are about to discuss does so and offers a reasonably
detailed, if speculative, account of how the child analyses incoming speech
and then produces a particular pattern of output.

Maratsos and Chalkley (1980) argue that while a child may begin with a
semantically-based system, such a system provides an inadequate basis for
learning the rules of grammar. They argue that languages include rules that
are highly specific and even idiosyncratic and rules that are general (though
often subject to many exceptions). Their model attempts to encompass both
these types of rules in principle but they specifically attempt to account for
general rules. They argue that a child's production model may begin as a
semantically based system but eventually comes to be based on form-class
distinctions. There are two key points to be considered here.

Let us assume that the point at which this discussion begins is a child with a
variety of limited-scope rules of the type discussed by Braine (1976). We
know from the evidence of Brown (1973) and others that the child will
progressively acquire a variety of morphemes that will gradually bring his
speech into line with adult speech. Maratsos and Chalkley argue that
children will initially learn these morphemes on an item-by-item basis. A
child may, for example, hear a variety of words used with -ed to denote
pastness. Many of these same words will be used with -s to denote generic
present. From these particulars the child could notice that some terms have
correlated distributional patterns. (Many of the terms that have correlated
distributional patterns will probably already be grouped by limited scope
formulae.) The distributional patterns could thus suggest a new basis for
grouping: those terms that share distributional patterns belong to the same
class. A corollary to this is that hearing a novel term used in one of the
relevant contexts will be sufficient to (a) signify its form-class, and (b)
predict its other possible occurrences.

Maratsos and Chalkey's argument thus claims that form classes derive
from the analysis by the child of distributional and semantic properties of
words. Thus, the concepts of NOUN, VERB etc., which, they argue, under-

lies the mature production system, are not primitive concepts that the child starts with and gradually elaborates but rather these concepts are the outcome of, and are defined by, the distributions into which particular words enter. Put another way: A verb is not a word that combines with -ed, -s, etc. to denote particular meanings but rather words that combine with -ed, -s etc. to denote these meanings are verbs. It is important to emphasise that Maratsos and Chalkley's argument does include both distributional and semantic criteria for the formation of form-classes. The semantic criteria are necessary for several reasons: (a) they are necessary at the input level in that the child must be able, on the basis of meaning, to determine what the reference of a word is (although Maratsos and Chalkley have relatively little to say about this issue); (b) they are necessary in order to specify such rules as "add -ed to denote pastness' in that pastness is a semantic concept and, in order to acquire the rule, the child must have access to this concept independently of the morpheme that denotes pastness; and (c) they are necessary to avoid the confusions that would occur if one were to analyse the morpheme -s without reference to meaning as it can be used to denote plurality, possession and third-person generic present.

Maratsos and Chalkley offer some detailed reasons as to why a model such as theirs is preferable to other alternatives. They argue that form-classes cannot be clearly defined semantically because if we consider verbs and adjectives, then both classes include terms that denote actions and states and yet form-class errors (applying the operations of one class to a member of the other) are rare. On the other hand errors of overregularization within form-classes are more common implying (a) the members of the class are psychologically homogenous, (b) the form-class is not semantically defined and (c) the observed behaviour of the child must be attributed to the use of a productive rule and cannot be reduced to item-by-item learning.

The implication of this is that the child's production model may begin as a semantically-based system but as development progresses other regularities take precedence as the criterial basis for the operation of production rules – in particular Maratsos and Chalkley would argue, regularities of distribution. If the initial system is semantically-based then the relative rarity of form-class errors where general semantic categories such as action and state cross form-class boundaries indicates that ACTION and STATE may be too broad a characterization of the underlying structure of two-word utterances. As we have discussed above, the child's system may be organized by categories of a more limited scope.

One evident difficulty in integrating the proposals of Maratsos and Chalkley with the research on two-word utterances discussed earlier is that the transition between the initial organization of the child's system and its organization in terms of form-classes is not discussed in any detail. The emphasis of the Maratsos and Chalkley argument is entirely on individual lexical items without any consideration of how the uses of these items are already being controlled by limited scope formulae. While it may be that one type of organization is simply abandoned in favour of another, it is worth investigating the possibility that the earlier structural organization has a role to play in the transition to later structural organization. As there are no relevant data that we know of, the following account is a speculative possibility, no more.

Limited-scope formulae may form prototypes around which a new grammatical category will develop.* Specifically, the lexical items that are most commonly used in a limited-scope formula may be the ones to which a grammatical morpheme is first added. Thus, for example, a child might learn to use -ed initially with a selected range of verbs as Bloom *et al.* (1980) have suggested. Having learnt this, the child might observe that in the speech of other people the use of -ed is not confined to the particular words to which he first attached it. This observation may force the child to gradually enlarge the definition of the limited scope formula and, eventually, to internally reorganize the formula so that participation in the grammatical regularities of the category becomes the defining criterion of membership. (This process is but one possibility. There are many others.)

However, Maratsos and Chalkley argue that grammatical categories cannot have a prototypical structure. As no detailed theory exists that argues that grammatical categories have a prototypical structure, their argument is one of principle against what they perceive to be the main assumptions of any possible prototype theory of grammatical structure. They assume that a prototype theory of grammatical structure would consist of major categories such as NOUN, ADJECTIVE, VERB, and so on. These major categories might initially be formed around core members. For example, action terms might be core verbs and state terms might be core adjectives. A further assumption is that each lexical item within a category is labelled as to how good a member it is of its category. Maratsos and Chalkley argue that such a semantic characterization of form-classes is inadequate. Their principal argument is that there will be considerable semantic overlap between the VERB and ADJECTIVE category as many verbs denote states and many adjectives denote actions. Thus, it will be impossible to sort "bad" terms into the appropriate category on a semantic basis. This should lead to a certain amount of misclassification and thus to production errors. Maratsos and Chalkley claim that the production errors that should occur on this account, do not, in fact, occur. (Maratsos and Chalkley offer two further objections but these depend crucially on the validity of the objection stated above. As we are concerned to dispute this objection we will not pursue their further objections.)

Granting, for the moment, the assumption that action and state would, respectively, be the semantic prototypes of a VERB and ADJECTIVE category, then the overlap between the categories is problematic to the extent that terms in the overlapping area are in productive use by children and are not misclassified (as evidenced by production errors). However, this

---

* De Villiers (1980) has also argued for a prototype theory of grammatical categories. Her account is rather different from the account discussed here.

only establishes that a radical semantically-based prototype theory will not work. It does not establish that no prototype theory will work. There are a number of other possibilities, among which are the following: children's grammatical concepts have prototypical organization, but these concepts cover a smaller range than the adult form-class category and, as we suggested, may initially develop from an existing limited-scope formula. It is an empirical issue whether, in fact, grammatical morphemes are first acquired for existing limited scope formulae and whether these formulae are overlapping or not. If no such overlap exists then the child will not initially encounter any temptation to misapply a rule across form-class boundaries. Thus, in development, the "action category" might initially consist of several subcategories that are only later integrated to form the adult ACTION category. Evidence for such a process would be the limited application of some grammatical rule by the child to a particular subcategory when the rule could legitimately be applied more generally. This, in fact, seems to happen (see Bloom *et al.*, 1980; Slobin, 1981). In addition, a developed prototypical model of form-classes could be entertained if it were considerably more sophisticated than the option considered by Maratsos and Chalkley. What their argument establishes is that there is no single semantic feature common to all members of a category. However, prototype theory explicitly countenances the lack of such a feature. Thus, it is doubtful that the objection to a prototype-based account of grammatical development is telling.

We have seen, thus far, the problems that are encountered in attempting to specify the nature of a production model for language development. The earliest model that the child uses seems best summarized by the limited-scope formulae discussed by Braine (1976). These formulae may consist of individual word patterns or of semantic category patterns. Where there is evidence for the latter it is important to discover both the scope of the semantic category that the child is using and the origin of this category in non-linguistic cognition. Little progress has been made to date on the latter issue.

Limited-scope formulae may persist well beyond the initial stages of word combinations – witness Bloom *et al.*'s (1980) finding that verb inflexions are initially acquired for selective populations of verbs. However, beyond the earliest stages of language development the detailed evidence that is necessary to formulate a production model runs out. Many particular issues have been explored in the literature but, with the exception of the model discussed by Maratsos (1978) and Maratsos and Chalkley (1980), little serious attempt has been made to integrate the many issues into a coherent account of language acquisition. The model developed by Maratsos and Chalkley offers an account of form-class development that may have considerable advantages over other alternatives. Prototype theory also offers some tantalizing possibilities, especially if limited-scope formulae are seen as prototypes for the addition of grammatical morphemes.

F. Input for Grammatical Development

There is little consistent evidence on the role that input language plays in the development of grammatical competence. There are two basic research paradigms that can be used to study this issue: naturalistic observation of mother–child speech and intervention studies in which an experimenter attempts to affect some aspect of language development.

Naturalistic observation raises a number of issues to which little serious theoretical attention has been paid. To begin with, there is a great variety of possible relations between the input a child receives and the output that results. In the absence of a theory of the state relations that mediate between input and output it is difficult to know where the research should begin. It can begin by "fishing" of course. This simply involves computing every possible correlation between input and output. Like all fishing expeditions, something usually turns up. The difficulty is in knowing what to make of it. In the absence of a theory of how input relates to output (i.e. how learning takes place) fishing expeditions are likely to turn up a lot of old boots.

A second problem that hinders progress in this area is knowing what the relevant temporal interval is between input and output. Some studies measure both variables contemporaneously. Some leave long gaps (up to six months or more) between measuring input and correlating it with output. Is it a reasonable assumption in the latter case that the input variable initially measured has operated uniformly throughout the interim period? This simply is not known. There has also been little research on the timing of relevant input although it is a reasonable assumption that this is another crucial factor. Presumably exposure to complex grammatical input is of little relevance to a new-born baby in his eventual mastery of these constructions. But, if that is the case, when does such input become relevant? It is possible to take at least two positions on this issue. The first is that within some definable time-period the more input of a particular sort, the more output of that sort. A second position is that quantity of input is unimportant; it is the timing and relevance of the input that is crucial. The positions impose somewhat different theoretical and empirical requirements. The former requires no more than the correlation of the relevant variables (assuming, of course, that one has a theory of what these are). It is the implicit position adopted by much research on input. The latter requires a specification of when and why particular inputs may be crucial. This is a far from easy task and understandably there is little that can be said about this possibility at the moment.

If we consider naturalistic studies of input-output relations in grammatical development then the results are thin indeed. Brown, Cazden, and Bellugi (1969) demonstrated that neither positive reinforcement (in the form of approval) nor punishment (in the form of disapproval) had any effect on the acquisition of syntax in the three children they studied. They did however, find a weak relation between expansions and grammatical development. At

3 years old, the two children who acquired language most quickly had mothers who used expansions more frequently than the mother of the child whose age-related development was slowest. A study of 15 mother–child pairs by Newport *et al.* (1977) is indicative of the strengths and weaknesses of correlational techniques. The study measured development in the children's speech over six months. The data were obtained from two observations, one at the beginning, the other at the end of the period. On the first observation, measures were taken of the speech of both mother and child. On the second observation, measures of the children's speech only were taken. Newport *et al.* used careful statistical techniques to control for differences in age and initial level of language development of the children. They found no correlations between various measures of "propositional content" in the child's speech and the measures of the mothers' speech employed. They did, however, find correlations between the development of some grammatical morphemes in the child's speech and measures of the mothers' speech.* In particular, there was a strong correlation between the number of auxiliaries per verb phrase in the children's speech and the number of Yes–No questions in the mothers' speech. Newport *et al.* suggest that input language may affect the acquisition of parts of the grammatical system that are specific to a particular language, such as the auxiliary system in English, but may have relatively little effect on more universal aspects of structure and content. These conclusions might be cautiously entertained at present. The failure to find correlations between measures of propositional content in the children's speech and the input language could be due to the measures used rather than the absence of any such relation. Further, the long interval between the two measures raises issues of effects that may have been present over a shorter period and issues of the nature of the intervening input to the children concerned. Presumably it was not the input on that particular day, six months previously, that was important in the Newport *et al.* study but without any data on the variance and the invariance of the input in the intervening period it is difficult to begin the construction of a model of learning with any degree of confidence.

Probably the first intervention study was that carried out by Cazden (1965). She studied 12 children in the age-range 29 to 37 months. The performance of two experimental groups were compared with a control group who received no intervention. In one of the experimental groups the experimenter consistently expanded the child's utterances. In the other group, well-formed sentences other than expansions were presented in reply to each utterance by the child. Each child was seen individually for about 30 minutes over 60 sessions. There was little evidence of a significant improvement in either of the experimental groups. However, intervention by other experimenters has had a more positive effect. Nelson, Carskaddon, and Bonvillian (1973) provided children with "recast sentences". A recast sentence is a response to a child's utterance that preserves the underlying

* There were also weak correlations between Yes–No questions in the mother's speech and the MLU of the child's speech.

semantic relations in the child's utterance but changes the form of the utterance. An example offered by Nelson *et al.* (1973) is that *The bunny chased fireflies* might receive the reply *The bunny did chase fireflies, didn't he?*

Nelson *et al.* found that 3-year-olds who received recast sentences scored higher on all five post-test measures of syntactic development than a "new sentence" group who received short grammatical responses that specifically excluded the content words of the child's utterances and a control group who received no intervention. In particular, the children who received recast sentences scored significantly better than the other groups on tests of auxiliary constructions and of verb use as measured by the mean number of verb elements per verb construction. (It should be noted that these two measures are not independent.) As Newport *et al.* (1977) have also found a correlation between auxiliary constructions in child speech and adult input, it seems that the development of this construction, at least, may be strongly dependent on input.

Nelson (1977) performed a similar experiment, but only certain syntactic constructions were provided in the recast sentences. A group of twelve 2½-year-olds whose speech lacked both complex questions and complex verb-forms was selected. Each child participated in five one-hour experimental training sessions over a two-month period. Half of the children received recasts in the form of complex questions and half received recasts that introduced complex verb forms. The children who heard complex questions in the recast sentences acquired new forms of questions and the child who heard complex verb forms in the recast sentences aquired new verb forms. Thus, intervention, in this case, led to the successful acquisition of particular syntactic forms that were not previously present in the children's speech. The results of these studies do not necessarily bear directly on the normal process of acquisition. Children, in their everyday environment, probably do not receive the same intensive input as was provided in this experiment. On the other hand, the studies do demonstrate that the acquisition of particular constructions can be facilitated by increasing the everday exposure to these constructions by a relatively small amount of additional intensive exposure. This finding again raises the issue of what sort of model of input–output relations is necessary to explain language aquisition. Would carefully chosen (we are assuming the existence of some relevant criteria) bouts of intensive exposure lead to more rapid acquisition than a slow steady diet of continuous exposure? It is disturbing that there is so little discussion of this issue or (we reiterate) of the discourse relations between input and output.

IV. Conclusion

Our concern in this chapter has been to discuss key issues in lexical and grammatical development. The main focus of our discussion has been the types of state models that have been hypothesized to account for the observed output. A number of general remarks can be made about these models.

The Chomskyan revolution in linguistics and psycholinguistics led to the construction of powerful generative models of grammatical development and of lexical development. In recent years it has become evident that the child operates with a much more piecemeal system than was previously envisaged. Semantic Feature Theory proposed a few parsimonious principles in order to account for lexical development. Unfortunately, the issues are considerably more complex and less homogenous than the theory envisages. We have traced in some detail, the variety of issues that confront a theory of reference. Even in this restricted area of the lexicon there are considerable unresolved issues of how the sense and denotation of a word are established by a child. If we consider words that refer to actions, rather than to objects, then there is an even greater dearth of relevant evidence and, more importantly, of relevant theory. This is unfortunate, both because of the emphasis on action in many theories of cognitive development and because of the central and complex role of verbs in sentence construction. If there is one domain of the lexicon that, above all others, requires more investigation, it is the domain of action reference.

The literature on dimensional adjectives has long been a source of intense investigation. The initial impetus came from Semantic Feature Theory but in this area too the theory has been found wanting. Carey's (1978b) model may provide a renewed focus for experimentation. The model regards the discovery of the relevant dimensions as the primary psychological problem in acquiring dimensional adjectives. Carey argues that dimensional adjectives may be used appropriately for certain entities, without the child fully understanding to which dimensions reference is being made. However, this unanalysed pairing of word and objects may aid the child in later discovering the relevant dimensions for a particular term. Much remains to be clarified and explored in relation to these ideas.

Models of grammatical development have, typically, paid little attention to individual lexical items. However, Braine's (1976) limited scope formulae, which often involve a grammatical rule for combining a specific word with an element from some larger set, suggest that grammatical privileges are frequently learnt for single lexical items. This constitutes a radical departure from earlier models of word combinations. One issue that still faces theories of early word combinations is the appropriate level of generality for characterizing the more general categories in Braine's formulae. Is there, for an example, an ACTOR category, all of whose members have the same grammatical privileges in the child's production system? Or, is the category called 'actor' a series of smaller subcategories, each with different (or perhaps overlapping) grammatical privileges?

A further issue to which we have drawn attention is the discovery of form classes by the child; in particular the form class VERB. Maratsos and Chalkley (1980) argue that the child initially learns inflexions for "verbs" on a word-by-word basis and then discovers that there are regularities in this lexical system. Specifically, the child discovers that inflexions have correlated privileges of occurrence in that a word to which the inflexion -ed can be added in one context, will take the inflexion -s in another context and (possibly) -ing in a further context. Much empirical detail is required before this proposal can be evaluated properly. Bloom et al.'s (1980) claim that inflexions initially code aspect rather than tense indicates that there are many issues to be resolved about the acquisition of inflexions and their role in the linguistic system.

The frequent discrepancy between tests of comprehension and production in lexical and grammatical development also suggests that the child's representation of the linguistic system is much more polymorphous than has often been assumed. One issue that requires more careful consideration in state models is how linguistic and contextual factors interact in determining the production and comprehension of utterances. It is evident enough that such an interaction occurs but a principled account of the details is lacking at present. In the absence of such an account it is impossible to have a complete characterization of how cognitive processes control and exploit communication.

Lexical and grammatical development are not separate processes. A child in learning words has to learn the meaning of a word and its role in the grammatical system. How these processes overlap and interact has received far too little attention. However, the increasingly prominent role of the lexicon in both formal and developmental models of grammar will, it is to be hoped, lead to a more integrated theory of language development.

A model of language development should contain both a description of the changes that occur in the child's system over time and an explanation of those changes. At present much remains to be discovered about these issues. Descriptions are never theoretically neutral and it is for this reason that we have paid considerable attention to the production models that have been hypothesized to account for the observed output. But, in addition to a model that accounts for some given output, one also needs an explanation of how the child's system changes over time. Change can be accounted for in a number of ways: by maturation, by reduction to some other developing system (but this merely moves the issue of explaining change one step backwards in the equation), or by developmental processes that are autonomous to the domain in question. Regardless of what balance will exist among these factors in a complete model of language change, the environment in which a child lives and grows will have crucial effects on development. Put at its simplest, a child must receive some relevant input before producing related output. Even if other processes play a considerable role in selectively sensitizing the child to particular inputs at particular times, the environment will still play a crucial role in change. It is in relating input to output that our knowledge of change is weakest at present. This is unfortunate not just because of the lacuna that it creates in explanations of change, but also because models of language intervention crucially require a knowledge of the relevant manipulatable environmental variables. Despite a relative profusion of studies of the characteristics of parental speech there has been little attempt to construct other than the most simple-minded models of the environment and of input–output relations. The key to such a model lies, we feel, in the interrelations among the changing characteristics of parental speech, the changing sensitivities of the child to input, and the discourse context in which new structures are introduced to the child.

References

Amidon, A. and Carey, P. (1972). Why five-year-olds cannot understand *before* and *after*. *Journal of Verbal Learning and Verbal Behavior*, **11**, 417–423.

Anglin, J. M. (1979). The child's first terms of reference. *In* "Symbolic Functioning in Childhood", (N. R. Smith & M. B. Franklin, eds.) Erlbaum, Hillsdale, New Jersey.

Atkinson, M. (1982). "Explanations in the Study of Child Language Development". Cambridge University Press, Cambridge.

Barrett, M. D. (1978). Lexical development and overextension in child language. *Journal of Child Language*, **5**, 205–219.

Barrie-Blackey, S. (1973). Six-year-old children's understanding of sentences adjoined with time adverbs. *Journal of Psycholinguistic Research* **2**, 153–165.

Berlin, B. and Kay, P. (1969). "Basic colour terms: Their universality and evolution". University of California Press, Berkeley.

Bierwisch, M. (1970). Semantics. *In* "New Horizons in Linguistics", (J. Lyons, ed.) Penguin, Harmondsworth.

Black, M. and Chiat, S. (1981). Psycholinguistics without 'psychological reality'. *Linguistics* **19**, 37–61.

Bloom, L. (1970). "Language development: Form and function in emerging grammars". MIT Press, Cambridge, Massachusetts.

Bloom, L. (1973). "One Word at a Time". Mouton, The Hague.

Bloom, L., Capatides, J. B. and Tackeff, J. (1981). Further remarks on interpretive analysis: In response to Christine Howe. *Journal of Child Language*, **8**, 403–411.

Bloom, L., Lifter, K. and Hafitz, J. (1980). Semantics of verbs and the development of verb inflection in child language. *Language*, **56**, 386–412.

Bloom, L., Lightbown, P. and Hood, L. (1975). Structure and variation in child language. *Monographs of the Society for Research on Child Development*, **40** (2, Serial No. 160).

Bowerman, M. (1978). The acquisition of word meaning: An investigation into some current conflicts. *In* "The Development of Communication", (N. Waterson & C. Snow, eds). Wiley, Chichester.

Bowerman, M. (1981). Language development. *In* "Handbook of Cross-cultural Psychology: Developmental Psychology", (H. C. Triandis and A. Heron, eds) Vol. 4. Allyn & Bacon, Boston.

Braine, M. D. S. (1963a). The ontogeny of English phrase structure: the first phase. *Language*, **39**, 1–13.

Braine, M. D. S. (1963b). On learning the grammatical order of words. *Psychological Review*, **70**, 323–348.

Braine, M. D. S. (1976). Children's first word combinations. *Monographs of the Society for Research in Child Development*, **41**, (1, Serial No. 164).

Brewer, W. F. and Stone, J. B. (1975). Acquisition of spatial antonym pairs. *Journal of Experimental Child Psychology*, **19**, 299–307.

Brown, R. (1958). How shall a thing be called? *Psychological Review*, **65**, 14–21.

Brown, R. (1965). "Social Psychology". The Free Press, Glencoe.

Brown, R. (1973). "A First Language". Harvard University Press, Cambridge, Massachusetts.

Brown, R. and Bellugi, U. (1964). Three processes in the acquisition of syntax. *Harvard Educational Review*, **34**, 133–151.

Brown, R., Cazden, C. and Bellugi, U. (1969). The child's grammar from I to III. *In* "Minnesota Symposium on Child Psychology", (J. P. Hill, ed.) Vol. 2. University of Minnesota Press, Minneapolis.

Brown, R. and Fraser, C. (1963). The acquisition of syntax. *In* "Verbal Behavior and Learning: Problems and Processes", (C. Cofer and B. Musgrave, eds). McGraw-Hill, New York.

Bruner, J. (1975a). From communication to language. *Cognition*, **3**, 255–287.

Bruner, J. (1975b). The ontogenesis of speech acts. *Journal of Child Language*, **2**, 1–19.

Bullowa, M. (ed.) (1979). "Before speech: The Beginning of Interpersonal Communication". Cambridge University Press, Cambridge.

Campbell, R., Bowe, T. and Dockrell, J. (in press) The relationship between production and comprehension and its ontogenesis. *In* "Language and Language Acquisition", (F. Lowenthal, J. Condier and F. Vandanne, eds). Plenum, New York.

Campbell, R. and Wales, R. (1970). The study of language acquisition. *In* "New Horizons in Linguistics", (J. Lyons, ed.) Penguin, Harmondsworth.

Carey, S. (1978a) *Less* may never mean "more". *In* "Recent Advances in the Psychology of Language", (R. N. Campbell and P. T. Smith, eds). Plenum, New York.

Carey, S. (1978b) The child as word learner. *In* "Linguistic Theory and Psychological Reality", (M. Halle, J. Bresnan, and G. A. Miller, eds). MIT Press, Cambridge, Massachusetts.

Cazden, C. B. (1965). Environmental assistance to the child's acquisition of grammar. Unpublished doctoral dissertation, Harvard University.

Cazden, C. B. (1968). The acquisition of noun and verb inflections. *Child Development*, **39**, 433–488.

Chafe, W. (1970). "Meaning and the Structure of Language". University of Chicago Press, Chicago.

Chomsky, C. (1969). The Acquisition of Syntax in Children from Five to Ten. MIT Press, Cambridge, Massachusetts.

Chomsky, N. (1957). "Syntactic Structures". Mouton, The Hague.

Chomsky, N. (1959). Review of "Verbal Behavior" by B. F. Skinner. *Language*, **35**, 26–58.

Chomsky, N. (1965). "Aspects of the Theory of Syntax". MIT Press, Cambridge, Massachusetts.

Chomsky, N. (1968). "Language and Mind". Harcourt, Brace, & World, New York.

Clark, E. V. (1970). How young children describe events in time. *In* "Advances in Psycholinguistics", (G. B. Flores d'Arcais and W. J. M. Levelt, eds). North-Holland, Amsterdam.

Clark, E. V. (1971). On the acquisition of the meaning of *before* and *after*. *Journal of Verbal Learning and Verbal Behavior*, **10**, 266–275.

Clark, E. V. (1972). On the child's aquisition of antonyms in two semantic fields. *Journal of Verbal Learning and Verbal Behavior*, **11**, 750–758.

Clark, E. V. (1973a). What's in a word? On the child's acquisition of semantics in his first language. *In* "Cognitive Development and the Acquisition of Language", (T. E. Moore, ed.) Academic Press, New York.

Clark, E. V. (1973b). Non-linguistic strategies and the acquisition of word meanings. *Cognition* **2**, 161–182.

Clark, E. V. (1974). Some aspects of the conceptual basis for first language acquisition. *In* "Language Perspectives: Acquisition, Retardation, and Intervention", (R. L. Schiefelbusch and L. L. Lloyd, eds). Macmillan, London.

Clark, E. V. and Garnica, O. K. (1974). Is he coming or going? On the acquisition of deictic verbs. *Journal of Verbal Learning and Verbal Behavior* **13**, 559–572.

Clark, R., Hutcheson, S. and Van Buren, P. (1974). Comprehension and production in language acquisition. *Journal of Linguistics*, **10**, 39–54.

Comrie, B. (1977). "Aspect". Cambridge University Press, Cambridge.

de Villiers, J. G. (1980). The process of rule learning in child speech: A new look. *In* "Children's Language", (K. E. Nelson, ed.) Vol. 2. Gardner Press, New York.

de Villiers, J. G. and de Villiers, P. A. (1973). A cross sectional study of the development of grammatical morphemes in child speech. *Journal of Psycholinguistic Research*, **3**, 267–278.

Dixon, R. M. W. (1979). Ergativity. *Language*, **55**, 59–138.

Dockrell, J. (1981). The child's acquisition of unfamiliar words: An experimental study. Unpublished Ph.D. thesis, University of Stirling.

Donaldson, M. and Balfour, G. (1968). Less is more: A study of language comprehension in children. *British Journal of Psychology*, **59**, 461–471.

Donaldson, M. and Wales, R. J. (1970). On the acquisition of some relational terms. *In* "Cognition and the Development of Language", (J. R. Hayes, ed.) Wiley, New York.

Eilers, R. E., Oller, D. K. and Ellington, J. (1974). The acquisition of word-meaning for dimensional adjectives: The long and short of it. *Journal of Child Language*, **1**, 195–204.

Fillmore, C. (1968). The case for case. *In* "Universals in Linguistic Theory", (E. Bach and R. Harms, eds). Holt, Rinehart, & Winston, New York.

Gentner, D. (1975). Evidence for the psychological reality of semantic components: The verbs of possession. *In* "Explorations in Cognition", (D. A. Norman and D. E. Rumelhart, eds). Freeman, San Francisco.

Gentner, D. (1978). On relational meaning: the acquisition of verb meaning. *Child Development*, **49**, 988–998.

Gleason, J. B. and Weintraub, S. (1978). Input language and the acquisition of communicative competence. *In* "Children's Language", (K. E. Nelson, ed.) Vol. 1. Gardner Press, New York.

Glucksberg, S., Hay, A. and Danks, J. H. (1976). Words in utterance contexts: Young children do not confuse the meanings of *same* and *different*. *Child Development* **47**, 737–741.

Goldin-Meadow, S., Seligman, M. and Gelman, R. (1976). Language in the two-year old. *Cognition*, **4**, 189–202.

Golinkoff, R. M. (1981). The case for semantic relations: Evidence from the verbal and non-verbal domains. *Journal of Child Language*, **8**, 413–437.

Gordon, P. (1977). Partial Lexical Entry and the Semantic Development of *more* and *less*. Unpublished B.Sc. thesis, University of Stirling.

Grieve, R., Hoogenraad, R. and Murray, D. (1977). On the young child's use of lexis and syntax in understanding locative instructions. *Cognition*, 235–250.

Grieve, R. and Stanley, S. (1980). Less obscure? Pragmatics and 3- to 4-year-old children's semantics. Unpublished manuscript. Department of Psychology, University of Western Australia, Australia.

Halliday, M. A. K. (1975). *Learning how to mean*. Edward Arnold, London.

Harrison, B. (1972). "Meaning and Structure". Harper & Row, London.

Hoogenraad, R., Grieve, R., Baldwin, P. and Campbell, R. N. (1978). Comprehension as an interactive process. *In* "Recent Advances in the Psychology of Language", (R. N. Campbell & P. T. Smith, eds). Plenum, New York.

Hopper, P. J. and Thompson, S. A. (1980). Transitivity in grammar and discourse. *Language*, **56**, 251–299.

Howe, C. J. (1976). The meaning of two-word utterances in the speech of young children. *Journal of Child Language* **3**, 29–48.

Howe, C. (1981). "Acquiring Language in a Conversational Context". Academic Press, London and New York.

Huttenlocher, J. (1974). The origins of language comprehension. *In* "Theories in Cognitive Psychology", (R. L. Solso, ed.) Erlbaum, Potomac, Maryland.

Hymes, D. (1971). Competence and performance in linguistic theory. *In* "Language Acquisition: Models and Methods", (R. Huxley and E. Ingram, eds). Academic Press, London and New York.

Johnson, C. N. and Wellman, H. M. (1980). Children's developing understanding of mental verbs: Remember, know, and guess. *Child Development*, **51**, 1095–1102.

Karmiloff-Smith, A. (1979). "A Functional Approach to Child Language". Cambridge University Press, Cambridge.

Katz, J. J. and Fodor, J. A. (1963). The structure of a semantic theory. *Language*, **39**, 190–210.

Kay, D. A. and Anglin, J. M. (1982). Overextension and underextension in the child's expressive and receptive speech. *Journal of Child Language*, **9**, 83–98.

Kay, P. (1975). Synchronic variability and diachronic change in basic color terms. *Language in Society*, **54**, 610–646.

Kripke, S. A. (1972). Naming and necessity. *In* "Semantics of Natural Language", (D. Davidson and G. Harman, eds). Reidel, Dordrecht.

Kuczaj, S. A. (1977). The acquisition of regular and irregular past tense forms. *Journal of Verbal Learning and Verbal Behavior*, **16**, 589–600.

Kuczaj, S. A. and Maratsos, M. P. (1975). On the acquisition of *front, back*, and *side*. *Child Development*, **46**, 202–210.

Labov, W. (1973). The boundaries of words and their meanings. *In* "New Ways of Analyzing Variation in English", (E. N. Bailey and R. W. Shuy, eds). Georgetown University Press, Washington.

Leopold, W. (1939–49). "Speech Development of a Bilingual Child", (4 vols). Northwestern University Press, Evanston, Illinois.

Lewis, M. M. (1936). "Infant Speech". Routledge & Kegan Paul, London.

Lock, A. (ed.) (1978). "Action, Gesture and Symbol: The Emergence of Language". Academic Press, London and New York.

Lyons, J. (1978). "Semantics", Vol. 1. Cambridge University Press, Cambridge.

McCawley, J. (1968). The role of semantics in a grammar. *In* "Universals in Linguistic Theory", (E. Bach and R. Harms, eds). Holt, Rinehart & Winston, New York.

McNeill, D. (1966). Developmental psycholinguistics. *In* "The Genesis of Language", (F. Smith and G. A. Miller, eds). MIT Press, Cambridge, Massachusetts.

McNeill, D. (1970). "The Acquisition of Language". Harper & Row, New York.

McShane, J. (1979). The development of naming. *Linguistics* **17**, 879–905.

McShane, J. (1980). "Learning to Talk". Cambridge University Press, Cambridge.

McShane, J. (1981). How do children learn verbs? *Working Papers of the London Psycholinguistics Research Group,* **3**, 40–45.

Maratsos, M. (1978). New models in linguistics and language acquisition. *In* "Linguistic Theory and Psychological Reality", (M. Halle, J. Bresnan, and G. A. Miller, eds). MIT Press, Cambridge, Massachusetts.

Maratsos, M. P. and Chalkley, M. A. (1980). The internal language of children's syntax: The ontogenesis and representation of syntactic categories. *In* "Children's Language", (K. E. Nelson, ed.), Vol. 2. Gardner Press, New York.

Miller, G. A. (1977). "Spontaneous Apprentices: Children and Language". Seabury, New York.

Miller, G. A. and Johnson-Laird, P. N. (1976). "Language and Perception". Cambridge University Press, Cambridge.

Miscione, J. L. Marvin, R. S., O'Brien, R. G. and Greenberg, M. T. (1978). A developmental study of preschoolchildren's understanding of the words "know" and "guess". *Child Development,* **49**, 1107–1113.

Murphy, C. M. (1978). Pointing in the context of a shared activity. *Child Development,* **49**, 371–380.

Nelson, K. (1973). Structure and strategy in learning to talk. *Monographs of the Society for Research in Child Development,* **38**, (1–2, Serial no. 149).

Nelson, K. E. (1977). Facilitating children's syntax acquisition. *Developmental Psychology,* **13**, 101–107.

Nelson, K. E., Carskaddon, G. and Bonvillian, J. D. (1973). Syntax acquisition: Impact of experimental variation in adult verbal interaction with the child. *Child Development,* **44**, 497–504.

Nelson, K., Rescorla, L., Gruendel, J. and Benedict, H. (1978). Early lexicons: What do they mean? *Child Development,* **49**, 960–968.

Newport, E. L., Gleitman, H. and Gleitman, L. R. (1977). Mother I'd rather do it myself: Some effects and non-effects of maternal speech style. *In* "Talking to Children", (C. E. Snow and C. A. Ferguson, eds). Cambridge University Press, Cambridge.

Ninio, A. (1980). Ostensive definition in vocabulary teaching. *Journal of Child Language,* **7**, 565–573.

Ninio, A. and Bruner, J. (1978). The achievement and antecedents of labelling. *Journal of Child Language,* **5**, 1–15.

Palermo, D. S. (1973). More about less: A study of language comprehension. *Journal of Verbal Learning and Verbal Behavior,* **12**, 211–221.

Palermo, D. S. (1974). Still more about the comprehension of "less". *Developmental Psychology,* **10**, 827–829.

Pinker, S. (1979). Formal models of language learning. *Cognition,* **7**, 217–283.

Postal, P. M. (1966). Review Article: Andre Martinet: "Elements of general linguistics". *Foundations of Language,* **2**, 151–186.

Putnam, H. (1975). The meaning of "meaning". *In* "Language, Mind and Knowledge", (K. Gunderson, ed.) Minnesota studies in the philosophy of science, Vol. 7. Minneapolis: University of Minnesota Press.

Richards, M. M. (1976). *Come* and *go* reconsidered: Children's use of deictic verbs in contrived situations. *Journal of Verbal Learning and Verbal Behavior*, **15**, 655–665.

Richards, M. M. (1979). Sorting out what's in a word from what's not: Evaluating Clark's semantic features acquisition theory. *Journal of Experimental Child Psychology*, **27**, 1–47.

Rosch, E. (1978). Principles of categorization. *In* "Cognition and Categorization", (E. Rosch and B. B. Lloyd, eds). Erlbaum, Hillsdale, New Jersey.

Rosch, E. and Mervis, C. B. (1975). Family resemblances: Studies in the internal structure of categories. *Cognitive Psychology*, **7**, 573–605.

Rosch, E., Mervis, C., Gray, W., Johnson, D. and Boyes-Braem, P. (1976). Basic objects in natural categories. *Cognitive Psychology*, **8**, 382–439.

Schieffelin, B. S. (1979). A developmental study of word order and casemarking in an ergative language. *Papers and Reports on Child Language Development*, **17**.

Schlesinger, I. M. (1971). Production of utterances and language acquisition. *In* "The Ontogenesis of Grammar", (D. I. Slobin, ed.) Academic Press, New York and London.

Schaffer, H. R. (ed.) (1977). *Studies in mother–infant interaction*. Academic Press, London, and New York.

Schwartz, S. P. (1979). Natural kind terms. *Cognition*, **7**, 301–315.

Shatz, M. (1978). On the development of communicative understandings: An early strategy for interpreting and responding to messages. *Cognitive Psychology*, **10**, 271–301.

Skinner, B. (1957). "Verbal Behavior". Appleton-Century-Crofts, New York.

Slobin, D. I. (1970). Universals of grammatical development in children. *In* "Advances in Psycholinguistics", (G. B. Flores d'Arcais and W. J. M. Levelt, eds). North-Holland, Amsterdam.

Slobin, D. I. (1981). The origins of grammatical encoding of events. *In* "The Child's Construction of Language", (W. Deutsch, ed.) Academic Press, London and New York.

Snow, C. E. and Ferguson, C. A. (eds), (1977). "Talking to Children". Cambridge University Press, Cambridge.

Thomson, J. R. and Chapman, R. S. (1977). Who is 'Daddy' revisited: The status of two-year olds' overextended words in use and comprehension. *Journal of Child Language*, **4**, 359–375.

Townsend, D. J. (1976). Do children interpret "marked" comparative adjectives as their opposites? *Journal of Child Language*, **3**, 385–396.

Trehub, S. E. and Abramovitch, R. (1978). Less is not more: Further observations on nonlinguistic strategies. *Journal of Experimental Child Psychology*, **25**, 160–167.

Vorster, J. (1975). Mommy linguist: the case for motherese. *Lingua*, **37**, 281–312.

Vygotsky, L. (1934). "Thought and Language", (Trans. E. Hanfman and G. Vakar). MIT Press, Cambridge, Massachusetts, 1962.

Wales, R. J. and Campbell, R. (1970). On the development of comparison and the comparison of development. *In* "Advances in Psycholinguistics", (G. B. Flores d'Arcais and W. J. M. Levelt eds). North-Holland, Amsterdam.

Warden, D. (1981). Children's understanding of *ask* and *tell*. *Journal of Child Language*, **8**, 139–149.

Wellman, H. M. and Johnson, C. M. (1979). Understanding of mental processes: A developmental study of "remember" and "forget" *Child Development*, **50**, 79–88.

Wexler, K. and Culicover, P. N. (1980). *Formal principles of language acquisition.* MIT Press, Cambridge, Massachussetts.

Wieman, L. (1976). Stress patterns of early child language. *Journal of Child Language,* **3**, 283–286.

Wilcox, S. and Palermo, D. (1975). "In", "on" and "under" revisited. *Cognition,* **3**, 245–254.

White, T. G. (1982). Naming practices, typicality, and underextension in child language. *Journal of Experimental Child Psychology,* **33**, 324–346.

II

Production of Language in Non-speech Modalities

3

The Organization of Movement in Handwriting and Typing

P. Viviani   *CNRS*
C. Terzuolo   *University of Minnesota*

I. Introduction

Some of the mechanisms subserving language production appear to be specifically designed for this purpose, inasmuch as they seem to have no other function. This contrasts sharply with the situation in written production of language, which utilizes motor mechanisms that, from the phylogenetic point of view, evolved for quite different purposes. The problem then arises of how the system of principles and constraints which are specific to language come to terms with the set of principles and constraints of these motor mechanisms.

Two main forms of written language production have evolved so far, namely handwriting and typing, Morse code being closely related to the latter. Handwriting research has mainly focused on the kinematics of the hand and finger movements, the levels of approach ranging from detailed simulations of handwriting by biomechanical models, to the formulation of general functional principles. Only indirect evidence has so far been provided for the involvement of linguistic factors in the organization of handwriting, mainly from the analysis of lapses and spelling errors. Moreover, it is only recently that early work on errors (Bawden, 1900) has been revisited from a quantitatively satisfactory viewpoint (e.g. Wing and Baddeley, 1978). In typing instead, interest in linguistic problems has predominated from the very inception of research in this field (Bryan and Harter, 1897, 1899; Book, 1908). In particular, the imprint on the sequence of keypressings by the linguistic nature and content of the message has been investigated on the basis of both the temporal aspects of the sequence and the incidence of typing errors.

The organization of this chapter necessarily reflects the situation just outlined. However, emphasis will mostly be placed on those principles of motor organization which are either common to both forms of written production of language, or appear to be of particular relevance *vis-à-vis* the central control of movement. The notion of *invariance* will be the key concept and the leading theme in much of what follows. Almost all principles of motor organization to be considered express the conservation of some quantity relevant to the description of the movement, across changes in some other quantities. Thus, in handwriting, the two main kinematic parameters of the movement, namely the shape of the trajectory and the velocity of execution, covary in such a way as to leave the angular velocity approximately invariant over finite intervals (Isogony Principle). Furthermore, the relative timing of the dynamical events in the course of the movement is invariant across large changes in total duration (Time–Homothetic behaviour) and the relative size of different portions of the trajectory is preserved when the overall size is intentionally varied (Motor Equivalence). Finally, handwriting shares with other intentional fast movements the property of Isochrony, that is the built-in tendency to increase the speed of execution as a function of the linear extent of the movement's trajectory, so as to keep its total duration roughly constant.

Invariance is ubiquitous also in typing movements. The most striking example is the experimental observation that to each word corresponds a time sequence of keystrokes which is highly characteristic of the operator but does not depend on the context. Time–Homothetic behaviour will emerge again in the case of typing: while the total duration of the sequence of keystrokes for a given word may vary within relatively large limits, the set of ratios between interstrokes intervals (motor engram) is always kept invariant. A third form of invariance is remarkably similar to that found in articulatory movements: it expresses the independence of the final (target) spatio-temporal positioning of the fingers with respect to the initial conditions.

All these issues will be discussed in some detail in relation to the linguistic nature of the skills. Several topics will instead be partially or totally neglected. We will not consider any of the numerous simulation studies in handwriting (Eden, 1962; Denier van der Gon, Thuring and Strackee, 1962; Vredenbregt and Koster, 1971; Yasuhara, 1975; Hollerbach, 1980a,b) nor the biomechanical description of the hand and fingers (e.g. Wing, 1978). Reaction Time studies in typing (Sternberg, Monsell, Knoll and Wright, 1978; Ostry, 1980) and their bearing on language processing and motor programming, as well as the analysis of typing errors (MacNeilage, 1964; Shaffer and Hardwick, 1969) will only receive a cursory mention. Finally, we will deal exclusively with the fully developed skills and disregard completely the learning process (Bryan and Harter, 1897, 1899; Book 1908; Freeman, 1914; Dvorak, Merrick, Dealy and Ford, 1936; Søvik, 1975; Van Galen, 1980).

II. Biomechanical and Control Aspects

A. Handwriting

Handwriting movements result from the coordinated action of many muscles and joints, and each aspect of the movement (size, speed, slant, pressure, etc.) is potentially relevant to the performance. Detailed understanding of this coordination may be years to come, expecially if one considers the large number of individual postural variations. Wing (1978) has recently provided a summary of some facts relevant to this subject, as well as a simplified formal framework for the description of the forearm–wrist–fingers system. Here we will adopt a strictly phenomenological viewpoint, by considering handwriting as the response of an otherwise unspecified biomechanical system to efferent motor commands.

From the purely kinematic point of view, handwriting is a continuous movement which, unlike typing, shows no well-defined segmentation. However, from the very inception of handwriting studies it was recognized that this apparent continuity conceals a discrete underlying structure, much as the continuous articulatory–acoustic output of speech may be thought of as possessing an underlying discrete structure. To quote Freeman (1914) "... a letter is represented to us, not as a uniform whole, but as composed of certain subordinate units". In a subsequent section, we will review some evidence which demonstrates unequivocally the existence and the nature of such units. However, since in recent years a number of authors (cf. Kugler, Scott Kelso and Turvey, 1980; Scott Kelso et al., 1980) have chosen to emphasize the essentially continuous-kinematic aspects of skilful and fast movements (including handwriting), we begin by presenting an overview of this approach. Then, we will discuss the criticism in which it incurs.

1. The Spring-Mass view

The continuous-kinematic view of handwriting derives from the simple intuition that movement is essentially oscillatory in nature and that curvilinear trajectories result from the composition of two basically harmonic, orthogonal vectors (see for instance Denier van der Gon and Thuring, 1965). Clearly this is an empirical hypothesis, quite independent of the issue of the nature of the central processes that control the movement. In actual fact, such a view has become deeply associated to a particular conception of the control mechanisms, which several authors (e.g. Kugler, Scott Kelso and Turvey, 1980) have recently proposed as a general organizational principle of the motor system. This view, which originates from a series of seminal papers by Feldman and coworkers (Asatryan and Feldman, 1965; Feldman, 1966a,b), postulates that the behaviour of a group of muscles acting as unit ("Coordinative Structure"; see Turvey, Shaw and Mace, 1978) is functionally equivalent to that of a spring-mass-dashpot system with several degrees of freedom (see Feldman 1974 a, b, and also Bizzi et al., 1978). Voluntary changes in the velocity and direction of the movement would then be achieved by modulating the setting of the system's parameters (stiffness and resting length), while the energy flux to the system (forcing function) would not depend explicitly on time but rather on properties intrinsic to the system's design. According to this view, stability – the property of producing a bounded response to a finite input – is always a built-in feature of the push–pull arrangement of agonist and antagonist muscles.

Hollerbach (1980a,b) has provided a detailed characterization of this view in the particular case of handwriting: "Handwriting production is viewed as a constrained modulation of an underlying oscillatory process. Coupled oscillations in horizontal and vertical directions produce letter forms, and when superimposed on a rightward, constant velocity, horizontal sweep, result in spatially separated letters. Modulations of the vertical oscillation is responsible for control of letter height, either through altering the frequency or altering the acceleration amplitude. Modulation of the horizontal oscillation is responsible for control of corner shape through altering phase and amplitude". In such a framework the logic and constraints specific to the mechanisms of language production would be translated into modulations of the movement dynamics compatible with the oscillatory nature of the system.

Strictly speaking, the Spring-Mass view does not preclude the possibility that the underlying control processes possess a discrete structure, and one could in fact postulate that the centrally imposed modulations are of a discrete, step-like nature. However, when real samples of movement are thus analysed, the control signals necessary to duplicate the experimental records turn out to be essentially continuous (see, for instance, Teulings and Thomassen, 1979). Conversely, if one hypothesizes step changes in the parameter modulation to mimic actual writing traces with Lissajou trajectories* (Denier van der Gon, Thuring and Strakee, 1962; McDonald, 1966), the dynamical aspects of the movement are not those to be found in actual records.

In conclusion, discontinuity and segmentation are not emerging properties of the Spring-Mass representation. The following section summarizes some experimental evidence suggesting instead that discontinuity and segmentation are indeed characteristic features of handwriting, and more generally of natural writing-like movements.

2. Differential properties and the Isogony Principle

An interesting problem in the study of handwriting is the relation between the geometrical and dynamical aspects of the movement. A priori, one would not predict any specific and reproducible dependency of the tangential velocity on the trajectory of the movement. However, since the first

* Whenever the motion of a point in the plane results from the composition of two harmonic functions, the point is said to follow a Lissajou trajectory.

recording of handwriting by Binet and Courtier (1893) it became apparent that some relation exists (Fig. 1). A series of recent experiments (Viviani and Terzuolo, 1982; Viviani and McCollum, 1983; Lacquitaniti, Terzuolo and Viviani, 1983a, b) have demonstrated that, at all regular points of the trajectory, the time courses of the tangential velocity V and of the radius of curvature r are strikingly similar (Fig. 2(A)). Indeed, the proportional law $V(t) = k\, r(t)$ provides a satisfactory first order approximation to the data. Since, by definition, the ratio $V(t)/r(t)$ is the angular velocity $d\alpha(t)/dt$ (in absolute value), these results demonstrate a surprisingly general characteristic of writing movements: segments of trajectory which encompass equal angles tend to be executed in equal times. For obvious reasons the name Isogony Principle was suggested to describe this differential property of the movement. The validity of the principle extends to other forms of spontaneous finger movements not directly related to language (see later).

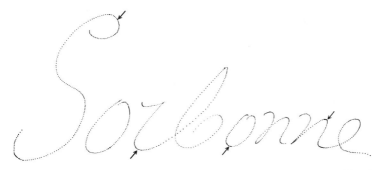

FIG. 1. The earliest dynamic recording of handwriting. Unpublished recording of the dynamics of handwriting obtained by Binet at the end of last century. Binet used a modified version of Edison pen which burned the paper with a spark every 5 ms. Velocity can be estimated by the inverse of distance between successive points. Notice that marked decelerations occur at points of higher curvature. (Courtesy of the Binet Archives, Paris).

A closer analysis of the angular velocities in spontaneous writing brings to the light another interesting characteristic of these movements. As shown by the examples in (B), (C) and (D) of Fig. 2, the absolute value of the angular velocity (slope of the curves $\alpha = \alpha\,(t)$) is not really constant throughout the movement. Rather, it jumps several times, and quite abruptly, from one approximately constant value to another. As a rule, all figural landmarks of the trajectory produces one of these step-like changes in angular velocity. However, they also occur between landmarks where the trajectory is perfectly continuous. These abrupt changes clearly suggest a segmentation of the movement in identifiable units of actions. Since angular velocity resumes both the dynamic and figural aspects of the trajectory, such segmentation is likely to reflect a discontinuity in the spatio-temporal organization of the motor commands rather than a discontinuity of the resulting kinematic parameters.

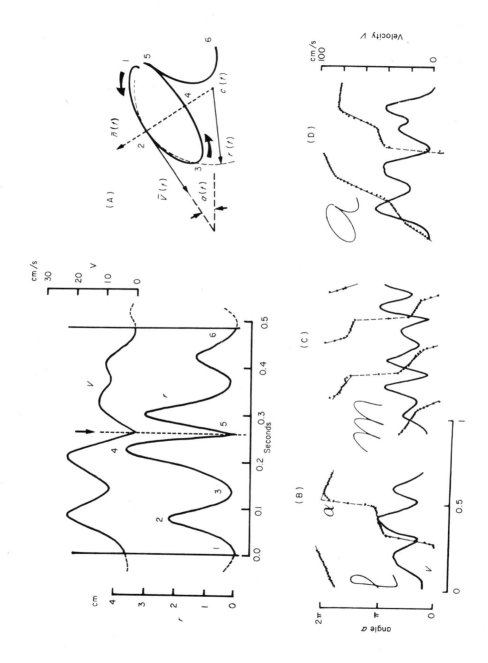

Both the Isogony Principle and the step-like modulation of the angular velocity are difficult to reconcile with the Spring-Mass philosophy. In fact, the stated aim of this approach is to show that control and coordination of movement are emerging properties of those synergic relations among muscles which can be identified with a force-driven oscillatory system (Scott Kelso *et al.*, 1980). There can be no doubt that a properly driven Spring-Mass system may exhibit both the characteristics of handwriting described above. Actually, it is even possible that, in some particularly simple instances (see below), the required driving commands be quite similar to the real ones. In general, however, we do not see how the Isogony Principle, the segmentation of the movement into units of motor action, as well as other general properties of natural, writing-like movements to be discussed shortly could emerge from the postulated synergic relations, without invoking *ad hoc* modulations of the setting for the system's parameters which would be almost as complicated as the behaviour itself. In this case, the desired controlled dissipation of the body's degrees of freedom would not be achieved.

3. *Global properties of free movements*
The Isogony Principle describes a local (differential) property of continuous hand and finger movements. Other, more global properties of these movements will now be briefly reviewed. The first relation that needs to be mentioned is the so-called Fitts' Law (Fitts, 1954) which states that movement time (MT) is a logarithmically increasing function of the ratio between the amplitude of the movement (A) and the required accuracy (W):

$$MT = K_1 + K_2 \log_2 (2A/W).$$

More recent results (Welford, 1968; Schmidt *et al.* 1979) somewhat revise this formulation, but it is questionable whether much theoretical significance should be attached to any specific functional relationship between the

---

FIG. 2. Relationship between figural and dynamical aspects of handwriting. The instantaneous radius of curvature $r(t)$ and the modulus of the tangential velocity $V(t)$ completely describe the figural and dynamical aspects of the movement respectively, while the time course of the angle $\alpha(t)$ of the tangent to the trajectory resumes both these aspects. These three quantities are identified on the example of trajectory shown in (A). The quantities r and V (left panel) were calculated from the instantaneous coordinates $x(t)$ and $y(t)$ recorded by the digitizing table. The relevant result shown in this figure is the great similarity between the time course of r and V. Numbers on the trajectories permit to identify the corresponding dynamic events. Notice the presence of a singularity in the movement: the cuspid (point 5), where the tangential velocity goes to zero. In panels (B), (C) and (D) the curves labelled V represent the modulus of the tangential velocity for the indicated letter. Dots (●) show the values (module 2π) of the angle $\alpha(t)$. The solid lines interpolating the data points are theoretical predictions. (- - -) correspond to points of discontinuity of the movement (as in (B) and (C), or fast transitions for which no reliable prediction could be made (as in (A)). In all cases it is obvious that the slope of $\alpha(t)$ undergoes step changes which clearly identify discrete segments of the movement (from Viviani and Terzuolo, 1982).

above parameters. In the present context, we rather wish to emphasize a qualitative implication of these findings, namely the (apparently automatic) compensatory action whereby the speed of execution increases with the distance to be travelled (Bryan, 1892; Stetson and McDill, 1923). Roughly speaking, this implies a built-in tendency to make the execution time less variable than movement size, especially for large movements (see Fig. 3(A)). Such a tendency, referred to as the Isochrony Principle, was originally studied in the case of simple, unidimensional movements. However, it also applies to many other motor performances as sharply different as saccadic eye movements (Yarbus, 1967; Stark, 1968), head rotations (Zangemeister, Lehman and Stark, 1981a,b) and to the writing of isolated letters, as Freeman (1914) noted almost 70 years ago (Fig. 3(B)) (cf. also Wing, 1978). In the specific case of complex writing-like movements, the Isochrony and Isogony Principles interact in a subtle way (Viviani and McCollum, 1983). Thus, for instance, in the drawing of a folded-up Figure Eight (Fig. 4(A)) the tangential velocity depends on both the curvature of the trajectory and the linear extent of the two circles that form the pattern. In particular, the isochronic component of the velocity is an amazingly regular function of the linear extent (Fig. 4(B) and (C)). It is certainly tempting to suppose that such an exquisite regulatory principle must have a teleonomic value for us. Unfortunately, we are still unable to figure out what life would be like if this ubiquitous mechanism did not exist. We would like to remark, however, that Isochrony is no more an emerging property of Mass-Spring Systems than either Isogony or segmentation, discussed previously.

Another important global property of human movements is the phenomenon of Motor Equivalence (Bernstein, 1967; Hebb, 1949; Lashley, 1951; Merton, 1972) that is, the well-known fact that the form of a letter or word is invariant over considerable changes in its overall size (Fig. 5), even when different sets of joints and muscles are involved. This behaviour can be termed "Space–Homothetic" since, as in the case of the homothetic transformation of geometry, it implies that the relative sizes of all trajectory components are invariant across changes in absolute size. It also indicates that the trajectory components are represented in a quite abstract manner and that the intended form is specified as an invariant relation between these abstract representations. A second, complementary aspect of structural invariance in continuous movement is illustrated by the following observation. If one intentionally varies the speed of writing while keeping constant the size of the letters, the duration of each portion of the movement is scaled in direct proportion to the total duration (Fig. 6). Thus, the representation of the movement does not specify the absolute timing for each movement component but rather the (abstract) ratios between the duration of these components. The homothetic behaviour in the time domain illustrated in Fig. 6 follows from the fact that these ratios are invariant. When writing the same letter or word in different sizes, both the above homothetic behaviours can be observed. In fact, as predicted by the Isochrony Principle, any

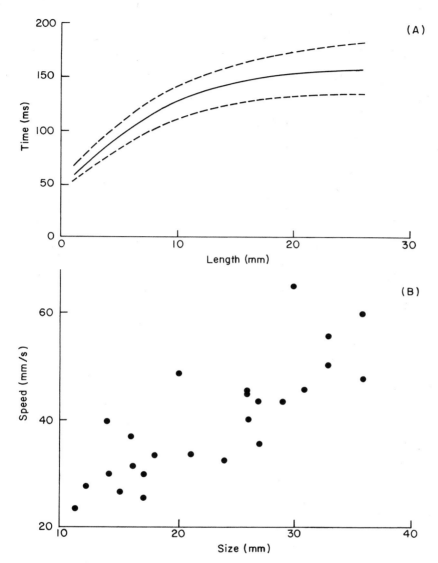

FIG. 3. Demonstration of the Isochrony Principle. (A) The case of simple rectilinear movements: the subject draws 100 vertical strokes whose length varies between 2 and 25 mm. On the abscissa the length and on the ordinate the duration of the movement. The average (——) and the variance (- - -) demonstrate that duration increases far less than linearly as a function of movement extent, being almost constant above 15 mm. (redrawn from Michel, 1971). (B) The case of complex handwriting movements. The data points demonstrate that, in writing the letters of the alphabet, the average speed (ordinate) is proportional to the length of the trajectory (abscissa). The data points have been calculated from the results of Table II in Freeman, (1914).

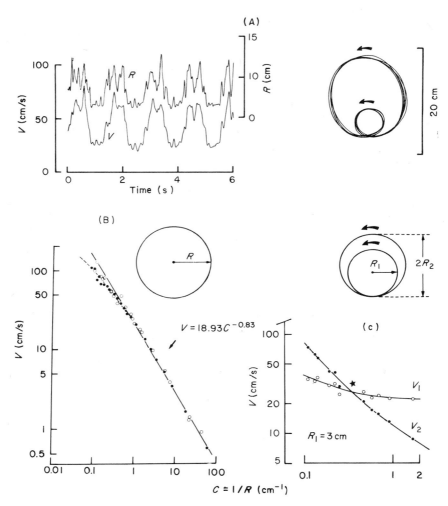

FIG. 4. Interaction of local and global effects on drawing velocity. In (A) are shown typical measurements of the radius of curvature (R) and of the tangential velocity (V) for the illustrated Figure Eight pattern. Velocity depends both on the local curvature of the trajectory and on the linear extent of the two loops that compose the Figure Eight. The latter dependency is demonstrated in greater detail in (B) where it is shown that the average velocity in the drawing of circles is an exquisitely precise function of the circle's size. The data in (C) relate to an experiment in which one loop of the Figure Eight was kept constant (R_1 = 3 cm), while the other (R_2) was varied. The results demonstrate that the velocity in both the variable and the constant loop depends on the total linear extent of trajectory (from Viviani and McCollum, 1983).

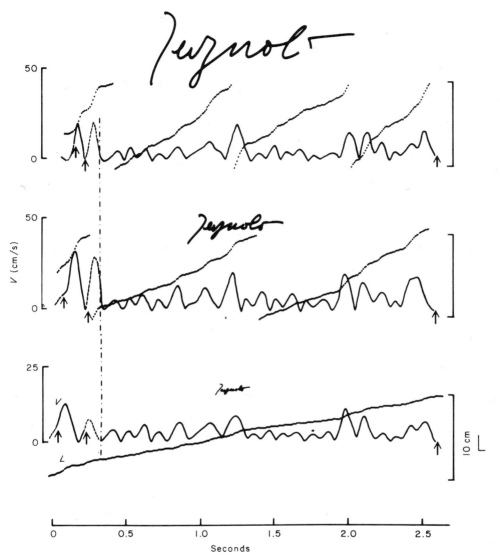

FIG. 5. Motor equivalence in handwriting. The signature of a given individual is easily recognizable whatever its size and despite the fact that different joints and muscles may be involved. (. . .) in each diagram (L) represents the linear extent of the movement as a function of time (the upper signature is roughly four times as large as the bottom one). (——) represents the tangential velocity of the movement (*V*). (- - -) indicates the points where the pen was not touching the paper. (—·—·—·) indicates the dynamic event used to align the tracings. Arrows delimit the first isolated letter of the signature. The examples shown illustrate a case in which the Isochrony Principle applies strictly: the total duration of the movement is kept constant by increasing proportionally the writing speed. Notice also that the timing of each segment of the motion is invariant (from Viviani and Terzuolo, 1980a).

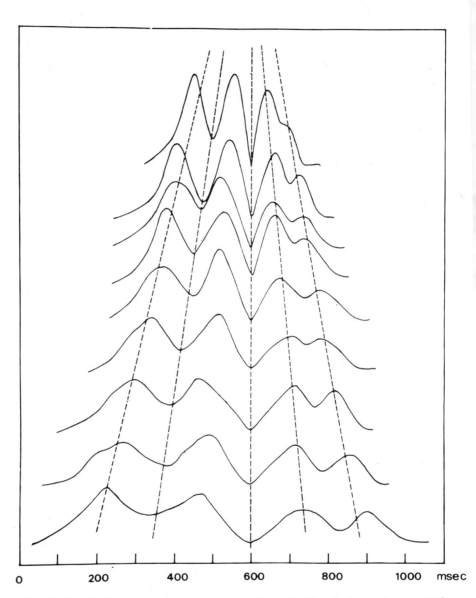

0   200   400   600   800   1000   msec

FIG. 6. Homothetic behaviour in the time domain for handwriting. Each record represents the modulus of the tangential velocity for the same letter and the same subject of Fig. 2(A). The subject was instructed to intentionally modify the writing speed while keeping constant the size of the letter. When the total duration of the movement decreases, the instantaneous values of the velocity increase proportionally in such a way as to leave invariant the ratios among the times of occurrence of the major features of the profile. This is demonstrated by ranking and scaling the records as in Fig. 14(B). The lines interpolating the times of occurrence of the major features all have a common origin (from Viviani and Terzuolo, 1980a).

increase in size generally entails less than proportional increases in movement time (Fig. 7). Instances of overcompensation may occur, in which a
larger letter is actually written in a shorter time than a smaller one (see for
instance letter I in Fig. 7). In all cases, however, both principles of homothetic invariance are simultaneously and independently satisfied
(Braitenberg, 1965; Viviani and Terzuolo, 1980a).

4. *The effects of external constraints*
So far we have only considered the case of spontaneous, unimpeded movements. In what follows, we will discuss some results concerning the effects of
various kinds of external constraints.

Since handwriting – like all movements – is the result of motor commands
acting upon a biomechanical system, the simplest question that can be asked
is the effect of changing some physical parameters of this system. We are
aware of no specific study of the modifications that may result in handwriting
from changes in the mass of the system. However, Fitts, as well as Schmidt
and his coworkers, studying comparably fast and accurate movements,
concluded that relatively large changes of the mass can be adequately
compensated for by correlative changes in motor commands. Experiments
on typing soon to be described also lead to the same conclusion. These
results contrast with the effects of changing artificially the frictional forces
(Denier van der Gon and Thuring, 1965), which results into appreciable
reduction of the movement size (movement time is instead unaffected). In
the face of these somewhat contradictory findings, it is difficult to accept the
occasional claim (cf. Wing, 1978), that such experiments can prove or
exclude the involvement of sensory feed-back in the control of handwriting.

Constraints of a more complex and abstract nature arise when the format
of the movement is externally imposed. Freeman (1914) found that if the
size of the letters is constrained by two parallel lines (as in the early years of
school practice) the shape is unaffected, but the tempo is appreciably
slowered. Barnard and Wright (1976) reported a similar effect when people
are forced to write in spaced character format, using block capitals. Wing
(1979) contrasted different ways of marking the character format. A most
extreme form of constraint has been recently considered (Viviani and
Terzuolo, 1982). Subjects were asked to copy scribbles previously drawn
extemporaneously. The execution time under these conditions, as expected,
is greatly increased (10-fold increases are typical). However, according to
the time-honoured distinction between free movements and movements
under strict visuo-motor guidance (Pew, 1974; Denier van der Gon and
Wieneke, 1969; Van der Tweel, 1969; Paillard, 1980) one would also have
expected a profound change in the dynamic structure of the movement.
Instead we found that the Isogony Principle is still valid and that the motion
is segmented in exactly the same units as in free drawing (Fig. 8). Furthermore, it can be shown (Viviani and Terzuolo, 1982) that the principle is valid
even in the extreme case in which a form is drawn using a template. The
segmentation of the movement is again the same as the one observed when

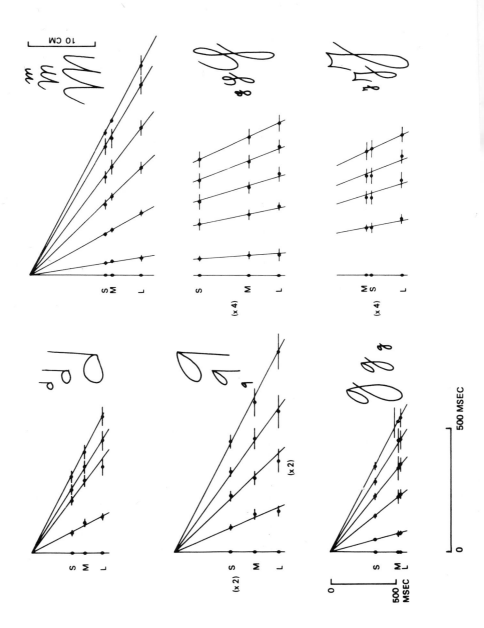

the same form is drawn freely, despite the speed difference in the two cases. This proves that the principle cannot be the consequence of purely mechanical factors and must therefore pertain to the logic of the central control processes *per se*.

B. Typing

1. *Target invariance*

The basic event in typing is the movement leading each finger to its target key. However, the picture which emerges during continuous operation is vastly more complex than a purely serial succession of such basic events. In fact – as in speech, where the articulatory movements required for a sequence of phonemes overlap in time (Perkell, 1969) – in professional typing a considerable amount of overlap does occur between successive basic events. Generally, each finger starts its aiming movement well before the preceding letter has been typed (Fig. 9(A)). Thus, because of the obvious biomechanical constraints, the trajectory of a finger cannot be specified independently of what other fingers are, or will be doing. Rumelhart and Norman (1982) have recently presented a formal model for this complex interaction. Fortunately, a characteristic property of these complex movements simplifies considerably their description. The analysis of the finger movements with a high-speed camera (Gentner, Grudin and Conway, 1980) or with chronometric measurements (Jordan, 1981) demonstrates in fact that, despite the "coarticulatory" effects mentioned above, the spatial and temporal goals to be achieved by each finger are specified much more rigidly than the necessary intermediate steps (Fig. 9(B)). Quite remarkably, the relative ordering of the times to target bears little relation to the relative ordering of the initiation times. This property of "Target Invariance" (cf. Bernstein, 1967), common to virtually all coordinated actions (Paillard, 1946), enables the amount of relevant information for describing the temporal aspects of the motor sequences to be drastically reduced. Since the spatial aspects are uniquely specified by the text, via the keyboard design, we can in fact assume that the intended motor sequence is satisfactorily described by the actual temporal sequence of keypressings.*

* Of course, this is an idealization because absolute target invariance is never achieved.

FIG. 7. Space–time invariance in handwriting. Data from two subjects (left and right column). Each diagram compares the results for three greatly different sizes of the same letter (shown along side). The horizontal rows of dots represent the timing pattern established on the basis of a proper choice of feature in the time course of the tangential velocity (see Fig. 6). Horizontal bars encompass ± 1 standard deviation. The patterns were scaled vertically, and lines with a common origin were interpolated (as in Fig. 14(B)) to demonstrate the presence, also in this case, of homothetic behaviour in the time domain. Vertical scales have been adjusted to enhance the differences in total duration. Note that the variability of the time of occurrence of each feature increases far less than linearly with the rank order of the feature in the sequence (from Viviani and Terzuolo, 1980a).

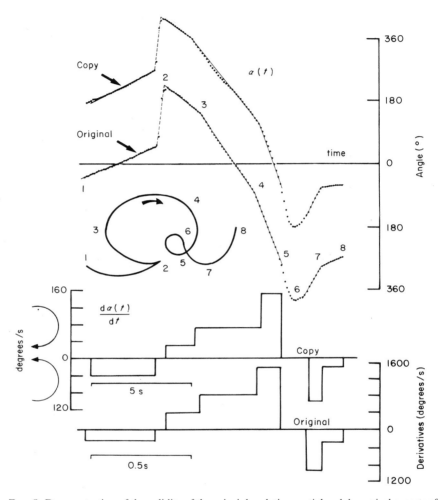

FIG. 8. Demonstration of the validity of the principle relating spatial and dynamical aspects of movement also in the case of visual guidance. The two upper plots demonstrate the similarity of the changes in $a(t)$, between an extemporaneously drawn scribble (curves labelled Original) and the same scribble copied by the same subject under careful visual guidance (curves labelled Copy). The two lower plots represent the slopes of the theoretical lines interpolating the phase angle curves $a(t)$. Notice that the execution time for the copy was about ten times longer than for the original. The time scales for the two curves labelled Copy were compressed accordingly, to facilitate the comparison. The similarity between free and visually guided drawing extends even to the short time interval (from points 5 to 7) when the phase angle $a(t)$ could not be reliably fit by straight lines (from Viviani and Terzuolo, 1982).

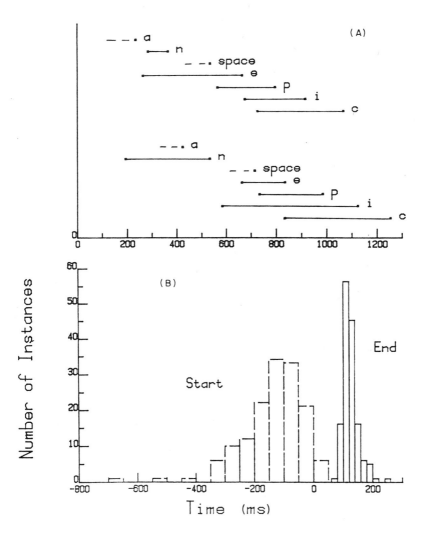

FIG. 9. (A) Relative timing of keystrokes for the sequence ". . . an epic . . ." on repeated typing of the same sentence. The left ends of the horizontal lines represent the initiation time of the keystrokes, and the right ends of the lines represent the time of the keypresses. Initiation times were not measured for the letter *a* and the *space* bar; this is indicated by the dashed lines to the left of the keypress times. Note that successive keypresses are more regularly timed than the corresponding initiations. In two cases, although the keys were pressed in the proper order, the keystrokes were initiated out of order: in the first sentence the *e* keystroke was initiated before that of *n* in the previous word; in the second sentence the keystrokes for the word *epic* were initiated in the order *i, e, p, c*. (B) The distribution of starting and ending times of keystrokes, measured relative to the time of the previous keypress. Most keystrokes overlap, with the second finger movement starting before the keypress at the end of the previous movement. The starting times of movements show much more variability than the ending times (from Gentner, Grudin and Conway, 1980).

This can readily and accurately be studied by measuring the time intervals between keypressings on the typewriter of a digital computer.

2. *Timing of the strokes*

A professional typist averages seven or eight keystrokes per second, which corresponds to intervals of 120–140 ms between successive letters. Choice reaction times for single letters are instead of the order of 300 ms (Quastler and Brabb, 1956; Hayes and Halpin, 1978). Therefore, actual typing cannot be construed as a sequence of individual perpectuo-motor events. The apparent regularity of the rhythm has suggested (Shaffer, 1978) that a professional typist may strive to pace the finger movements by some metronomic mechanism analogous to that supposedly used to produce repetitive tapping (Michon, 1967; Wing and Kristofferson, 1972, 1973). Shaffer (1978) reports that a slight negative correlation exists between successive intervals, which would agree with one possible interpretation of the pace-keeping hypothesis (Wing and Kristofferson, 1972; Wing, 1980). Gentner (1982) finds instead either no correlation (86% of the cases) or a significantly positive one. The discrepancy may be due to different amounts of rate modulation in the typing sequences. In any case, a quantitative analysis of the interstroke intervals shows the presence of profound and systematic rate modulations (Fig. 10) which – although not fatal to the pace-keeping hypothesis – deprive it of much of its explanatory appeal. Consequently, in what follows we will describe some of the biomechanical and control aspects of the task without committing ourselves to any theoretical framework.

Since the early work of Coover (1923) and Lahy (1924), it is known that the intervals between keypressings executed with fingers of different hands (alternations) are shorter on average than the intervals between keypressings involving fingers of the same hand. Figure 11 provides a more recent quantitative description of this effect from Terzuolo and Viviani (1980). The left and middle panels in this figure represent the interval distributions for all pairs of letters typed with the same hand (SH) and with different hands (DH), respectively. The right panels contrast the distributions for pairs typed with the same finger (SF) and different fingers (DF) of the same hand. Purely biomechanical factors are, most likely, responsible for setting both the average and the minimum interval when the same finger is used. In fact, the viscoelastic properties of the tissues certainly limit the rate at which any given finger can be raised and lowered. Biomechanical constraints are also present when different fingers of the same hand are involved, but these constraints seem too mild to account for the average interstroke intervals (see, however, Rumelhart and Norman, 1982). Instead, it is likely that the limiting factors in this case are the central and neuromuscular control mechanisms, as also suggested by reaction time studies (Sternberg *et al.*, 1978). Finally, the rate in pure alternations (as in typing the word HANDI-WORK) is obviously only limited by these control factors. The higher rate observed in this case suggests that motor commands dispatched to different hands can be made to overlap in time more than those dispatched to

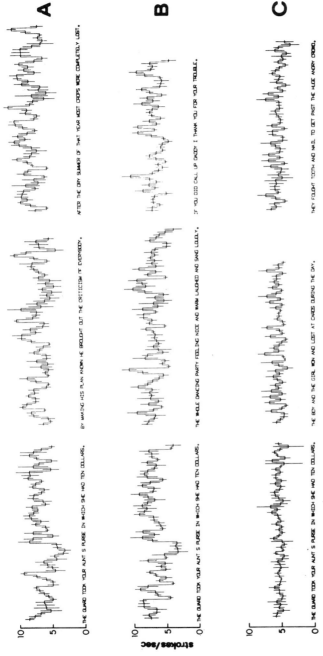

FIG. 10. Modulation of the instantaneous typing rate. The data shown are averages of the instantaneous typing rate (inverse of the interval between strokes) for three sentences and for each of three subjects. Averages and standard deviations (vertical bars) were calculated from at least twenty trials. Note the considerable differences in individual performances when typing the same text (leftmost column) and, for the same subject, when typing different texts (from Terzuolo and Viviani, 1980).

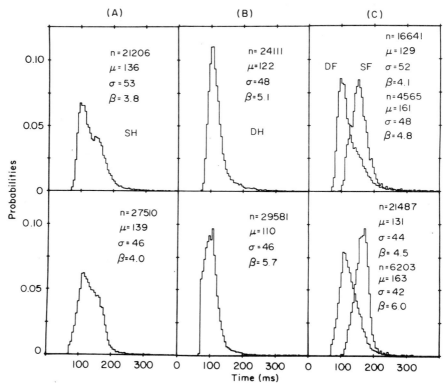

FIG. 11. Distribution of time intervals between strokes. The interval distribution for all pairs of consecutive letters are shown for two subjects. SH: pairs of letters typed with the same hand (left and right). DH: pairs of letters typed using both hands. In the last column, the rightmost distributions (SF) correspond to all pairs of letters typed with the same finger. The other distributions (DF) refer to pairs of letters typed with different fingers of the same hand. Time intervals from any letter to a space and from a space to any letter are not included. Values in the ordinate are probabilities; time scale in ms; n = sample size; μ, σ, and β indicate mean, standard deviation and Pearson's skew coefficient of the distributions, respectively (from Terzuolo and Viviani, 1980).

different fingers of the same hand. Thus, keyboard design affects in several ways the distribution of the time intervals between keypressings.

3. *Load compensation*

The absolute amount of force necessary to activate the keys has a rather modest effect on both the overall rate and the timing of the sequences. Most expert typists using today's electric typewriters average 65 to 75 words per minute, a rate which was well within human possibilities already at the time of the mechanical typewriters.* In fact, the limiting factor with the old

---

* A well-known world champion in the Thirties could type more than 100 words a minute.

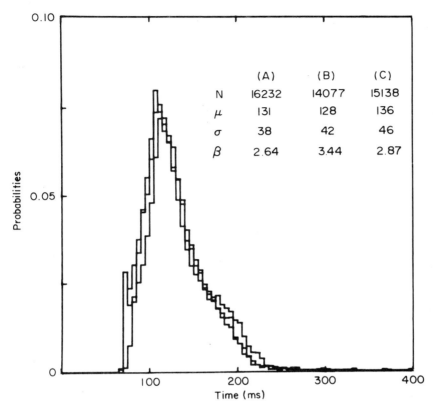

	(A)	(B)	(C)
N	16232	14077	15138
μ	131	128	136
σ	38	42	46
β	2.64	3.44	2.87

FIG. 12. Compensation for load changes. The figure compares the time interval distribution for normal typing with analogous distributions obtained (in the same subject) when the mass of the fingers is increased to two and three times the normal value. The three distributions are indistinguishable. The parameter of the distribution for the three cases are given in the inset: (A) normal; (B) doubled mass; (C) tripled mass (from Terzuolo and Viviani, 1980).

machines was mostly the necessity of preventing the bars from getting tangled up. Thus, striking force seems to be a free parameter of the motor plan that can be regulated independently of the temporal organization. The extent to which force commands can be modulated for compensatory purposes has been investigated by altering experimentally the mass of the fingers (Terzuolo and Viviani, 1980). Quite remarkably, the interstroke interval distributions are unaffected when the mass of all fingers is increased progressively up to three times the normal value (Fig. 12). Moreover, the structure of the typing sequence, which is characteristic of the sentence and the typist (see Fig. 10 and later), is also unchanged. The compensatory properties of the motor control system are actually even more impressive. Highly asymmetric modifications of the mass such as when only the fingers of one hand are loaded, result in relatively modest rate changes and again do not modify the structure of the sequences. Only when the mass of just one finger is increased to four times its normal value, did we observe a change in the timing structure; this change, however, remains localized.

4. *Role of sensory inputs*

While the temporal structure of a typing sequence is internally specified (see later), the implementation of the movement is normally accompanied by an array of exteroceptive and proprioceptive sensory afferences (cf. Stelmach, 1978). Their possible role was investigated in a series of experiments in which some of these afferences were selectively suppressed (Terzuolo and Viviani, 1980). In these experiments the right hand was allowed to operate as usual, while the operating conditions of the left hand were modified in various ways. Touch and pressure exteroceptive information was eliminated by asking the operator to perform the usual finger movements with the hand hovering just above but not touching the keys. All the subjects readily adjusted to this rather unusual condition which, they claimed, was not disrupting the normal exercise of the skill. In fact, in the case of words which necessitate the use of both hands, suppression of the touch and pressure exteroceptive information from the left fingers produced a profound modification of the temporal sequence: even those intervals typed with the right hand were affected. If the proprioceptive information from the joint and muscle receptors are also eliminated, by intentionally suppressing the movement of the left fingers, some further slight disruption occurs which, however, is difficult to quantify. Thus, normal movement is mostly contingent upon the presence of touch and pressure information. The conclusion is further supported by the observation that if one systematically blocks all the keys acted upon by the left hand the performance is altogether normal. Earlier data on the role of sensory inputs were reviewed by Alden, Daniels and Kanarick (1972).

III. Linguistic Factors in Typing

A. Words Are the Basic Units of Motor Action

1. *Single transition probabilities*

The most elementary feature of a typing sequence is the interval between two successive strokes. This interval is not constant, and we have shown in a preceding section that part of the variability is implicit in the fact that the fingers are used according to a scheme which, in professional typing, is uniquely defined with respect to the keyboard. As originally shown by Lahy (1924), another systematic component of the variability depends on the relative frequency of digrams (ordered pairs of letters) in the language. More specifically, recent experiments (Terzuolo and Viviani, 1980) have shown (Fig. 13(A)) that the frequency-dependent component of the

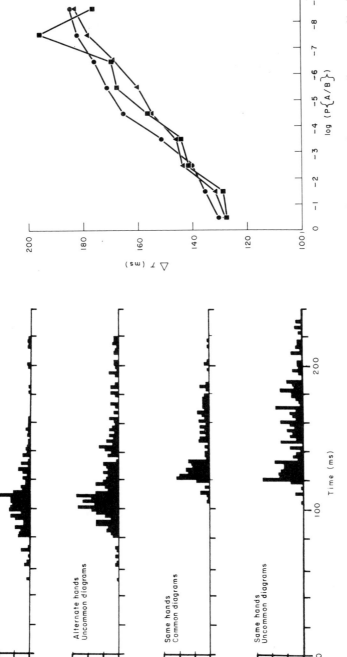

(B)

(A)

FIG. 13. Relative frequency of digrams and typing rate. (A) Distribution histograms of transition times for common and uncommon digrams typed by the same hand or with both hands. Over and above the strong alternation effect (cf. Fig. 11), the results indicate that the transition times for uncommon digrams are more scattered and longer than those for common digrams (from Fox and Stansfield, 1964). (B) A more specific analysis of the frequency effect. The data points represent the average transition times for all digrams contained in a prose text, as a function of the conditional transition probabilities. Each symbol identifies a subject. The abscissa is scaled logarithmically and inverted to provide a measure of information. The data for all digrams whose frequency falls between two successive values of the abscissa were pooled together, and the data point was arbitrarily placed at the mid-point between the extreme values of the mean. Note that the sample size decreases from the most frequent to the least frequent class (from Terzuolo and Viviani, 1980).

TABLE I

Two-letter transitions are context dependent[†]

Digram	$P(a/b)$	Word	T (ms)
AN	0.212	Thank	146.7 (10.94)
		Ran	94.1 (4.17)
HE	0.519	Pushed	95.4 (6.67)
		He	160.1 (52.71)
DI	0.165	Disgust	91.7 (11.77)
		Addition	188.6 (30.07)
TE	0.113	Ten	95.2 (5.11)
		Matter	153.8 (12.87)
RI	0.093	Bring	87.1 (4.37)
		Criticism	156.9 (24.44)
IS	0.115	Discussed	108.5 (12.39)
		Criticism	190.5 (16.37)

[†]A few examples in one subject of the general finding that the typing time for any given digram depends on the word in which it is embedded. The averages and the standard deviations (in parentheses) are illustrative of the maximum differences normally observed. Notice that the examples shown have rather high conditional transition probabilities $P(a/b)$ (calculated from Mayzner and Tresselt, 1965) (modified from Terzuolo and Viviani, 1980).

interval between letters is a linear function of the amount of information of the digram (minus the logarithm of the conditional probability: see Mayzner and Tresselt, 1965). The frequency effect applies to all combinations of fingers and cannot be explained by the fact that most frequent digrams are typed by two hands (Grudin and LaRochelle, 1982). This result, however, must be qualified in two ways. First, the frequency effect is only present when the digram is embedded in real words or pronounceable pseudowords. Indeed we will show later that typing sequences for unpronounceable pseudowords are dramatically different from normal sequences. Secondly, averaging conceals the fact that some very uncommon digrams are nevertheless typed very fast (see Fig. 13(A) taken from Fox and Stansfield, 1964).

Another systematic effect on the interval between keypressings is the rank position order of the digram within the letter sequence. In the case of sequences of digrams that actually occur in English (Sternberg et al., 1978), of words, and of unpronounceable pseudowords (Ostry, 1980), it is found that the typing rate decelerates toward the middle of the sequence and then increases again toward to the end.

TABLE II.

Examples from one subject of trigrams whose time structure depends on the word in which they are included†

	R	T(ms)
ING	0.81–1.24	194–225
TEN	0.81–1.41	209–297
END	0.84–1.44	214–283
BRI	1.43–2	267–309
PRE	0.69–0.91	185–302
FOR	0.90–1.19	194–237
ESS	1.01–1.17	293–387
EVE	1.03–1.37	252–316
MON	1.10–1.45	242–357
GHT	0.93–1.39	207–243

† In column R is reported the range of variation (over a sample of words containing the trigram) of the ratio between the average of the second and the first interval in the trigram. Column T gives the range of variation for the average total duration of the trigrams. Values are calculated from averages based on 30 trials for each word. For all trigrams, the difference between the extreme values of the average total duration (column T) is significant at the 0.01 level or better. In many cases, however, the structure and duration of a trigram is very similar in different words (from Terzuolo and Viviani, 1980).

2. Higher units: the word pattern

Over and above the effects of keyboard design* and of digram frequency and position, the interval between two successive strokes varies significantly according to the word in which the pair of letters is embedded (Table I). Similar context-dependent effects are also observed for more complex features of the sequence, both in Morse code (Bryan and Harter, 1897) and typing (Book, 1908; Shaffer, 1978). Table II illustrates typical examples of such dependence in the case of successive pairs of intervals. The data now to be presented show that as far as the average timing is concerned, context effects do not cross word boundaries. As for the variability of digram duration, Gentner (1982) shows that context effects extend over three characters before and two after the digram, and may cross word boundaries.

The basic observation concerning the average timing is illustrated in Fig. 14. Panel (A) shows that the total duration of the motor sequence for a

* An extensive literature on keyboard design is available (cf. Kinkead, 1955; Klemmer, 1971; Alden, Daniels and Kanarick, 1972; Kroemer, 1972).

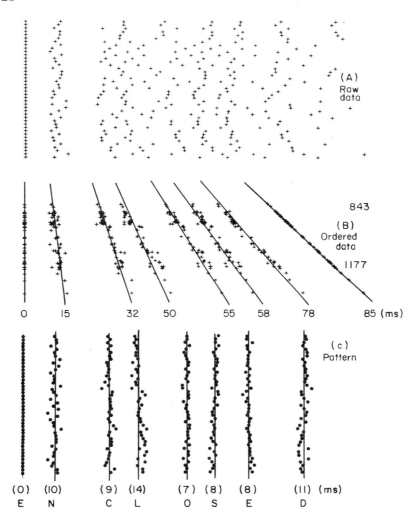

FIG. 14. Invariant structure of the motor sequence used to type a given word. In (A) are shown 42 instances of the motor sequence for the word ENCLOSED. Each symbol marks the time of occurrence of a keypressing. All sequences are aligned on the first letter (time zero). The data were obtained from one subject during a period of more than two years. The longest instances were obtained by adding a mass to the fingers. In (B), the same sequences presented in (A) are ranked according to their total duration and are spaced along the vertical axis by an amount equal to the difference between their durations. The durations of the shortest and the longest instances are given to the right (in ms). The lines that interpolate the homologous data points all have the same origin (not shown in the figure). Thus, the ratios of the time intervals between each pair of strokes are approximately constant in all instances. The standard deviations, across instances, of the times of occurrence of the corresponding event are indicated (in ms) below the data points. The dot symbols in (C) describe the pattern of the word. Each instance was

given word may vary considerably from trial to trial, as a consequence of both endogenous and contextual factors (see later). However, the ratios between all pairs of time intervals remain constant and independent from the total duration of the sequence. This is demonstrated by the fact that the best fit lines interpolating the times of occurrence of the same letter in each sequence have a common origin (Fig. 14(B)). Thus, as in the case of handwriting, the temporal structure of the sequence is invariant over large changes in typing rate (homothetic behaviour in the time domain) and can be extracted by linearly scaling to an arbitrary duration all instances of sequences for a given word (Fig. 14(C)). The structure which emerges is strikingly stable, as demonstrated by the residual standard deviations across trials of the time of occurrence of each stroke (Fig. 15). Even more important, however, is the fact that to almost every word corresponds a unique, characteristic sequence structure which is independent of the context. In fact, it makes no difference whether the word is part of a meaningful sentence or of a string of unrelated words.* Moreover, Grudin (1982) has presented evidence that the timing pattern found in words with transposition errors is close to that found in the same words typed correctly. Although some similarities between typists are present, each typist has his own exquisitely personal way of typing a given word.

These findings, as well as other general considerations, have suggested (Terzuolo and Viviani, 1979) that the word-specific invariant structure of the typing sequences exhibit the qualifying attributes of motor patterns (cf. Bernstein, 1967). Each instance of sequence is a unit of motor action which results from the coordination of subordinate units, made possible through learning and practice. Therefore, despite its uniqueness for any given individual, the word pattern reflects to some extent the general statistical properties of its constituents (digrams, trigrams, etc.). A specific mechanism whereby the properties of constituent subunits are reflected in the overall organization of the pattern will be illustrated in a subsequent paragraph. More generally, however, we observe that the low-level motor habits of any given individual, which influence the timing of small groups, can easily be

---

* Notice that also the average typing rate is the same for connected meaningful texts and lists of unrelated words (Shaffer and Hardwick, 1968).

---

homothetically transformed either by increasing or decreasing its actual duration in such a way that: (a) the average across all instances of the time of occurrence of each event in the sequence is the same before and after the transformation; (b) the variance of the time of occurrence across all instances and for each event of the sequence is the least. This procedure eliminates that part of the variability of the times of occurrence of each stroke which is due to differences in total duration.

For convenience, the time scale in (C) is the same as in (A) and (B). The pattern is, however, independent of absolute time. The values in parentheses below the dots represent the standard deviations (in ms) of the time of occurrence of the events in the pattern. A comparison with the analogous values in (B) shows that most of the variability in the typing sequences is due to differences in total sequence duration (from Terzuolo and Viviani, 1980).

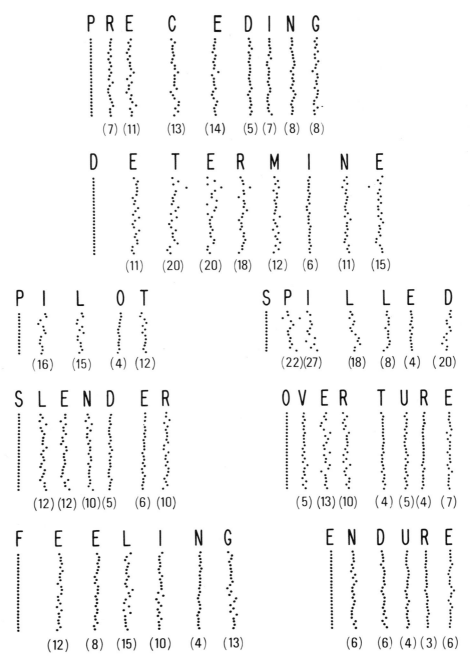

FIG. 15. Examples of patterns in three professional typists as in Fig. 14(C). The numbers below each letter indicate the standard deviation (in ms) across instances of the times of occurrence of the strokes (from Terzuolo and Viviani, 1980).

recognized in most word patterns containing these groups. Conversely, the significant context-sensitive differences observed in digrams and trigram (see Table I and II) are obviously attributable to the specificity of the pattern.

3. *The establishment of patterns*

For each real word there is a corresponding motor pattern. However, normally words are always preceded and followed by spaces, and there are reasons to believe that spaces cannot be treated like the other characters. In fact, the distributions of the time intervals which both precede and follow the typing of the space are quite different from the distributions of all other pairs, possibly because the space bar is the only key pressed by a rotatory movement of the thumb. Moreover, manipulation of the spaces affects both the average typing rate and the perceptual grouping of the input-string (Thomas and Jones, 1970; Pollatsek and Rayner, 1982). In any event, spaces certainly induce a segmentation of the motor output. Therefore, the first question to be asked is whether any sequence of letters encased between spaces is *ipso facto* translated into a patterned motor sequence. Experiments with random texts show that this is not the case. Consider a text obtained from a set of meaningful sentences by exchanging at random the letters among words while leaving the spaces as in the original. The result is a set of meaningless and often unpronounceable pseudowords with the same word-length and letter-frequency distributions of English. By analysing the typing of such texts it is immediately obvious that the trial-to-trial variability of the sequences is so high that no pattern can be detected. Thus, "patternability" seems an exclusive property of real words. The impossibility of organizing letter sequences into patterns has a clearly adverse effect on the perform-ance, and in particular on the typing rate. In the extreme condition of unspaced random sequences of consonants, Genest (1956) found that the rate falls to one third of the normal value. However, the performance is slightly better if vowels and spaces are introduced (Hershman and Hillix, 1965; Thomas and Jones, 1970). Furthermore, first-order approximation to the letter distribution of English are typed faster than completely random (zero-order approximation) pseudo-words (Shaffer and Hardwick, 1968) (but still much slower than normal texts). Typing rate is not the only parameter affected. Indeed, the digram interval distribution for normal and random texts are markedly different in both variance and skew, even when considering single letter pairs (see Fig. 16). In particular, the large skew of the distributions for the random texts is suggestive of a "searching process" whereby each finger movement would be elicited by the corresponding letter (cf. Shaffer, 1976). This contrasts with the seemingly global nature of the motor processes in the case of real words, where sequences of letters are typed with coordinated, arpeggio-like sequences of finger movements, as in piano playing (Shaffer, 1981). In this context, one may note that, already at the perceptual level, real words appear to be processed globally (Massaro, 1975; Massaro and Klitzke, 1977), whereas random strings of letters require

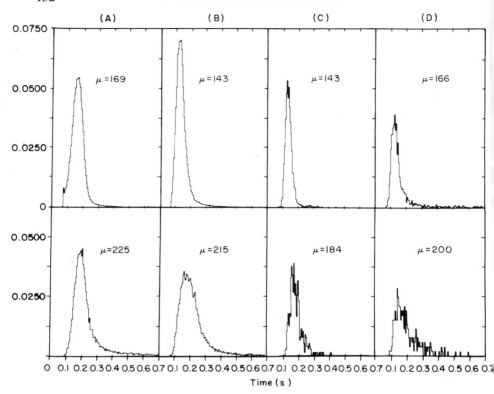

FIG. 16. Distribution of time intervals between strokes as a function of the nature of the text. (A) and (B): results in two subjects with a normal prose text (upper panels) and a random text (lower panels). The interval values for all digrams are pooled together. Notice the large differences in mean, variance and skew of the transition interval distributions (modified from Viviani and Terzuolo, 1980 b). (C) and (D) show the time interval distributions for two specific digrams as typed by one subject. The upper and lower panels correspond again to normal prose and random texts, respectively. These results demonstrate that the differences in the overall distributions ((A) and (B)) are not due to the pooling of data from different digrams, but are instead a specific consequence of the nature of the text (modified from Terzuolo and Viviani, 1982).

an independent processing of each component (Eichelman, 1970). Thus, the grouping principles in both the perceptual and motor representations seem to share some common aspects. In this context, it should also be mentioned that the performance of a motor sequence is much easier if the representation of the sequence obeys some principles of organization (Geoffroy and Norman, 1982).

To interpret the results obtained with random texts we must consider that pseudowords differ from real ones on at least three counts: the distribution of the transition probabilities, the lack of meaning (no lexical entry corresponds to the letter sequence), and the degree of pronounceability. Each of these aspects may be critical, or at least pertinent, for the establishment of a motor pattern, but the available evidence cannot yet resolve clearly among alternative hypotheses. However, several observations suggest that pronounceability may be a sufficient condition for assembling the individual motor acts. Genest (1956) found that CVC syllables are typed 1.36 times faster than unpronounceable CCC triples and, in general, pronounceable pseudowords yield faster rates (Thomas and Jones, 1970; Shaffer and Hardwick, 1968). This is in keeping with the fact that, whenever a pronounceable string of three or more letters is encountered in a random text, the typing rate suddenly increases and the intertrial variability decreases, so that an almost normal, patterned behaviour emerges. The significance of the letter sequence seems instead less critical to the establishement of a pattern. Although common words are typed faster than rare or abstruse ones (Genest, 1956), patterns can be observed even for some rare words that are easily pronounceable, but for which it is unlikely that a lexical entry has been established.

To conclude, we would like to remark that both spoken and written production of language share an intriguing property that we might call "Availability". Just as learning and practice in a language permit reading aloud, with normal tempo and intonation, a word that has never been pronounced before, so learning and practice in typing permits one to assemble and implement almost instantaneously a (pronounceable) word that has never been typed before. While it is reasonable to suppose that a permanently stored motor pattern exists for some of the more frequently occuring words, it seems very unlikely that the typist's skill results from the accumulation of a enormously large motor lexicon. We rather view this skill as the possibility of translating in real time the perceptual representation of a word into an abstract and invariant motor representation of the corresponding typing sequence.

4. *Pattern subunits*

An interesting feature of the motor organization at the word level is the presence of recognizable subunits within the pattern. Early chronometric studies of both Morse code (Bryan and Harter, 1897, 1899) and typing (Book, 1908) suggested that, in the course of learning, phonological syllables represent the first stage of organization of the motor skill, after the letter-by-letter stage. Not surprisingly, traces of this elementary segmentation persist even after higher stages are attained, especially when some difficulty prevents the use of the more developed skills. The analysis of transposition errors in typing (Shaffer, 1975) also points to the existence of a syllabic level of organization. However, syllables are not well-defined units in spoken or written English, and evidence can be found of subunits which encompass more than one syllable. This is particularly obvious in long, composite words where the segmentation sometimes coincides with the constituent morphemes. The analysis of the digram variability performed by Gentner (1982) may be taken to suggest that the average size of the subunits should not exceed four characters. The principles of coordination of the subunits within a pattern are instead far from obvious. Some insight into the matter can however be gained with the technique illustrated in Fig. 17. On the ordinate are reported the cumulated average intervals for the actual word-sequence. On the abscissas are indicated the cumulated average intervals for the corresponding digrams, calculated from a large corpus of

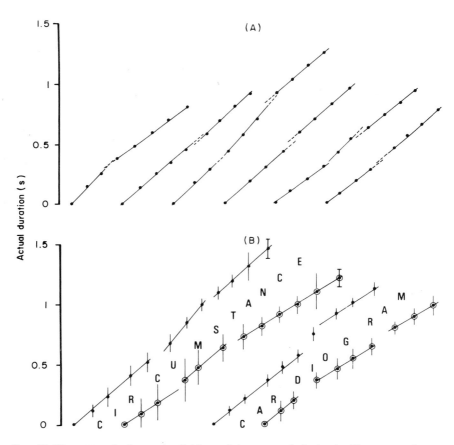

FIG. 17. The pattern for long polysyllabic words is composed of subunits. The pattern of some representative words is plotted against the sequence predicted by collating the average letter-to-letter transition times, using the same time scale for both vertical and horizontal axis. The words in (A) are from left to right: EARNINGS, EVERYBODY, CENSORSHIP, BRINGING, PRODUCTION, OVERTURE (two for each of three subjects). In (B) a comparison is provided for the same word in two subjects. Note that the subunits for long and uncommon words may be different in different subjects (from Terzuolo and Viviani, 1980).

words containing these digrams. In this representation any departure of the data points from a straight line indicates a specific feature of the pattern that cannot be attributed to differences in mean digram intervals. In the examples illustrated it can be seen that certain letter sequences within the words fall into distinct segments of lines, each of which can be taken to represent a subunit of the pattern. For some of the words only the slope of the segments changes, indicating that the corresponding letters are typed faster or slower than average. In other cases, successive segments run parallel, which implies the shortening or lengthening of just the interval connecting the segments.

This criterion of subunit identification certainly does not exhaust all the possibilities, and it may not even be the most significant one. Also, we cannot rule out the existence of other modalities of organization of the subunits, besides those illustrated in Fig. 17. We believe, however, that the very existence of these subunits is of theoretical importance for the comprehension of the control processes involved in typing.

5. Why a pattern?

It may be natural *a priori* to suppose that the aim of fluent typing is to press keys as regularly and evenly as possible, as though successive responses were paced by an internal metronomic beat (Shaffer, 1976). Since the evidence has proved quite damaging to this expectation, it is equally natural to speculate about the *raison d'être* of such highly structured and consistent syncopation of the motor output, which cannot be accounted for simply by mechanical factors. Historically, a leading theme in the quest for an interpretation has been the analogy with spoken language. As Bryan and Harter put it ". . . The telegrapher must acquire, besides letters, syllables, and words habits, an array of higher language habits, *associated with the combination of words in connected discourse* . . . the several [timing] values for a given character in different parts of the sentence . . . are not accidental variations from their average value . . . The operator *does not intend* to make the same character exactly alike in successive positions. *This internal representation corresponds to inflection in speech*" (our italics). Book (1908) strikes a very similar chord in his analysis of typing. Certainly the modulations in keying rhythm are reminiscent of the prosodic and inflectional profiles in speech. However, the analogy cannot be taken too literally because the suprasegmental features in speech have an expressive value and may be used to convey meaning, while this is unlikely in typing. It may be more fruitful, instead, to stress some principles of motor organization which are common to both typing and speaking (Kent and Minfie, 1977). Let us assume with Shaffer (1978) that syllables are coherent units of articulation, defined by an abstract timing pattern imposed on a group of invariant phoneme commands. The pattern is supposed to fix the time relationship among phonemes up to a linear transformation (Ohman, 1966, 1967), while absolute times are only specified at the execution stage to fix the tempo of speech and the rhythmic stress of the syllable. Then, a striking similarity appears between this view of speech motor patterns and the known properties of typing word-patterns. In particular, a common principle of organization emerges which involves two hierachical levels of control. While at the higher level the engram specifies the invariant definition of the unit of action, a flexible execution is achieved at the lower level by specifying the value of a free (dummy) timing parameter. Since it is unlikely that this flexibility of motor pattern is used in typing to convey expressive meaning, the question arises of its possible functional role. At the present stage only a tentative line of argument can be offered which goes as follows.

Some convincing evidence exists that in perception (e.g. Bever, Lackner and Kirk, 1969; Levy-Schoen and O'Regan, 1979), spontaneous production (e.g. Martin, 1970, Butterworth 1975; Butterworth and Goldman-Eisler 1977) and reproduction (e.g. Lindblom and Rapp, 1973; Klatt, 1975; Cooper, 1976) linguistic information is not processed at a uniform rate but rather by "chunks" of appropriate size. Since a considerable amount of looking-ahead occurs in typing (Butsch, 1932), we must also conclude that one or more input chunks are processed at some level while a past chunk is being translated into an actual motor sequence at some other level. The amount of temporal overlap between input and output can be estimated in several ways. Manipulation of preview (number of visible characters to the right of the one being typed) (Hershman and Hillix, 1965; Shaffer and Hardwick, 1970) demonstrates that more than six characters must be displayed to ensure a normal typing rate. Butsch (1932) remarked that the eye–finger span is about 1 second worth of typed characters, almost independently from the instantaneous rate. For skilled professionals this amounts to about eight characters. Finally, the analysis of typing errors (MacNeilage, 1964; Shaffer, 1976; Shaffer and Hardwick, 1969) shows that, although most transpositions occur within contiguous characters, the overlap can occasionally cross word boundaries as in the examples *fully of heavy* (full of heavy) and *forget me fnot* (forget me not) reported by Shaffer. Thus, even taking a conservative estimate, at least five or six characters are temporarily stored before execution. A good deal of the typist's skill must therefore consist of maintaining the correct serial order in this continuously updated queue.

According to one authoritative view (Shaffer, 1976) this task requires a memory buffer where changes in the input rate can be reabsorbed as fluctuations of the queue size, thus assuring a stable output rate. However, considering that the goal of a stable output rate is not pursued – or at least not attained – in professional typing, the hypothesis of a classical buffer operation is not too compelling. The available evidence is instead compatible with the "Cascade" mode of operation (McClelland, 1979), in which all the available storage is permanently occupied by successive transcoding stages of the input. The notion of pattern, with its characteristic homothetic behavior, fits rather nicely in this model. Indeed, since the implementation stage can regulate within large limits the total duration of a word sequence (cf. Fig. 14), it becomes possible to speed up the execution when the input processing is fast, and to stretch it out in time if the input processing is lagging behind. Thus, a non-uniform rate of input processing can be translated into a continuous (albeit modulated) output flow, without ever exceeding the available storage. At the same time, the pattern itself affords an efficient encoding of the word structure, which is independent of the input processing rate.

In conclusion, if one adopts the reasoning outlined above, the notion of pattern appears to be an optimal solution for a smooth input–output coordination in the presence of memory constraints.

B. Evidence of Higher Order Contextual Imprints in the Motor Prosody

So far we have considered the linguistic imprints on the motor sequences up to and including the word level. Indeed, a major aspect of this imprint is the very fact that words, which are a basic unit of description of the language, are at the same time the basic unit of motor organization in typing. In this final section we will consider how the internal representation of the sentence as a whole is reflected in the organization of the motor sequence.

The basic observation is that the typing sequence for a given typist and a given sentence is very reproducible – even over long time periods – and highly characteristic of the text being copied (Fig. 10). In other words, whole sentences exhibit the same structural stability already demonstrated at the word level. Consequently, the superordinate processes whereby the motor sequences corresponding to individual words are combined sequentially to form higher units of motor action are also remarkably stable. In the preceding section it was argued that these processes reflect the underlying modulation of the input processing rate and that they affect the only context-dependent parameter of the word patterns, namely their total duration. A quantitative description of this underlying modulation can be obtained by the following procedure.

(1) Generate a (scrambled) text in which all the words of the sentences to be studied are rearranged in a random order. We can suppose that a least organized input representation corresponds to this scrambled text, in which all contextual constraints have been eliminated.

(2) Calculate the average typing sequence for each word using both the original, and the scrambled text. Notice that the word's patterns are the same in both cases (see above). The total duration of each sequence – which is irrelevant *vis-à-vis* the pattern – may instead be influenced by the presence of contextual constraints.

(3) Match, for each word, the sequences of the scrambled text to those of the original text. The optimal letter-to-letter match (i.e. the match that minimizes the sum of the squares of the deviations between homologous events in the two sequences) is obtained by contracting or expanding homothetically the sequences for the scrambled text. One can then evaluate

differentially the word-to-word rate fluctuations which are specific to each sentence of the original text.

A set of 25 sentences was analysed with this procedure (Viviani and Terzuolo, 1980b). They were derived with minor modifications from those constructed by Bever, Lackner and Kirk (1969) to study the effects of syntax on perceived time relationships, and differed in the position of the main boundary between clauses. Figure 18 illustrates some typical results in three subjects. Each panel compares the word-to-word rate modulation profile for the same sentence in three professional typists. According to the adopted convention, values above the reference line indicate that the corresponding word was typed faster in the original text than in the reference condition (scrambled text). For some sentences the profile of word-to-word rate modulation was similar in different typists, as illustrated in (A), (B) and (C). For other sentences, however, individual differences were as large as in (D). Because the high stability of the whole-sentence sequences leaves no doubt that the rate modulation reflects the internal organization of the input, these results demonstrate that such organization is not uniquely determined by the text, but depends also on the typist's attitude and idosyncratic habits. An interesting question in this respect is the possible role of the syntactic structure of the sentences in determining the input processing rate. Indeed, syntactic relationships are the most obvious constraints among words in connected discourse and it was observed (Genest, 1956) that points of syntactical difficulty are typed slower than normal. In some cases we observed in fact a deceleration of the average typing rate corresponding to the main clause boundaries of the sentence. However, no consistent trend emerges when all the sentences are considered. This may be due to several factors. The phrases used–while semantically simple–are syntactically difficult, and cultural differences may therefore come into play. Also, copy-typing from a written text may not be ideally suited to pursue this line of investigation because the degree of understanding of its structure remains uncertain. This methodological difficulty could be overcome by using previously memorized sentences.

In any event, even if each sentence had a consistent rate profile in all subjects it would still be impossible to infer the internal representation on the syntactic constraints, given the absence of a specific model for their effects on the input processing rate. Therefore, we do not see that a definite answer can be given to the question raised above on the basis of currently available experimental evidence.

IV. Conclusions

The central problem in the study of vicarious means of language production such as handwriting and typing is the adaptation of the motor mechanisms subserving these skills to the system of principles and constraints specific to

(A)

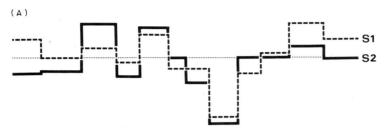

THEY FOUGHT TOOTH AND NAIL TO GET PAST THE HUGE ANGRY CROWD+

(B)

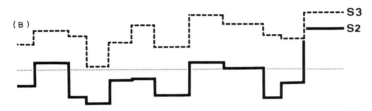

IN ORDER TO SEE OUT THE SMALL CHILD PUSHED UP THE WINDOW+

(C)

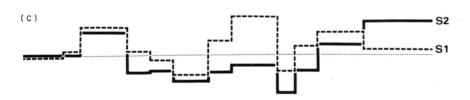

HIDING MY FRIENDS HAT THE SMALL BOY LAUGHED AT HIS STRANGE PREDICAMENT+

(D)

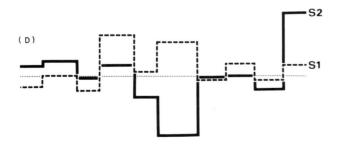

NOT QUITE ALL BRAND NEW CHAIRS WERE SOLD THAT DAY+

FIG. 18. Word-to-word rate modulations in connected prose depend on the text. Fully explained in the text (from Viviani and Terzuolo, 1980b).

language. Quite obviously, the facts and speculations presented in the preceding sections are but a very partial contribution to the analysis of this problem. Moreover, the experimental findings are not yet as closely knit as one might wish. Thus, rather than attempting a premature synthesis, we will conclude by emphasizing just one theoretical issue already hinted at in discussing the functional significance of typing engrams.

The issue in question is that of the specific properties that the motor mechanisms should possess in order to convey linguistic information as effectively as they do. Accuracy and speed are obviously necessary for writing and typing; yet they are not distinctive of these skills, for many other finger movements are just as accurate and fast. Likewise, resolution in both space and time domains is as good in typing and writing as in several other manual skills. Finally, the phenomenon of Motor Equivalence, so strikingly present in handwriting, is also present in virtually all voluntary movements and possibly is the most general property of motor control. It thus appears that, in order to isolate those specific aspects of the control logic which make writing movements so successfully adapted, we must hark back to language, and more specifically to its fundamentally discrete nature. To be sure, typing and writing movements are quantitatively continuous, like all other finger movements. There is, however, a difference in the nature of the information upon which motor planning is based. The schemata of action involved in, say, pointing, aiming or grasping rely upon kinesthetic, visual and endogenous information whose flow is, *prima facie*, continuous. In language-related movements instead, the information inflow is essentially discontinuous inasmuch as it reflects the discrete nature of the linguistic string. This fact poses some specific demands to the logic of the motor control.

First of all, we must admit that, in the course of learning, we develop a repertoire of stereotyped motor habits corresponding to the most elementary units of linguistic information. In handwriting, these elementary habits may be identified with the letters and, in typing, with the most frequently occurring digrams and trigrams. Secondly, provision must be made in the control system for assembling, in real time, long chains of low-level habits to form superordinate units of motor action which correspond to increasingly large chunks of information. Parsimony would further require that the result of the assembling be itself a stereotyped motor habit largely independent of the context, and, indeed, the existence of motor engrams supports this view. Thirdly and lastly, the structural rigidity of these high-order motor habits should be complemented with the capability of modulating the tempo of the movement. We argued in fact that the possibility of regulating the total duration of the motor sequence, without changing its structure, is instrumental in reconciling a non-uniform rate of input processing with a continuous output flow. The reality of such regulating mechanism was demonstrated in the case of both typing and handwriting.

We would like to conclude with a general remark. It should be clear that all the properties which, supposedly, are specific to writing movements also apply – *et pour cause* – to articulatory movements. This would tend to sharpen the conceptual distinction between language-related movements and all other forms of voluntary motricity. Such a distinction, however, rests upon an unspoken assumption that must be spelt out clearly. It is a fact that the information inflow and outflow which guide movements such as pointing, aiming or grasping is – as we record it – essentially continuous. If we make the further assumption that the *internal representation* of this information is also continuous, then Occam's razor would indeed prevent us from bestowing the planning of these movements with the specific properties discussed above. However, the information recorded externally may very well be as sharply different from its internal representation as the air pressure waves are different from the phonemes they carry. For all we know, it cannot be ruled out that this internal representation shares with language some of its distinctive features. If this were the case, the properties that – we surmised – are specific to language-related movements, would instead pervasively apply to all movements, and would emerge as soon as we had a knowledge of the internal representation comparable to our knowledge of language.

Acknowledgements

The preparation of this chapter was partly supported by ATP – INSERM 1650 – 5169 Research Grant and NIH Grant NS – 15018.

References

Alden, D. G., Daniels, R. W. and Kanarick, A. F. (1972). Keyboard design and operation: a review of the major issues. *Human Factors*, **14**, 275–293.

Asatryan, D. and Feldman, A. (1965). Functional tuning of the nervous system with control of movement or maintenance of a steady posture. 1. Mecanographic analysis of the work of the joint on execution of a postural task. *Biofizika*, **10**, 925–935.

Barnard, P. and Wright, P. (1976). The effects of spaced character formats on the production and legibility of handwritten names. *Ergonomics*, **19**, 81–92.

Bawden, H. H. (1900). A study in lapses. *Psychological Review Monograph Supplements*, **3**, 1–121.

Bernstein, N. (1967). "The Coordination and Regulation of Movements". Pergamon Press, New York.

Bever, T. G., Lackner L. R. and Kirk R. (1969). The underlying structures of sentences are the primary units of immediate speech processing. *Perception and Psychophysics*, **5**, 225–234.

Binet, A. and Courtier, J. (1893). Sur la vitesse des mouvements graphiques. *Revue Philosophique*, **35**, 664–671.

Bizzi, E., Dev, P., Morasso, P. and Polit, A. (1978). Effect of load disturbancies during centrally initiated movements. *Journal of Neurophysiology*, **41**, 542–556.

Book, W. F. (1908). "The Psychology of Skill". Montana Press, Missoula.

Braitenberg, V. (1965). A note on the control of voluntary movements. *In* "Cybernetics of Neural Processes". (E. R. Caianello, ed.) CNR, Rome.

Bryan, W. L. (1892). On the development of voluntary motor ability. *American Journal of Psychology*, **5**, 125–204.

Bryan, W. L. and Harter, N. (1897). Studies in the physiology and psychology of the telegraphic language. *Psychological Review*, **4**, 27–53.

Bryan, W. L. and Harter N. (1899). Studies on the telegraphic language; the acquisition of a hierarchy of habits. *Psychological Review*, **6**, 345–375.

Butsch, R. L. C. (1932). Eye movements and the eye–hand span in typewriting. *Journal of Educational Psychology*, **23**, 104–121.

Butterworth, B. (1975). Hesitation and semantic planning in speech. *Journal of Psycholinguistic Research*, **4**, 75–87.

Butterworth, B. and Goldman-Eisler, F. (1977). Recent studies in cognitive rhythm. *In* "Temporal Aspects of Speech", (A. W. Siegman and Feldsteins, eds). Erlbaum, New York.

Cooper, W. E. (1976). Syntactic control of timing in speech production: a study in complementary clauses. *Journal of Phonetics*, **4**, 151–171.

Coover, J. E. (1923). A method of teaching typewriting based on a psychological analysis of expert typing. *National Education Association Addresses and Proceedings*, **61**, 561–567.

Denier van der Gon, J. J. and Thuring, J.Ph. (1965). The guiding of human writing movements. *Kybernetik*, **2**, 145–148.

Denier van der Gon, J. J., Thuring, J.Ph. and Strackee, J. (1962). A handwriting simulator. *Physics in Medicine and Biology*, **6**, 3, 407–414.

Denier van der Gon, J. J., and Wieneke, G. H. (1969). The concept of feedback in motorics against that of preprogramming. *In* "Biocybernetics of the Central Nervous System", (L. D. Proctor, ed.) pp. 287–296. Little, Brown & Co., Boston.

Dvorak, A., Merrick, N. L., Dealy, W. L. and Ford G. C. (1936). "Typewriting Behavior". American Book Co., New York.

Eden, M. (1962). Handwriting and pattern recognition. *IRE Transactions on Information Theory*, **IT-8**, 160–166.

Eichelman, W. H. (1970). Familiarity effects in the simultaneous matching task. *Journal of Experimental Psychology*, **86**, 275–282.

Feldman, A. G. (1966a). Functional tuning of the nervous system with control of movement or maintenance of a steady posture–II. Controllable parameters of the muscles. *Biofizika*, **11**, 565–578.

Feldman, A. G. (1966b). Functional tuning of the nervous system with control of movement or maintenance of a steady posture–III. Execution by man of simplest motor tasks, *Biofizika*, **11**, 766–775.

Feldman, A. G. (1974a). Change of muscle length due to shift of the equilibrium point of the muscle-load system. *Biofizika*, **19**, 534–538.

Feldman, A. G. (1974b). Control of muscle length. *Biofizika*, **19**, 749–753.

Fitts, P. M. (1954). The information capacity of the human motor system in controlling the amplitude of the movement. *Journal of Experimental Psychology*, **47**, 381–391.

Fox, J. G. and Stansfield, R. G. (1964). Digram keying times for typists. *Ergonomics*, **7**, 317–320.

Freeman, F. N. (1914). Experimental analysis of the writing movement. *Psychological Review Monograph Supplement*, **17**, 1–46.

Genest, M. (1956). L'analyse temporelle du travail dactylographique. *Bulletin du Centre d'Etudes et Recherches Psychotechniques*, **5**, 183–191.

Gentner, D. R. (1982). Evidence against a central control model of timing in typing. *Journal of Experimental Psychology: HPP*, **8**, 793–810.

Gentner, D. R., Grudin, J. and Conway, E. (1980). Finger movements in transcription typing, *Occasional papers of the Center of Human Information Processing*, U.C. San Diego, **4**.

Geoffroy, A. and Norman, D. A. (1982). Ease of tapping fingers in a sequence depends on the mental encoding. *ONR Technical Report no. 8203*.

Grudin, J. T. (1982). Central control of timing in typing. *ONR Technical Report no. 8202*.

Grudin, J. T. and LaRochelle, S. (1982). Digraph frequency effects in skilled typing. *CHIP Technical Report no. 110*.

Hayes, V. and Halpin, G. (1978). Reaction time of the fingers with responses measured on a typewriter keyboard. *Perceptual and Motor Skills*, **47**, 863–867.

Hebb, D. O. (1949). "The Organization of Behavior". Wiley, New York.

Hershman, R. L. and Hillix, W. A. (1965). Data processing in typing. *Human Factors*, **7**, 483–492.

Hollerbach, J. M. (1980a). An oscillation theory of handwriting. *M.I.T. Artificial Intelligence Laboratory Internal Report*, AI-TR, 534.

Hollerbach, J. M. (1980b). An oscillation theory of handwriting. *Biological Cybernetics*, **39**, 139–156.

Jordan, M. I. (1981). The timing of endpoints in movement. *CHIP Technical Report no. 8104*.

Kent, R. D. and Minfie, F. D. (1977). Coarticulation in recent speech production models. *Journal of Phonetics*, **5**, 115–133.

Kinkead, R. (1955). Typing speed, key rates and optimal keyboard layouts. Proceedings of the 19th Annual Meeting of the Human Factors Society 159–161.

Klatt, D. H. (1975). Vowel lengthening is syntactically determined in a connected discourse. *Journal of Phonetics*, **3**, 129–140.

Klemmer, E. T. (1971). Keyboard entry. *Applied Ergonomics*, **2**, 2–6.

Kroemer, K. H. E. (1972). Human engineering the keyboard. *Human Factors*, **14**, 51–63.

Kugler, P. N., Scott Kelso, J. A. and Turvey, M. T. (1980). On the concept of coordinative structures as dissipative structures: I Theoretical lines of convergence. *In* "Tutorials in Motor Behavior", (G. E. Stelmach and J. Requin, eds) pp. 3–48. North-Holland, Amsterdam.

Lacquaniti, F., Terzuolo, C. and Viviani, P. (1983a). The law relating kinematic and figural aspects of drawing movements *Acta Psychologica*, in press.

Lacquaniti, F., Terzuolo, C. and Viviani, P. (1983b). Global metric properties and preparatory processes in drawing movements *In* "Preparatory States and Processes", (S. Kornblum and J. Requin, eds), in press.

Lahy, J. M. (1924). Motion study in typewriting. *Studies and Reports*, Series J. International Labour Office, Geneva, 1–63.

Lashley, K. S. (1951). The problem of serial order in behavior. *In* "Cerebral Mechanisms in Behavior", (L.A. Jeffress, L. A., ed.), pp. 112–36. Wiley, New York.

Levy-Schoen, A. and O'Regan, K. (1979). The control of eye movements in reading. *In* "Processing of Visible Language I", (P. A. Kolers, M. E. Wrolstad and H. Bouma, eds). Plenum, New York and London.

Lindblom, B. and Rapp, K. (1973). Some temporal regularities in spoken swedish. *Papers from the Institute of Linguistics*, University of Stockholm, Publication 21.

McClelland, J. L. (1979). On the time relations of mental processes. An examination of systems of processes in cascade. *Psychological Review*, **86**, 287–330.

MacNeilage, P. F. (1964). Typing errors as clues to serial ordering mechanisms in language behaviour. *Language and Speech*, 7, 144–159.

McDonald, J. S. (1966). Experimental studies of handwriting signals. *RLE Technical Report no. 443, MIT.*

Martin, J. G. (1970). On judging pauses in spontaneous speech. *Journal of Verbal Learning and Verbal Behaviour*, 9, 75–78.

Massaro, D. W. (1975). Primary and secondary recognition in reading. *In* "Understanding Language: An Informations Processing Analysis of Speech Perception, Reading and Psycholinguistics". (D. W. Massaro, ed.) Academic Press, New York and London.

Massaro, D. W. and Klitzke, D. (1977). Letters are functional in word identification. *Memory and Cognition*, 5, 292–298.

Maysner, M. S. and Tresselt, M. E. (1965). Tables of single-letters and digrams frequency counts for various word-length and letter-position combinations. *Psychonomic Monographs Supplement*, 1, 13–22.

Merton, P. A. (1972). How we control the contraction of our muscles. *Scientific American*, 226, 30–37.

Michel, F. (1971). Etude expérimentale de la vitesse du geste graphique. *Neuropsychologia*, 9, 1–13.

Michon, J. A. (1967). "Timing in Temporal Tracking". Soesterberg, The Netherlands: Institute for Perception RVO-TNO.

Ohman, S. E. G. (1966). Coarticulation in CVC utterances: Spectographic measurements. *Journal of the Acoustical Society of America*, 39, 151–168.

Ohman, S. E. G. (1967). Numerical model of coarticulation. *Journal of the Acoustical Society of America*, 41, 310–320.

Ostry, D. J. (1980). Execution-time movement control. *In* "Tutorials in Motor Behavior", (G. E. Stelmach and J. Requin, eds), North-Holland, Amsterdam.

Paillard, J. (1946). Quelques données psychophysiologiques rélatives au declanchement de la commande motrice. *L'Année Psychologique*, 28–47.

Paillard, J. (1980). The multichannelling of visual cues and the organization of a visually guided response. *In* "Tutorials in Motor Behavior", (G. E. Stelmach and J. Requin, eds) pp. 259–280. North-Holland, Amsterdam.

Perkell, K. (1969). "Physiology of Speech Production: Results and Implications of a Quantitative Cineradiographic Study". MIT Press, Cambridge, Massachusetts.

Pew, R. W. (1974). Human perceptual-motor performance. *In* "Human Information Processing: Tutorials in Performance and Cognition", (B. H. Kantowitz, ed.) Erlbaum, New York.

Pollatsek, A. and Rayner, K. (1982). Eye movement control in reading: the role of word boundaries. *Journal of Experimental Psychology: HPP*, 8, 817–833.

Qualster, H. and Brabb, B. (1956). Human performance in information transmission, Part, 5: The force of habit. Illinois University Control Systems Laboratory, Report R-70.

Rumelhart, D. E. and Norman, D. A. (1982). Simulating a skilled typist: a study of skilled cognitive-motor performance. *Cognitive Science*, 6, 1–36.

Schmidt, R. A., Zelaznik, H., Hawkins, B., Frank, J. S. and Quinn, J. T. (1979). Motor-output variability: A theory of the accuracy of rapid motor acts. *Psychological Review*, 1979 86, 415–451.

Scott Kelso, J. A., Holt, K. G., Kugler, P. N. and Turvey, M. T. (1980). On the concept of coordinative structures as dissipative structures: II Empirical lines of convergence. *In* "Tutorials in Motor Behavior", (G. E. Stelmach and J. Requin eds) pp. 49–70. North-Holland, Amsterdam.

Shaffer, L. H. (1975). Control processes in typing. *Quarterly Journal of Experimental Psychology*, **27**, 419–432.

Shaffer, L. H. (1976). Intention and performance. *Psychological Review*, **83**, 375–393.

Shaffer, L. H. (1978). Timing in the motor programming of typing. *Quarterly Journal of Experimental Psychology*, **30**, 333–345.

Shaffer, L. H. and Hardwick, J. (1968). Typing performance as a function of text. *Quarterly Journal of Experimental Psychology*, **20**, 360–369.

Shaffer, L. H. and Hardwick, J. (1969). Errors and error detection in typing. *Quarterly Journal of Experimental Psychology*, **21**, 209–213.

Shaffer, L. H. & Hardwick, J. (1970). The basis of transcription skill. *Journal of Experimental Psychology*, **84**, 424–440.

Søvik, N. (1975). "Developmental Cybernetics of Handwriting and Graphic Behavior". Oslo, Universitetsforlaget.

Stark, L. (1968). "Neurological Control Systems, Studies in Bioengineering". Plenum, New York.

Stelmach, G. E. (1978). "Information Processing in Motor Control and Learning". Academic Press, New York and London.

Sternberg, S., Monsell, S., Knoll, R. L. and Wright, C. E. (1978). The latency and duration of rapid movement sequences: comparison of speech and typewriting. *In* "Information Processing in Motor Control and Learning", (G. E. Stelmach, ed.) Academic Press, New York and London.

Stetson, R. H. and McDill, J. A. (1923). Mechanism of the different types of movement. *Psychological Monograph*, **32**, 18–40.

Terzuolo, C. A. and Viviani, P. (1979). The central representation of learned motor patterns. *In* "Posture and Movement" (R. Talbot and D. R. Humprey, ed.). Raven Press, New York.

Terzuolo, C. A. and Viviani, P. (1980). Determinants and characteristics of motor patterns used for typing. *Neurosciences*, **5**, 1085–1103.

Teulings, J. L. H. M. and Thomassen, A. J. W. M. (1979). Computer-aided analysis of handwriting movements. *Katholieke Universiteit Nijmegen Internal Report*, 79FU16.

Thomas, E. A. C. and Jones, R. G. (1970). A model for subjective grouping in typewriting. *Quarterly Journal of Experimental Psychology*, **22**, 353–367.

Turvey, M. T., Shaw, R. and Mace, W. (1978). Issues in a theory of action: Degrees of freedom, coordinative structures and coalitions. *In* "Attention and Performance VII", (J. Requin, ed.) Erlbaum, Hillsdale.

Van der Tweel, L. H. (1969). Designated discussion of Denier van der Gon & Wieneke's paper. *In* "Biocybernetics of the Central Nervous System", (L. D. Proctor, ed.) pp. 297–304. Little, Brown & Co, Boston.

Van Galen, G. P. (1980). Handwriting and drawing: a two stage model of complex motor behavior. *In* "Tutorials in Motor Behavior", (G. E. Stelmach and J. Requin eds) pp. 567–578. North-Holland, Amsterdam.

Viviani, P. and Terzuolo, C. A. (1980a). Space-time invariance in learned motor skills. *In* "Tutorials in Motor Behavior", (G. E. Stelmach and J. Requin, eds) pp. 525–533. North-Holland, Amsterdam.

Viviani, P. and Terzuolo, C. A. (1980b). Engrammes moteurs dans le traitement de l'information linguistique. *In* "Anticipation et Comportement", (J. Requin, ed.) pp. 455–471. CNRS Ed., Paris.

Viviani, P. and Terzuolo, C. (1982). Trajectory determines movement dynamics. *Neuroscience*, **7**, 431–437.

Viviani, P. and McCollum, G.(1983). The relation between linear extent and velocity in drawing movements. *Neuroscience*, in press.

Vredenbregt, J. and Koster, W. G. (1971). Analysis and synthesis of handwriting, *Philips Technical Review*, **32**, 73–78.

Welford, A. T. (1968). "Fundamentals of Skill". Methuen, London.

Wing, A. (1978). Responses timing in handwriting. *In* "Information Processing in Motor Control and Learning", (G. E. Stelmach, ed.) pp. 153–172. Academic Press, New York and London.

Wing, A. (1979). The slowing of handwritten responses made in spaced character format. *Ergonomics*, **22**, 465–468.

Wing, A. (1980). The long and short of timing in response sequences. *In* "Tutorials in Motor Behavior", (G. E. Stelmach and J. Requin, eds) North-Holland, Amsterdam.

Wing, A. and Baddeley, A. D. (1978). Spelling errors in handwriting: a corpus and a distributional analysis. *In* "Cognitive Processes in Spelling", (U. Frith, ed.) Academic Press, London and New York.

Wing, A. and Kristofferson, A. B. (1972). The timing of interresponse intervals. *Perception & Psychophysics*, **13**, 455–460.

Wing, A. and Krisofferson, A. B. (1973). Response delays and the timing of discrete motor responses. *Perception & Psychophysics*, **14**, 5–12.

Yarbus, A. L. (1967). "Eye Movements and Vision". Plenum, New York.

Yasuhara, M. (1975). Experimental studies of handwriting process. *Rep. Univ. Electro-Comm.* **25-2** (Sciences & Technics Sect.), 233–254.

Zangemeister, W. H., Lehman, S. and Stark, L. (1981a). Simulation of head movement trajectories: model and fit to main sequence. *Biological Cybernetics*, **41**, 19–32.

Zangemeister, W. H., Lehman, S. & Stark, L. (1981b). Sensitivity analysis and optimization for a head movement model. *Biological Cybernetics*, **41**, 33–45.

4

Lexical Slips of the Pen and Tongue: What they tell us about Language Production

W. H. N. Hotopf,　　　*London School of Economics and Political Science*

I. Introduction

The cybernetic approach, when it first developed in psychology, was mainly concerned with the application of information theory to different psychological processes; for example, the concept of feedback and its relation to purposive behaviour, the measuring of channel capacity and such questions as whether the human operator functioned more like a digital or an analogue computer. In the 1960s, however, there began to develop more interest in understanding performance from the point of view of its initiation. An influential book that publicized this approach was Miller, Galanter and Pribram's *Plans and the Structure of Behavior* (1960). This book stressed the concept of the "plan", which played the same part for the human operator as the program, with its associated notion of commands ordered within it, did for the computer. The authors' descriptions of plans, the examples they gave of them, were rather large and general except in the case of rules for generating sentences derived from Chomsky (1957) whose *Syntactic Structures* had appeared three years earlier and lent great confidence to their approach.

But where programs and their associated commands were described in the analysis of motor skills, including the skills of speaking, these were never presented as more than inferences from the correct skilled behaviour shown. Their status was initially like that of the atom or gene before scientists became acquainted through further research with the actualities of these entities. In recent years, however, the concept of a program has received some embodiment through the study, not so much of skilled behaviour *per se*, as of faults in skilled behaviour.

An early indication of the potentialities of these for throwing light on the commands, from which skilled behaviour issues, was given by one who

LANGUAGE PRODUCTION VOL. 2
ISBN 0-12-147502-6

already in 1917 had argued the case for motor programming. This was Lashley's classic paper, *The problem of serial order in behavior* (1951), where he showed how the slips he had made in typing might indicate how this approximately skilled behaviour had, below the level of consciousness, been planned. Lashley used the few slips he reported for purposes of illustration, but the hint was taken up first by MacNeilage (1964) in a systematic study of slips of the typewriter; by MacKay (1969, 1970), who used the two great classic collections of slips of the tongue and related errors by Meringer (Meringer and Mayer, 1895; Meringer, 1908) to throw light on the planning of speech, though perhaps with undue disregard of Meringer's own theoretical excursions; and by Fromkin whose 1971 paper represented a fulfilment of the sporadic demonstration over the years by linguists (e.g. Wells, 1951; Simonini, 1956; Hockett, 1967; Fry, 1969) of how slips of the tongue testified to the validity of linguistic concepts in the analysis of language. How this approach to the concept of planning has developed on the part of these and other linguists and psychologists is shown by two recent collections of papers on slips of the tongue, both edited by Fromkin (1973, 1980).

Another approach that promises to reveal the planning processes upon which language production depends is the study of another kind of error of a much more severe kind than slips of the tongue or pen, namely, the forms of language derangement of aphasics. Though such evidence is not the concern of this chapter, similarities between slips and aphasic symptoms have been noted at least from the time of Meringer, whose co-author in his first (1895) book, Mayer, intended to follow it up with a study of the errors of aphasics from this point of view, a study which, however, never materialized. But it is in the sphere of writing that this connection has been most made manifest. In fact it might be said that the first published attempts at detailed study of slips of the pen were, in their authors' views, studies of agraphia. Thus Lecours (1966) studying the diary of Lee Harvey Oswald inferred from his slips a case of developmental dysgraphia, Potter (1980) considered a similar possibility in the case of Spooner from his diaries, whilst Chedru and Geschwind (1972), showed that many cases previously attributed to pure agraphia were in fact the consequences of confusional disorders, to which writing was peculiarly vulnerable. However, properly to evaluate slips of this kind as pathological, it is necessary to have some conception of types of slip and their relative frequency that "normal" people produce and this has recently been done both for groups of subjects (Hotopf, 1968, 1980a; Nauclér, 1980; Wing and Baddeley, 1980) and for individual writers reporting on their own collected slips (Ellis, 1979; Aitchison and Todd, 1981). The errors of aphasic patients however contrast with slips committed by normals not only in severity but also in frequency. Therefore, whereas it is easy to measure the deficiencies of aphasics experimentally by designing tests in the light of theories constructed to account for their deficiencies, slips of the tongue, pen and typewriter are too rare for this approach to be fruitful. Instead, apart from one experimental line of attack by Baars, Motley and MacKay (1975; see also Motley, 1980; Baars, 1980), all the evidence concerning slips has come from observing slips committed in the course of daily activities. This is, however, in consonance with linguists' preference for studying language as used in normal settings. Viewing language as a highly complex system, it is not necessarily believed that frequency is an essential criterion of significance. Any mistake, even if only a rare one, shows the system at work and has to be accounted for; the exception proving (or testing) the rule. Though such an attitude has not found favour amongst psychologists, I believe it is worth exploring as a possibility in the study of language performance. What follows is an essay in applying this philosophy. It is based on some 20 years spare time collecting of slips, noting of errors of absent-mindedness or perception and self-observation of processes accompanying these events.

II. Summary with Elaborations of Previous Position

Slips of the pen have in general been treated as though they differed little from slips of the tongue. In an earlier report on slips of the pen (Hotopf, 1980a) hereafter referred to as SP, I showed however that though this was largely true as regards the types of slips that occurred, it was not the case when their relative frequency was taken into account. I will first briefly summarize my previous study (SP), though with some elaborations of points which for reasons of space could not be dealt with fully in it.

A. Description of the Samples and Types of Slip at Lexical Level

The strategy of my research was to collect a number of samples systematically so as to be able to determine the relative frequency of the different categories of slips. This yielded four samples of slips of the tongue and three of slips of the pen.† One of each was of my own slips. The speech sample I shall refer to as the Author's S-sample and the writing sample as the Author's 1st W-sample. The other three speech samples were the Daily Life S-sample, collected over a period of two years and including only slips personally observed by me, but not including my own slips; the Meringer S-sample, consisting of all the slips listed in his two books (Meringer and Mayer, 1895; and Meringer, 1908) but categorized according to my own classificatory scheme; and the Conference S-sample, which consisted of slips noted from tape-recordings of unscripted lectures given to students by eight speakers at a psychology conference. The other two writing samples were the Monograph W-sample which was of slips from the writing of a draft of part of a Ph.D. thesis in psychology; and the Group W-sample which was

---

† For details of these samples and how they were collected, Hotopf (1980a) should be consulted.

derived from examination scripts in a psychology examination (Examination W-sub-sample) or from the writing of an answer to a question on the use of force in punishment by psychology graduate students pressed to write fast under distraction conditions (Distraction W-sub-sample).

I have since then assembled three further systematic samples. Two of these are samples of my own slips, consisting of 392 slips of the typewriter (Author's T-sample) and 298 slips of the pen (Author's 2nd W-sample).

The third sample is derived from the forty scripts analysed by Wing and Baddeley (1980) for spelling mistakes, which they have kindly placed at my disposal (Wing and Baddeley W-sample). The Wing and Baddeley scripts were analysed independently by two judges for certain types of slips in order to increase the number of these where in my earlier collected samples they were rather small. In addition to these three systematically collected samples, I have added to my non-systematic collection certain additional slips which were of particular theoretical interest. In what follows, any statistics I may give will be based on the samples described in SP unless the contrary is indicated. Examples may be drawn both from the systematic and the unsystematic collections. Where these are typing slips, this will of course be indicated.

Most slips are either of single words or base forms or of individual phonemes or letters. Therefore, for the purposes of exposition, two levels† were distinguished – lexical, including phrases and bound morphemes, and phoneme/grapheme, which included syllables, phonetic features, parts of letters, punctuation marks and the like. The categories in which the different slips were classified should be regarded as hypotheses or options for hypotheses, since it was considered possible that they betrayed or might betray different causal agencies. Once the category was determined, however, as far as possible a mechanical procedure was devised to allocate a slip to a category, even though this sometimes went contrary to intuition. This procedure also meant that some slips received a dual and even, in a few cases, a triple classification. Though sometimes two factors may well have been combining to cause a slip, there were, as we shall see, cases where the relationship may have been fortuitous. It was hoped, however, that the signal-to-noise ratio in the data would be sufficiently large for meaningful correlates of the category in question to be determined (see Hotopf (1980b) for an illustration of this).

B. Categories of Lexical Slip

I shall now introduce very briefly a cast of the characters (categories of slips) that are relevant to this chapter. In the examples given below the target word is given in brackets immediately after the error word that constitutes the slip, and an asterisk indicates that the error was corrected as it was made.

† This classification should not be confused with a functional one whereby, for example at the lexical level, the accessing of word stems from the lexicon is considered a separate operation from morphological operations applied to them.

Anticipations

    (1) I do not see how the first* (second) paragraph follows from the first.

    (2) I am slowing (slowly) catching up . . .

Repetitions

    (3) Even to give to (the) response without gaining food.

    (4) After thirty years of using bothing* (both) approaches . . .

1–4 were all slips of the pen. These two categories occur with about equal frequency in speech and writing, relative to other categories of slips.

Transpositions

    (5)   . . . between an (a) conditioned stimulus and a (an) unconditioned response.

Though transpositions are not common amongst slips of the tongue, (5) was the only one that occurred in the three writing samples referred to in SP and it is a very odd one, the transposed items unusually widely separated. The Author's 2nd W-sample and the Wing and Baddeley W-sample had yielded three more transposition slips. All of these were of adjacent closed-class words such as "is it" (it is) and "the in" (in the). Of course an anticipation slip like (1) might have turned out to be a transposition slip had it not been immediately detected and thus corrected before proceeding further. Transposition slips were not multiply categorized. That is to say, if the transposed items, which substituted for one another, happened also to be related in one of the ways distinguished below, if, for example, the words mutually substituted were similar in sound or in meaning, they were only counted as cases of transposition.

One word omissions These were common amongst slips of the pen and rare amongst slips of the tongue. 90% of the former were closed-class words or auxiliaries.

Immediate repetitions of words These were non-existent amongst slips of the tongue but constituted about 6% of slips of the pen at the lexical level. 79% of these were closed-class words or auxiliaries.

Semantic group These are substitution slips where error and target word are similar in meaning. They constitute the largest group at the lexical level in two of my four systematically collected samples and the second largest in the other two. They are called Semantic group slips because they are either polar contrasts, error and target word being antonyms or standing in a converse relationship to one another, or are, to use Lyons' distinction, co-hyponyms of one another. The latter relationship ranges from tightly constricted groups like the names of days of the week and colour words to loosely constricted groups like food words or time words, as in

(6)   I bought it and put in chopped garlic* (chive)
(7)   When we meet the students next term* (week)

This category of slip, which is examined in more detail in Hotopf (1980b), though comparatively very common amongst slips of the tongue such as (6) and (7) is comparatively very rare amongst slips of the pen, as Aitchison and Todd (1981) have also found. Two other characteristics should be mentioned. The first of these is that error and target word tend to a signifi- cant degree to be of equal frequency and the second that grammatical morphemes, including null affixes in unmarked forms, are preserved in 99% of these slips. This, which is compatible with Garrett's (1975) distinction between syntactic frames with slots into which open-class words are inserted, suggest that the substitutions we have to deal with here are those of the base forms of words.

Within form class substitutions of closed-class words   These are substitutions of one closed-class word for another of the same form class, as the next two examples of slips of the tongue show,

(8)   . . . fling back my (your) aggression . . .
(9)   If the unions were to come with* (to) us.

The closed-class words concerned are mainly pronouns and prepositions, plus articles in the German sample. They formed between 3–5% of the different samples of slips of the tongue. Amongst slips of the pen only prepositions occurred and nearly all of these were cases of dual classification so their occurrence amongst slips of the pen may be fortuitous and not represent a genuine category. As slips of the tongue this category was similar to that of semantic group slips in preserving syntactic distinctions. Thus all pronoun slips, as well as those involving articles in German, preserved case.

Structural similarity   These slips, hereafter referred to as "structural", are ones where error and target are similar to one another visually and acousti- cally. Examples amongst slips of the pen are "surge" (search), "that" (than), "a number" (another), "could" (good). Structural slips of the pen also include *homophones* and *quasi-homophones*, which are pairs of words which in most dialects sound identical. Examples of these are "their" (there), "referents" (reference), "two" (to, too), "weight" (wait), "write" (right), "scene" (seen), "are" (our), and "sought" (sort).
  Structural slips are the second commonest slip both in speech and in writing. However their nature differs in the two production situations. Of 312 cases amongst slips of the tongue, 94.9% of target and error word pairs were open class words and 3.2% closed-class word pairs. Amongst 136 cases taken from all five systematically collected slips of the pen, 39.7% were open-class word and 56.6% closed-class word substitutions. In only 4.2% of the structural substitutions amongst slips of the tongue was the form class of

target and error different,† whilst amongst slips of the pen the proportion was as high as 57.3%. Closed-class words therefore figure much more prominently amongst structural slips in writing than in speech and so do changes of syntactic form class. This latter finding is not due solely to the greater proportion of closed-class words amongst these slips in writing, since whereas only 3% of open-class words differ in form class in speech, 27.8% of these differ in writing, the corresponding proportions amongst closed-class word being 40% and 81.8%.

As with semantic group errors, these slips were also examined for evidence of preservation of grammatical morphemes. Amongst English and German slips of the tongue these averaged 95% and, amongst slips of the pen, 92.7%. Once again, then, substitutions at the lexical level appear to be of base forms of words.

Blends These are slips which seem generally to arise from competition or indecision concerning two alternative formulations with the result that parts of both words or phrases are combined in a new form; for example, "spawking" from "speaking" and "talking". Though not common amongst slips of the tongue, they do not occur at all in any of my samples of slips of the pen, systematic or otherwise, nor do they occur in the Aitchison and Todd (1981) corpus of slips of the pen.

Stem Variants These are cases where the error word has the same stem as the target but a different morphological form. Examples are:

(10)   . . . the psychoanalysis (psychoanalyst) might . . . suggest to his patient . . .
(11)   . . . the high correlation between difference (different) intelligence tests . . .
(12)   Many experiments are still been (being) carried out . . .
(13)   e.g. it (its) specifity (specificity)
(14)   . . . Scientic (Scientific) knowledge his* (has) reach (reached) to (too) large a volume

The above examples, which were all slips of the pen, suggest that different factors may have been operating to produce slips of this category. For instance, (11) is a case of anticipation of a bound morpheme, and (12), (13) and (14), which also contain other categories of slip, may well be structural slips. Indeed in nearly all stem variants, error and target word are visually or acoustically similar to one another, but this type of slip, though rare amongst slips of the tongue, is so common amongst slips of the pen that it was thought worth classifying it separately. Once this decision had been made slips like

---

† Where a word belongs to a number of different form classes then, if one of these was the same as that of the other member of the pair, they were counted as the same form class. Thus the common structural slip of the pen interchanging "that" and "than" was always counted as same form class substitution.

(15)   . . . the beginning and end is* (are) retained

had of course also to be included. In the case of (13) (it specifity) and (14) (reach to), however, an additional factor of context appears to have been at work as though these were graphic transcriptions of elisions of one of two successive consonant phonemes at word or morpheme boundaries according to the principle of geminate reduction (Oshika *et al.*, 1975). If this interpretation is correct, (13) and (14) are slips at the grapheme as well as at the lexical level. If to these are added closely similar cases were the word-final consonant was closely similar to the following word-initial consonant as in

(16)   Little Albert was condition (conditioned) by J. B. Watson
(17)   . . . were also suppose (supposed) to effect (affect) the personality.

the proportion such slips form among stem variant slips of the pen is 11.7%.

The differences in relative frequency of the different categories of slips at the lexical level both in speech and in writing are set out in Table I opposite. It can be seen that, relative to one another, structural, anticipation and repetition slips were about equally frequent in speech and in writing; that transpositions, blends, semantic group slips and closed-class substitutions within the same form class were relatively more frequent in speech than in writing; and that the reverse was the case with stem variants, immediate repetitions, omissions of single words and, within the above categories, changes in form class.

Unfortunately, it was not possible to apply statistical tests to the data since the different types of slips were, except in the author's samples and the monograph W-sample, produced by a relatively large number of different individuals who were of course not the same as between the S- and W-samples. However, the differences between speech and writing were consistent over a number of different samples including S-samples differing in the language (German and English) and period (late 19th and mid 20th century) over which they were collected.

This information does not however tell us what is the absolute likelihood of different types of slip in speech and in writing. To calculate this we need to know their frequency in relation to the number of words produced. Fortunately, this information is available for the Conference S- and Group W-samples. Six speakers in the former and all writers in the latter sample produced approximately 47 350 and 35 200 words, respectively. Frequencies in relation to total output for the main categories of slips are shown in Table II. There were some slips with a dual classification in which case half a slip was allotted to the two categories in question.

It is evident from the table that the types of slips that were more frequent relatively to one another in writing than in speech, were also more frequent in terms of total output, and that semantic group slips, all of which were cases of dual categorization in the W-sample, were of roughly half the frequency in writing than in speech.

The major difference between Tables I and II lies in the absolute frequency of structural slips. These whether of open- or of closed-class words were

TABLE I

Percentages of different types of slip at the lexical level

Mode of Discourse	Speech				Writing		
	Author's	Daily life	Meringer	Conference	Author's 1st & 2nd	Group	Monograph
Sample Number of Slips in Sample	103	307	852	154	112	271	105
Category of Slip							
A. Equally frequent							
Structural	29.8	26.3	24.5	11.7	42.0	20.6	17.1
Anticipations†	3.8	6.8	11.0	17.5	16.1	9.6	11.4
Repetitions	8.6	13.6	8.9	28.8	9.8	12.1	16.2
B. More frequent in speech than writing							
Transpositions	3.8	4.5	9.6	2.0	0.9	0.4	0.0
Blends	1.0	1.9	11.8	5.2	0.0	0.0	0.0
Semantic group	34.6	27.9	15.3‡	13.1	2.7	3.3	0.9
Closed-class word substitutions within form class	3.8	3.2	4.6	2.6	0.9	2.2	2.9
C. More frequent in writing than speech							
Stem variants	1.0	2.9	3.9	6.5	4.5	22.9	25.7
Immediate repetitions	–	–	–	–	2.7	7.3	1.9
One word omissions	1.0	1.0	2.0	7.8	17.9	17.2	14.3
Changes of form class§	2.9	9.5	7.3	14.6	53.2	36.6	40.3
D. Other Classes	12.4	11.3	7.4	5.2	2.7	3.7	9.5

† One word omissions are excluded from this category.

‡ This proportion is probably an underestimate since Meringer was not fully aware of this category when collecting the first of his two collections (see Hotopf, 1980b).

§ These cut across category boundaries and do not therefore contribute to the above percentages.

substantially more frequent in writing than in speech. The difference may partly be due to the unusually low relative incidence of structural slips in the Conference sample as shown in Table I in comparison with all other samples whether of writing or of speech. However, the difference in incidence of structural slips in Table II is so great that it is doubtful whether they would, as regards open-class words, have been reduced to equality even if the incidence of these slips in the Conference sample had been the same as that in the other S-samples.

TABLE II

Relative percentages of different categories of lexical slips† per number of words spoken or written in the Conference S- and Group W-samples

Category of Slip	Sample Conference	Group
Structural‡ (closed-class words)	0.018	0.054
Structural‡ (open-class words)	0.009	0.058
Anticipation	0.036	0.050
Repetitions	0.061	0.064
Semantic group	0.028	0.013
Stem variants	0.019	0.146
Changes of form class	0.021	0.151

† Slips belonging to two categories were counted as half a slip in each cateogory.
‡ Homophone slips excluded.

It might be objected that comparing the main W-sample with only the Conference S-sample leads to an underestimation of the distributional differences between writing and speech. For all the categories save one (blends) in Table I, where there is a marked difference in incidence between writing and speech, the Conference S-sample is more similar than the other S-samples to the W-samples. But the reason for this is probably that out of all the S-samples the Conference is the one most comparable to the W-samples and particularly to the Group W-sample. Like most of the W-samples, the Group sample is based upon long monologues dealing with abstract questions in psychology, requiring complex thought processes. Its language should therefore be in a similar register along a number of dimensions to that of the Conference sample, in contrast to the conversation, including the making of requests, on concrete matters of daily life or the dialogue of committee meetings, examination and cross-examination in the law courts, television interviews, discussion in staff meetings and seminars and so on from which much of the heterogeneous material in the other S-samples derives. It is therefore probably no accident that the Conference sample was more similar than the other speech samples to the samples of writing, although as Tables I and II show there are still distributional differences between the two kinds of language production.

C. Basis of Distributional Differences between Slips in Speech and Writing

Two possible causes of the distributional differences in slips between speech and writing will be considered. These are differences in the type of language used in the two different language production situations and differences in the time taken in speech and in writing.

1. *Differences in the language used in speech and writing*
It is a widely held view that the language used in writing differs in certain respects from that used in speech, but so far as the author knows no systematic study of this at the level at which we are concerned has been carried out. Clearly, the kind of language used in speech will itself vary according to the subject matter, abstract or concrete, the speaker's familiarity with the ideas he is expressing, the relative formality or informality of the communication situation, the degree to which the communication is by intercourse or monologue and so on. Some idea of this can be obtained by comparing Fries's (1952) examples of telephone dialogue, Maclay and Osgood's (1959) examples of speakers' talking in seminars and Duncan and Fiske's (1977) transcription† of a discussion between psychotherapists concerning a patient.

But whatever the speech situation, save perhaps the most formal, speech is likely to show a greater freedom from the constraints of rules than is the case with writing. The following example is typical of many in the Conference S-sample, except perhaps that it is better formed than most.

(18)   I got the impression – not at the times (time), I was far too ingenuous thirty-five years ago but in retrospect – got the impression that the damage I did to the dogs in trying to automate conditioning, this was what I was trying to do, to introduce automatic methods of conditioning prematurely as it turned out – which upset the dogs very much indeed – that the damage I did to

---

† McNeill (1979) in criticizing Boomer and Laver (1968) and Fromkin (1971) for proposing the phonemic clause as the planning unit of speech and substituting his own much shorter unit, the syntagm, which he bases on Duncan and Fiske's transcripts, neglects the differences in modes of speech. Some of Fromkin's and certainly much of my Daily Life and Author's S-samples were based on speech more like Fries's telephone conversations. There is also of course a danger in identifying the planning unit with the words actually spoken. Speech may be broken off before the whole planning unit has been put into execution.

them was because their brains were acting as probability computers, that the the brain (brains) of these dogs were essentially probabilistic or statistical in in their attitude to stimuli, and that what I was presenting them with was a too tough a statistical problem. And the dogs, some of them, broke down and got into serious mental trouble and, which mimicked as you know the experimental neurosis, the type of breakdown we see in human beings – and it occurred to me some many years later . . .

(18) reveals the extempore quality of speech. If rules for scientific discourse were to be extracted similar to those proposed for storytelling (e.g. Rumelhart, 1975) then, as with storytelling and generative grammar, we would expect them to be exemplified far more in writing than in speech. But here there is a paradox. Slips of the pen at the lexical level are far more characterizable in terms of errors of syntax than slips of the tongue, as shown by the much greater proportion of changes of form class between target and error word, by the greater involvement of closed-class words in slips and by the greater proportion of changes in grammatical morphemes as shown by the differential frequency of stem variants. And when there is a departure from grammar in speech, this is not necessarily to be classified as a slip so much as a dereliction allowable in speech but not in writing. In (18) there are two instances of immediate repetitions of words ("the", "in"), but these are treated not as slips but as hesitations which serve the purpose of playing for time whilst deciding how to proceed or making a lexical choice (Maclay and Osgood, 1959; Beattie and Bradbury, 1979). Although similar to immediate repetition slips in writing in that, according to Maclay and Osgood, the proportion (80%) that are closed-class words is practically identical in both language production situations, there is no evidence that they serve any similar purpose in writing and, although permitted to himself by a speaker, they are not so by a writer.

There is one other respect in which the same forms are treated differently in the language of writing from the language of speech. Certain deviations in phonology are acceptable in speech but not in the orthography of the same words. Examples of this are (13) and (14) where in fluent speech according to the principle of geminate reduction one of two identical consonants at word boundaries is omitted. The conventions of writing do not however confer a corresponding licence. Therefore (13) and (14) count as slips. In addition to this (12), (16) and (17) are likely also to be instances of what Ross (1975) calls the principle of "lazy tongue"; further examples will be given in Part IV. Of course in handwriting our pens are also "lazy" but the two forms of motor activity have their own rules and these do not coincide in their realization of the same abstract forms. Put in another way, where the tongue is lazy the pen is not allowed to be.

2. Differential effect of time for lexical selection in speech and writing

The reason advanced in SP for the differences in error pattern between speech and writing lay in the interrelationship between the relative speed of speech and writing and the degree to which material was planned ahead. Because of the existence of structural slips, interpreted as cases of phonological similarity, and in the case of writing homophone and quasi-homophone slips and misspellings which were however phonetically correct, it was assumed that the input to writing was the same as that to speech. It was held that words were initially accessed from long-term memory in their phonological rather than in their graphological form and in that form were held in a buffer store prior to being produced overtly. In the case of writing this of course required a subsequent translation into a graphological code prior to instructions being issued to the motor system to realize these words in writing or, as the case may be, in typing.

The general position that, in writing, words are first of all accessed in phonological form has however been challenged. I shall consider the objection in Part III, but for the time being I assume the correctness of my position. My second reason for treating the initial input to speech and writing as the same was that the span ahead at which it was planned appeared to be the same in the two language production situations.

The span ahead of speech and writing can be gauged from the distance ahead at which anticipation slips at the lexical level operate. In the case of speech, there were 33 such errors in the Daily Life and Conference S-samples, with an average span of 7.8 syllables. † In the Meringer sample of 42 slips in German, the average span was 6.5 syllables. In writing, combining my Group W-sample with the Wing and Baddeley W-sample, there were 46 anticipation slips at the lexical level and the average span was 6.2 syllables. When this close similarity in the spans of speech and writing is taken into account with the fact that fast speech, including pauses, may proceed at the rate of close to 6 syllables a second (Lenneberg, 1967, p. 91) and writing under conditions of maximum speed (Hotopf, 1980a; c.f. also Newman and Nicholson, 1976) only 0.75 syllables a second, then it can be seen that the timing conditions under which we speak and write are very different. Presumably the reason why the span is approximately the same for the two activities is because this is required for syntactic planning on a clause by clause basis.

The implications for slips are twofold. The greater time available for lexical access should reduce the incidence of errors in lexical access and the longer period clauses will have to be held in buffer store, before being realised in overt motor behaviour, is more likely to result in their deterioration through short-term memory decay.

As for the first of these implications, we have seen that there are far fewer semantic group slips in writing than in speech and that blends are virtually non-existent in writing. The low incidence of transpositions at the lexical

† Hotopf (1980a) gives a more detailed account as to how the size of the span is estimated.

level could also be explained on the grounds that they are corrected before the full transposition is effected. As shown on p. 151, with the exception of the very odd example of (5), the actual cases of transpositions at the lexical level in writing were all of short and adjacent closed-class words. Only structural slips, which are commoner in writing than in speech, fail to fit into this scheme. I shall consider in Section IV other reasons than errors in lexical access for their occurrence in writing.

It is true, of course, that pauses and hesitations can be used in the course of speech for purposes of lexical access (Goldman-Eisler, 1968; Butterworth, 1980) which, according to Butterworth, when occurring within the executive phase of speech, average about half a second in length. Perhaps these did not occur in the fast speech upon which Lennenberg's calculation was based. However, the time available for pausing must in most speech-situations be limited by social pressure – fear of losing the stage to a rival speaker, losing one's hearer's attention and so on – whilst in writing as much time as is needed for accessing the word required is always available. Furthermore, it seems unlikely that the target words in semantic group and structural slips would be of the low predictability that characterizes words found after pauses. 70% of semantic group slips and 57% of structural ones in my heterogeneous English sample occur in speech on familiar and concrete matters and tend to be of high frequency involving, in the case of semantic group slips, groups such as food, time, meal and kinship words, names of days, months and countries, greeting terms and common ajectives of the kind that have polar opposites. One might suggest that, instead of a hesitation, the wrong word is selected and the paradigm of this situation (Hotopf, 1980b) is the calling of a member of a familiar group, like a family group, by the name of another member of the same group. Not hesitating, save perhaps in this latter situation, is on most occasions successful so that the tempo of speech is not compromised by a proliferation of pauses before the selection of open-class words. On the other hand, the much more deliberate process in writing, imposed by its mechanical constraints, enables unhurried selection of these words to be made.

The tendency for semantic group slips to occur mainly with concrete words may furthermore account for the lower incidence relative to the other speech samples of semantic group slips in the Conference S-sample. That there was however difficulty in accessing words in the time available was frequently suggested by the quality of the language used in the Conference S-sample. Instances of this are shown in the following example in the use of general words and phrases like "people", "and so on", "sort of" and "something", as well as repetitions of the same phrases.

(19)   . . . it wasn't developed by psychologists. Like information theory it
        was developed by engineers, physicists, people like that. People
        largely developed it in military and aviation contexts where people
        developing weapon systems and so on just wanted to know how
        long it what chance you would have of detecting these sorts of

targets so that you could do something about them. People concerned with aircraft navigation wanted to know whether you would be able to detect a particular sort of landmark when fl- approaching it at Mach two.

I give these examples because I believe they are characteristic of the spoken language when dealing with complex, relatively abstract matters, but not characteristic of the written language where more time can be taken in selecting the right word and varying the phrasing even when writing fast under pressure of time as with the Group W-sample. Fuller research on this difference is however clearly required.

3. *Short-term memory decay and attentional factors*

Although the slower process of writing allows more time for lexical access and better grammatical phrasing, the longer period that planned clauses and lexically accessed words have to be held in a buffer store before they are realized makes it more likely that they will be distorted as a result of the decay of short-term memory. Further, the passage from initial phonological coding to graphological coding followed by the activation of the relevant motor commands for realization of the individual letters in writing, should make considerable demands as regards distribution of attention, from which bound morphemes and closed-class words being shorter, generally unstressed and more predictable, since they are members of smaller sets, are more likely to suffer. This was shown in SP not only in their much greater tendency to be transformed than in speech, but also in closed-class words being much more likely to be omitted than open-class words or to be immediately repeated, which is equivalent to failure to notice that they had not been omitted. Such an interpretation suggests that the relative deterioration of syntax in writing errors is not due to some defect in a syntactic planning agency but is due to difficulties in performance. Even the preservation of membership in the closed-class word group, shown by the tendency of word substitutions, though changing form-class, to be confined either within the open-class or within the closed-class word groups, a characteristic shown for closed-class words in the reading errors of cases of deep dyslexia (Coltheart, 1980), does not necessarily bear witness to some kind of residual syntactic functioning. It could be accounted for both in terms of substitutions tending to be between words of equal frequency groups and as due to the tendency in sound pattern slips for target and error word to have the same initial phoneme. With regard to the first of these, all but one of the sixty most commonly occurring words, accounting for 42.5% of all word tokens according to Kučera and Francis (1967) norms, are closed-class words. Both words in 37 out of 40 closed-class word substitution pairs in my main writing sample were in this group and the four remaining words still fell within the top 60%, though this top 60% of word tokens only accounted for 0.8% of word types. As regards the second reason for closed-class words substituting for one another, about 90% of closed-class word structural slips of the pen start with the same phoneme. Of these, 40% are between words starting with the phoneme /ð/ which is unique to closed-class words, and 25% between words starting with the phoneme /i/ which is the initial phoneme for such very frequently occurring closed-class words as "it", "is", "if" and "in", but is the initial phoneme in only six English monosyllabic open-class words, as listed in the Concise Oxford Dictionary, including such infrequent words as "imp", "inn" and "itch".

D. Distributional Differences between Speech and Writing at the Phoneme/Letter Level

Further evidence that factors of attention and short-term forgetting may be responsible for errors is shown when we go from the lexical to the letter level. However, since we have not said anything yet about the difference between slips of the tongue and the pen at this level, let us first briefly describe the main differences at this level before relating these to differences at the lexical level.

1. *Nature of the differences*
At the phoneme level, slips are substitutions of error for target items, additions of error items, or omissions of target items. They are largely attributed to anticipations, repetitions and transpositions of items. Illustrations of some of these are given below. (20) is an example of substitution, in this case of a syllable, apparently due to repetition; (21) of an addition, which is an anticipation; and (22) another anticipation, this time leading to an omission.

(20)   'Irene Rowers.† What are the team's views about women playing crickers?' (cricket)
(21)   . . . for the abler ones to be in the [si:m]* C stream
(22)   . . . one would see [souʃaik]* social psychologists essentially.

The most frequent slip is a substitution‡ (67% in the Meringer S-sample; 77% in the Garrett/Shattuck–Hufnagel sample (Shattuck, 1975)). Of course these substitutions, at least as far as anticipations and repetitions are concerned, might have been due to chance. No satisfactory evidence disproving the null hypothesis is available. However, certain regularities in the interrelationship between items have been discovered which lend credence to the attribution of interaction between items. These are that the source of the error items (where the anticipation or repetition comes from) tends to be

---

† The surname of the lady in (20) was actually Rowell. This is an example of a characteristic of slips that often when one slip is made, another follows. In this case it seems likely that the two are related.

‡ Transpositions are included amongst substitutions; though strictly speaking double substitutions, each transposition is counted as only one.

within a syllable of the same stress, weak or strong, as the syllable within which the target item is (Boomer and Laver, 1968); the items that interact (source of error and target) are in the same position within syllables, initial, medial or final (Boomer and Laver, 1968; Fromkin, 1968; Nooteboom, 1969; MacKay, 1970); and source and target items are likely to be similar as regards voice and manner, though not place, of articulation (MacKay, 1970).

Substitutions at the letter level are rare in my data. Others rate the proportion higher. This depends to a large degree on decisions concerning the level at which the slips are believed to occur. In contrast to other analyses, I have counted as slips at the lexical level any cases where a substitution of letters leads to the creation of a new word. I shall advance a justification of this in Part IV. At the other end from the lexical is the part-letter level. In the Author's 2nd W-sample, as well as that of Ellis (1979) which like mine was also based on an analysis of his own slips, there were a number of cases where an addition or an omission of a stroke forming a letter gave the appearance of a letter substitution. Such omissions or additions of strokes led to such confusions as w's with u's, m's with n's, n's with m's and i's, and u's and y's with undotted i's and j's and so on. These formed about 17% of the combined total (239) of all slips at the letter and part-letter level in the Author's 2nd W-sample. Such slips are obviously difficult to identify in the writing of others, such as the Group, and Wing and Baddeley W-samples. As for those substitutions where the error could be attributed to a second letter, which acts as the source for the error letter, occurring earlier or later than it, there was, in the few cases occurring in my data, little evidence of the operation of suprasegmental factors such as we have just noted in the case of speech errors. This can best be seen in the case of transpositions. These only formed between 2% to 8% of slips at the letter and part-letter levels in my different samples. If to them are added other slips from my total collection, 56 in all are available for study. In only 16.1% of these were the two transposed letters in the same position, initial, medial or final, within their syllables, whereas there were hardly any exceptions to this principle amongst slips of the tongue. The failure to conform to the *syllable position principle* in writing slips is probably because the span for letter transpositions in writing is very short, 82.1% of the cases being between adjacent letters, 80.4% of which were transpositions of a consonant with a vowel. It follows from this also that neither the principle concerning similarity of stress in the syllables containing the transposed letters, nor that concerning similarity of features in the transposed letters will have been manifested as they were amongst slips of the tongue.

It might be thought that this failure to show the influence of suprasegmental factors in slips of the pen at the letter level was strong evidence that the conversion from phonological to graphological code took place at least before the phonetic level of processing. However, as mentioned before, writers are often aware of covert speech accompanying their writing. I shall give evidence in Part IV of letter slips being detected before they were

committed which suggests that the representation had reached consciousness and could not therefore be characterized as abstract. The alternative
explanation may be once again that the slower process of writing gives more
time for the correct assembly of the representation, thus greatly reducing
errors at that stage.

2. *Attentional factors*

In writing, much the most common slip at the letter level, as all authorities
agree, is the omission of one or more letters either within a word; or between
adjacent words, resulting in two words being run into one another. Here
once again we get evidence suggesting that attentional factors may be at
work. The letters which tend to be omitted are to a significant degree those
which are not perceptually prominent, i.e. letters which are neither
ascenders nor descenders occurring in the middle rather than at the beginning or end† of exceptionally long words. When, however, perceptually
more prominent letters, i.e. those at the beginnings of words, were omitted,
then these errors were more likely to be detected and immediately corrected
than when they occurred in the middle of words.

In marked and paradoxical contrast to this, slips of the tongue tend to
involve the perceptually more prominent items. Thus, as Boomer and Laver
(1968; cf. also Nooteboom, 1969; MacKay, 1970; Fromkin, 1971; Garrett,
1975) have shown with regard to anticipation, repetition and transposition
slips, the word in the clause receiving primary stress is the one most frequently involved, whether as source of error or target, though chiefly the
former. Furthermore, interaction is most frequently between the strongly
rather than the weakly stressed syllables (Garrett, 1975) and word-initial
items figure much more prominently in slips than items in syllable-final or in
syllable-initial positions in later syllables (MacKay, 1970; Fromkin, 1971).
This relationship between slips of the tongue and attentional prominence
applies not only to substitutions but also to omissions. Whereas in writing,
the first two letters (which are the most prominent) formed only 22% of the
letters that were omitted, the corresponding proportion in speech amongst
the first two phonemes in the Meringer sample was 44%. The words within
which these omissions took place in the two samples were comparable in that
they were unusually long ones, 8.4 letters in both the writing and speech
samples. Greater difficulty might be expected in the realization of unusually
long words but clearly the mechanism causing slips in speech differs from
that responsible in writing.

So much then for the summary with elaboration of the findings published
in SP. The contrast between slips of the tongue and slips of the pen in terms

---

† This finding depends upon treating omissions of grammatical morphemes as slips at the
lexical rather than at the letter level. Evidence was presented in SP showing that letters at the
ends of words were more likely to be omitted when they formed morphemes (46.3%) than when
they did not (6.7%). There were also cases of similar changes in number, whether of nouns or
verbs, where what would normally be signalled by the omission of a morpheme were signalled
by a morphological change, as in "were" (was).

of relative weakness in lexical access versus relative weakness with closed-class words and bound morphemes and in obeying the constraints of form class has an appealing similarity to the dichotomy prominent in discussions of aphasia between word-finding difficulties with open-class words, characteristic of anomic aphasia on the one hand, and paragrammatic forms of aphasia on the other hand. However, as we have seen, lexical access appears to be less proficient in writing, as far as structural slips are concerned, than in speech, and the involvement of closed-class words and bound morphemes amongst slips of the pen is due not so much to defects in the computation of syntactic structure as to performance factors such as short-term forgetting and allocation of attentional resources. Where pathology is concerned, the similarity is less with aphasia than with confusional disorders, such as those shown by Chedru and Geschwind's (1972) patients, who manifested disturbances in attention and reduced short-term memory span. Their errors in writing as opposed to speech were indeed closely similar in nature to the slips in my own W-samples.

Meanwhile, rather than examining the similarities between aphasic symptoms and slips, the best contribution that the study of slips can make is to see what light they can throw on language production processes. In the rest of this chapter, I shall attempt to do this, first by considering criticisms of the view put forward in SP that the initial input to writing is phonological rather than graphological and, second, by considering whether the greater frequency of structural slips in writing than in speech can be attributed to other factors than faults in lexical access. The search for these other factors will throw further light on the production of language in writing.

III. Is Input to Writing at the Lexical Level Exclusively Phonological or Not?

In order to explain the paradoxical finding that there was a class of good readers who were poor spellers, it has been argued that whereas reading is mainly "by eye", writing is predominantly "by ear" (Frith, 1978, 1979, 1980). Part of the evidence for this was the occurrence of structural slips. Since these in speech were evidently due to phonological similarity between error and target words, it was assumed that this was also the case with structural slips in writing. I therefore argued (1968, 1980a) that, in writing, the semantic system initially accessed a lexicon which was phonologically ordered so that there had later to be a conversion of each word from its phonological to its graphological form. It has subsequently been objected that, though this may be so in the case of homophones (Ellis, 1979), it need not always or indeed predominantly be the case (Ellis, 1982). In support of this, rare cases of aphasia (about seven in all) where speech but not writing was disturbed are cited (Lhermitte and Derouesné, 1974; Hier and Mohr, 1977; Basso, Taborelli and Vignolo, 1978). Now it may seem obvious that, if speech but not writing is disturbed, then what is written correctly cannot first have been phonologically encoded. However, much depends upon the precise nature of the disability. What is common to a number of these cases is difficulty of lexical access in speech combined with phonemic paraphasia. But as we have seen, the slower pace of writing gives more time for lexical access – a fluent aphasic cannot, as it were, remain fluent and succeed in accessing open-class words, other perhaps than very common ones – whilst the kinds of error that are shown at the phoneme level in speech do not occur in writing. The latter could be due to the fact that conversion to a graphological code takes place before the phonetic level of representation is reached. Alternatively, as argued above, the longer time available makes it possible to avoid these errors. The evidence that would be decisive would be evidence that words, even in an unhurried naming situation, could not be accessed orally but could in writing. Here there is indeed a convincing case, reported by Hier and Mohr (1977), of a patient who could not speak the names of objects presented as pictures but was able to write them. But though this case shows what only a very doctrinaire attitude would be disposed to deny, that initial access of words through the graphological lexicon is possible, the question is whether this route would be much employed in clause production as opposed to naming. If the words, having been accessed, have to be held in a buffer store for a few seconds, as is likely to be the case in writing, then acoustic, as opposed to visual, coding will, according to the evidence from studies on short term memory, be the more durable. However, as stated above, I simply assumed in my earlier articles that structural slips in writing were manifestations of the same kind as structural slips in speech. It is time that this assumption was put to the test.

A. Procedure for Identifying Structural Slips by Phonemes or by Letters

The method by which structural slips had always been determined in my categorization of slips was the following. To be classified as a structural slip error and target word had to have the same number of phonemes in common as there were syllables in the longer words, provided these phonemes were in the same order in the two words. By that is meant that they should be in the same syllable (first, second etc.) and in the same position within that syllable. Phonemes in grammatical morphemes were not included in this count. Where there is a difference in number of syllables or number of consonants, dummy syllables or consonants are added to the word which is shorter than the other for the relevant item and arranged in any position which will favour a similarity judgement, except that the placing of the dummy consonant should not result in a cluster not permitted in English phonology. Now the same rule can be applied for graphological similarity, using letters instead of phonemes, and this should make it possible to compare degree of similarity using the two measures.

The following example illustrates how the procedure operates. A two-syllable error word, "function", was written instead of a three-syllable target word, "assumption". It is necessary therefore for at least three phonemes or letters to be identical and in the same position in the two words for the slip to be categorized as a structural one. If a dummy syllable is assigned as the first syllable in the error word, "function", this requirement is met, since the vowel in the second syllable and the last two phonemes in the third syllable of the two words are the same, and in the same position within the syllables. Similarly, five letters are the same and in the same position in the two words. The proportion of letters in common to total letters is greater than the proportion of phonemes in common to total phonemes.

Accordingly, a sample was drawn up for all pairs of words that satisfied both criteria – that for letter and that for phoneme similarity. The sample was not confined to slips occurring in systematically collected samples. However, no slips with a multiple categorization such as the example just given, which was also a repetition slip, were included, nor were stem variants, which were of course, except for irregular forms like "is" (are), always a pair that were visually and acoustically similar. Finally, no more than one occurrence of each kind of slip, such as the substitution of "their" for "there" or the reverse, was included in the sample.

Data. This procedure yielded three subsamples, two content word samples for slips of the pen and slips of the tongue, and one function word sample for the former only. The results are presented in Table III. It can be seen that in all three subsamples, there was not a great deal of difference between the two measures – indeed there were cases of letter being greater than

TABLE III

Relative proportions of phonemes and letters in common among structurally similar slips of the tongue of open-class words and slips of the pen of open-class words and closed-class words

Slips of the tongue	Slips of the pen	
	Open-class	Closed-class
Open-class words ($N = 66$)	words ($N = 74$)	words ($N = 36$)
Proportion of letters in common 0.601	0.669	0.613
Proportion of phonemes in common 0.650	0.711	0.523
t 2.597, p 0.02[†]	2.4145, p <0.02[†]	−1.58, N.S.

[†] 2-tailed tests were applied.

phoneme similarity in all three subsamples. Though phoneme, as measured by an unrelated t test, was significantly greater than letter similarity in the two content word subsamples, in the function word subsample the relationship was the other way round though not significant. Further, if homophones and quasi-homophones are removed from the content word subsample of slips of the pen, reducing the number of cases to 62 and the proportions for letters in common and phonemes in common to 0.649 and 0.668 respectively, the superiority of phoneme over letter similarity is no longer significant. Since there were of course no homophones in the speech sample, it is clear that by this measure phonological as opposed to graphological similarity was greater in the case of speech than in that of writing.

In considering these results two points should be made. First, as noted in the previous section, structural slips in writing differ as regards frequency of closed-class words and changes in form class from those in speech. This suggests that not all of them are due to errors in lexical access, a matter which we shall examine in the next section.

Secondly, although English, as opposed, say, to German, can in its orthography through the occurrence of homophones make one aware of the possibility of phonological input in writing, the difference between acoustic and visual representations of words is, as Table III shows, still only a very slight one. What is required are representations which differ considerably for the two modalities. A few examples of this are available. These are mainly of two kinds, those involving confusions between numbers and upper case letters, and those coming from private abbreviations of my own. The former qualify as slips at the lexical level because the names of the numbers and letters would be spoken if they were read out aloud.

(23)   ques (cues)
(24)   W.H.N.8. (W.H.N.H.)
(25)   3 (C)
(26)   28 (20A)
(27)   5 (9)
(28)   1:4 (1:1)
(29)   2o (to)
(30)   ⌣ (wf)
(31)   ⊙ (is)

In 23, which was a typing slip, the name of the letter "q" is sounded in the word. (24), (25) and (26) are straightforward cases of sound similarity of number and letter name words, and (27) of two number words. In (28), where the spoken form of the complete target was "a one for one share issue" the homophone "for" is realized as "4" and, being a digit, displaced one position and substituted for the digit, "1", and in (29) there is substituted for the first letter of "to" the number corresponding to the sound of the word, again involving a homophone. (30) and (31) are examples which depend upon a particular private shorthand I' use. In (30) "with" is substituted for "which" and in (31), "in" for "is".

Although there are only some 20 cases like those given above in my collection of slips, there are none which are pure cases of substitution based upon visual but not acoustic similarity. There are no cases of substitutions at the lexical level where the names of numbers or upper case letters would be spoken, such as, for example, "5" for "S", "S" for "8", "C" for "O", "E" for "F".†

In addition to this evidence and the occurrence of homophone and quasi-homophone slips, there are two other kinds of evidence suggesting that input to writing is initially phonological. The first, to which I have already referred, are those slips classified as stem variants where the last letter of a word is omitted in cases where in speech one would also expect it to be omitted because the next letter represents an identical or closely similar phoneme. (13), (14), (16) and (17) were examples of this. The second piece of evidence is substitution slips of the pen at the letter level where the misspelling is in accordance with the sound of the word. Examples given in SP include "ridgid" (rigid) and "needent" (needn't). These are slips inasmuch as the writer knows the correct spelling of the word, and though strictly speaking at the letter level, count as slips at the lexical level on the theory that they are due to the sound of the word as a whole. They might be described as non-word homophones. I will deal with these in more detail in Section IV.

So much for the evidence concerning initial input to writing. Because of the close correspondence between phonology and orthography, we have been forced to rely on rather small samples of a variety of different types. The evidence seems to me to favour the conclusion that input in continuous writing is phonological, if not acoustically coded, though obviously stronger evidence is desirable. Experimental evidence might be obtained by teaching subjects some symbol system which segments differently from present orthography but such a system would have to be very highly practised to yield trustworthy conclusions and this may be difficult to bring about. An alternative approach would be to study slips in shorthand; not shorthand taken down from dictation but from spontaneous writing, such as Bernard Shaw used.

IV. Causes of Structural Slips of the Pen

Two related issues arise with regard to structural slips of the pen. These are whether they are due to factors other than errors in lexical access and to what extent these other factors are ones causing these slips to occur because of visual rather than acoustic similarity. That the latter might be the case is suggested by the evidence of Table III where we saw that error and target word were more similar to one another phonologically amongst slips of the

---

† Evidence will however be presented in Part IV, Sections F and G, that some structural slips not due to faults in lexical access may be due to visual rather than acoustic similarity.

tongue, which are regarded as being due to errors of lexical access, than amongst slips of the pen. That causes other than errors in lexical access may be operating with structural slips of the pen is what we would expect on the theory that more time is available for lexical access. Consequently, we would expect fewer structural slips of the pen than of the tongue, but, as Table II showed even with regard to open-class words, the opposite was the case. In this Part, I shall present evidence for five other causes for structural slips in writing. These, which occur at progressively later stages in the process of generation, are short-term forgetting, accessing the wrong spelling, access malapropisms in spelling, contextual influence, and visual feedback, and will be described in Sections C, D, E, F and G, respectively.

Identifying these other sources of structural slips throws light on how information is processed in the course of writing. I shall not therefore confine myself in this Part to describing these other sources but, in presenting them, I will refer to some current theories of language production. I will start by very briefly describing these theories in so far as they are relevant to my purposes in this Part.

A. How Language is Produced in Speech and Writing

Current theories of language production that arise from the study of slips postulate that the speaker's or writer's message in continuous speech, is set up clause by clause starting with a semantic structure for each clause. According to Fromkin (1971) and Fay and Cutler (1977) the semantic structure gives rise to a syntactic structure "with semantic and syntactic features specified for the word slots". Following this, words to fill the slots are accessed from what is described as a mental lexicon or dictionary. Butterworth (1980), on the other hand, believes that these processes do not occur in sequence but in parallel and that syntactic structure and lexical choice occur independently of one another. It may indeed be true that some words and even phrases may on occasion be accessed before syntactic structure, with slots for other not yet accessed words, is generated, and that this may require either a reaccessing of words or a regeneration of syntactic structure so that words and structure fit. However this would imply that syntactic structure and lexical access were interdependent, not independent of one another. The evidence for their being interdependent is that substitution slips of the tongue respect form class entirely in the case of semantic group slips and very largely for structural ones (see p. 153), and that what the form classes of the word stems are is in most cases unambiguous.

As regards selecting the words to fit into the syntactic structure, these are considered to be accessed in two stages from the mental lexicon. The first stage is semantic and the second phonological. Semantic slips which, according to my criteria (Hotopf, 1980b), are either polar contrasts or co-hyponyms, are regarded by most workers as being generally due to the change of a single semantic feature. It is worth noting, furthermore, that error words of the same form class as the target word and closely similar in meaning but with different subcategorization characteristics and selection restrictions practically never occur, which is further evidence for the controlling influence of syntactic structure over word choice. When the correct semantic entry in the lexicon is accessed, an address is found which contains a pointer to an address in the phonological part of the lexicon. Structural slips are then attributed to the speaker going slightly astray and accessing a neighbouring item in the phonological lexicon (Fromkin, 1971; Fay and Cutler, 1977). This explanation is backed by the claim that neighbouring items in actual dictionaries are similar to one another, and presumably distant items dissimilar – an extraordinary belief when one considers orthographically similar items like "bone" and "zone", which are about as widely separated as they can be.

On the basis of experimental evidence as well as evidence from slips of the tongue, the mental lexicon is believed only to list word stems. Grammatical and derivational morphemes which are not what Garrett calls "moribund", are regarded as affixed by rule procedures. Certainly the evidence concerned with the identity of grammatical morphemes for semantic group and structural slips, mentioned above (pp. 152 and 153), supports this. It is difficult to determine from current models how closed-class words are produced. However, as shown above (p. 152) substitution slips amongst closed-class words that respect form class also exist. It is as though these are selection errors within the classes of prepositions, pronouns, articles etc. When they occur, syntactic structure constrains their forms as it does that of open-class words, in the sense that error and target word are of the same case.

The stage at which word stems are accessed from the phonological part of the lexicon and placed into their slots in the syntactic structure, and morphemes are affixed to them or morphological transformations take place, is still at an abstract level. After the application of morphophonemic rules and as a result of pragmatic considerations, particularly the speed of speech and the speaker's attitude to the audience determining how clearly the speaker was going to enunciate (Lieberman, 1967; Oshika, Zue, Weeks, Nue and Aurbach, 1975; Cole and Jakimik, 1978), the final phonetic form of the clause is obtained. This is required, according to these models, to give the precise information required for the setting up of motor commands or motor schemata (Laver, 1980) for the realization of speech. The clause either in its fully specified phonetic form or as a string of the resulting commands is then held in buffer store awaiting articulation.

It is however not only the clause as a whole that is held in buffer store. Various early stages of it must similarly be held in storage after the program has advanced beyond them. This, according to Hockett (1967), Laver (1970, 1980), Baars, Motley and Mackay (1975), Baars and Motley (1976), Motley and Baars (1976) and Baars (1980), is necessary in order to account for pre-articulatory editing. The purpose of this is to correct errors in the program before they result in overt slips. This type of editing was first suggested by Hockett (1967) in his distinction between smooth error-free speech and blunderful speech like (18). The former was much more closely edited than the latter. In arguing for this view he referred to " 'thinking in words': the virtually unbroken inner flow of 'heard' speech from which we make certain selections to be spoken aloud" and added that he had "observed 'slips of the tongue' in my own inner flow, often caught and edited out before they could be mapped into overt speech by tongue and lips".† Again in justification of the notion of covert editing in speech he referred to our often "think(ing) of something, during a conversation, that we decide not to say".† I believe that slips identified in thinking, including that in which we are working out what to say, are not the same as slips identified in the actual program held in buffer storage prior to speech (see the next section). Nevertheless Laver (1970, 1980) took up the notion of covert editing and incorporated it in his model, agreeing with Hockett that slips identified in thinking (Laver, 1969) gave plausibility to this notion. Finally, experimental work in the eliciting of errors similar in form to slips has led to the view that more slips than are actually committed do in fact occur in the course of building up the program.

Dell and Reich (1980, 1981) oppose this view of editing on the grounds that a much simpler model could account for the phenomena in question. They claim that the intention to output a certain word will, by means of association with other words and their constituent syllables and phonemes, give rise to spreading activation through a relational network, thus sometimes causing other words, syllables, or phonemes to be output instead. Which will be output depends upon strength of association according to certain principles. Basically, this means that certain errors will be made more likely than others without having to postulate that these other errors are in fact first produced and then erased. However, as I shall show in the next section, covert slips, which are suppressed before overt articulation or writing, do occur, though this is of course not inconsistent with spreading activation also being a factor in the aetiology of slips.

So much for models of speech production. We however are concerned with writing. Therefore, given that words in writing are initially accessed from the phonological lexicon, we have to consider the stage at which there is a transition from a phonological to a graphological representation. Evidence will be presented later, in Section D, of the phonological representation having reached the phonetic level of specification before the translation is made. This may indeed mean that the program is in articulatory code, something that should not be surprising in view of common though informal testimony of the writer speaking to himself what he is writing, as he writes it. But it is not necessarily the case that the phonological program always reaches this level of specificity before being translated into a graphological form.

Since, as will be shown in Section F, anticipations at the letter level rarely exceed two words, I assume that no more than one or two words are taken at

---

† These quotations are from Hockett's article as published in Fromkin (1971, p. 118).

a time from the phonological buffer and converted into their graphological form. Since we are dealing with words, these will have to be accessed from the graphological lexicon but decomposed into stems and bound morphemes because that, according to the evidence of experimental studies (e.g. Gibson and Guinet, 1971; Snodgrass and Jarvella, 1972; Murrell and Morton, 1974; Taft and Forster, 1975, 1976) is how the graphological lexicon is arranged. We shall address this matter in Section D.

Just as in the formation of the fully specified phonological program there is a hierarchical process proceeding from the abstract to the final phonetically concrete form, so it has been proposed (Ellis, 1982) that there is a similar progression in forming the graphological program. This depends upon making a similar distinction with letters as with phonemes, the former being distinguished in analogy with the latter as either graphemes, allographs, or graphs. Evidence for this distinction comes from slips at the letter level when one form of a letter is substituted for another according to its context as in

(32)   Drays* (Drayton St. Leonards)

In (32) the grapheme "s" would have had in my writing the graphic form "f" in the target word but was rendered as "s" in the error word. Therefore we have here the anticipation of a grapheme rather than of a graph. In contrast to this, the most highly specified level at which slips of the pen occur is at the part letter level described above (p. 163) where, for example, omission of a stroke may convert an "m" into an "n", though whether slips such as these occur at the graphic level or are slips in motor programming is not always easy to decide.

The last stage in writing is seeing what one is writing as one is doing it. The function of this stage might be thought to be that of monitoring output, but though this may be the case it is also, as will be shown in Section G, itself a source of other slips of the pen.

B. Slips in Verbal Thinking and in the Phonological and Graphological Programs

It was pointed out in the previous section that Hockett and Laver had both experienced covert slips. However, they give no examples of these. Meringer in his two books gives a few examples and Hill (1972) also attests to their occurrence. The examples Meringer gives are of slips in verbal thinking rather than in the speech program. I give below some examples of slips in verbal thinking from my own collection.

(33)   On *Friday†* (Thursday) which for some reason I keep calling *Wednesday* (Friday)

(34)   It seems to be *raining* (snowing)

† Covert slips are indicated by italics.

(35)   It would be *tackling on* too much (tackling + taking on)
(36)   After all, if I'm going to *garages* (Gamages)
(37)   *BS* N.I. (PS N.I.)
(38)   . . . *one minute past ten* (ten minutes past one)
(39)   They *arther ei* (either are) . . .

The first example, which like (34), (35) and (39) was described by their author as occurring when she was talking to herself in subvocal speech, is a complicated one. It consists of two semantic group slips, one of which, "Friday", was also an anticipation slip. As for the others, (34) is also a semantic group slip, (35) is a blend, (36) and (37) sound pattern slips and (38) and (39) transpositions, at the lexical and the phonemic levels, respectively.

To be distinguished from covert slips in verbal thinking are slips in the program held in buffer store which when detected enable the speaker or writer to avoid making an overt slip. I will call those types of covert slips *suppressed slips.*

During the year or so in which I have attempted regularly to record suppressed slips I have only detected and thus prevented myself making six such slips in speech, all of which have been semantic group slips such as the following:

(40)   . . . *brush my teeth* (cut my nails)
(41)   . . . *magnifying glass* . . . (microscope)
(42)   The Weintraubs are living in San *Arbor* (San Francisco)

(40) is a semantic group slip of a verb phrase. In (42) the name of one town, Ann Arbor, the Weintraubs' home town, was substituted for another, a procedure facilitated by the fact that the first syllable of the target name contained the first syllable of the error name.

Two points can be made about these suppressed slips in the speech program. The first is their apparent rarity, which may be due to the short time span available for spotting them before they are realized. The second point is their confinement to errors of semantic group which is consistent with the notion that such a choice is likely to occur early in the construction of the linguistic program. There is however also evidence of slips being only partially committed and suppressed before they can be completed. This is particularly noticeable in transpositions. Meringer gives a number of instances of this, for example

(43)   Halt den Mund* *vor die Hand* (Halt die Hand vor den Mund)
       (Put your mouth* *in front of your hand* (Put your hand in front of
       your mouth))

The speaker in this case stopped herself before completing the transposition. Another example from my own collection is

(44)   I was on a Bailey* *at the old jury* (. . . jury at the Old Bailey)

As for other categories of slips at the lexical level, Meringer shows in a number of his examples that sometimes only the beginnings of error words in structural slips, anticipations and repetitions were spoken before the target word was substituted. Though I have observed the same phenomenon in my own slips I have not recorded it. Two examples of arrested structural slips, kindly placed at my disposal by David Fay, are the following

(45)   Since I was on *hospital* (holiday)
(46)   I always hear about him *bothering* (borrowing) from other people.

In the case of each of these slips only the initial consonant and vowel of the first syllable were spoken but the speaker testified as to the word he was about to say.

When we come to suppressed slips of the pen we find, not surprisingly in view of the slower realization of the program in writing, that these are more frequent. Altogether I have 42 cases at the lexical, letter and part-letter levels in my collection. Those at the lexical level include one example each of a blend, a semantic group slip and a transposition, slips which rarely occur overtly in writing.

(47)   *Merrett* (Garrett, derived from Merrill + Garrett)
(48)   . . . *kinaesthetic* (auditory)
(49)   5.2.80. (2.5.8).)

There are also structural slips such as the following, the first of which was reported by a woman in typing,

(50)   . . . unless you pay your arrears your *pregnancy* (tenancy) will be terminated
(51)   Unity can only be achieved in *science* (silence)

Whereas these slips appear to be due to errors in lexical access, most suppressed structural slips are due to short-term forgetting, as will be shown in Section C. There are however also cases of the kind we shall be dealing with in Section D, namely, homophones and phonetic misspellings as in (52) and (53).

(52)   *Wr-* (Ring) Nakeeran
(53)   *rephr-* (refrained)

Whereas (47), (48), (50) and (51) indicate errors in the phonological program, (52) and (53) are suppressed slips in the graphological program indicating now an awareness of what one is about to write before writing it.

It is not always easy to tell whether a structural slip is due to structural similarity, as can be seen from (54) and (55).

(54)   Let us look *as* (at) Figures 1 & 2
(55)   . . . *wat* . . . (was at)

(54) counts by my criteria as a structural slip. However, it could, like (55), be

due to the contextual influence of the next word, a running together of two words which in the case of (54) creates a new one.

In Section F we shall see that such anticipation with omission slips are more likely to form words than non-words.

That many suppressed slips at the letter level were of omissions, such as (54) and (55), is not surprising in view of their frequency amongst overt slips. The following are further examples

(56)   but controlled. It was . . . (but controlled it. It was . . .)
(57)   Aar (Agar)

(56) is a haplology (avoiding the immediate repetition of a form) at the lexical level; it is however a haplophony rather than a haplography because the form of the repeated item changes in writing. The first occurrence according to my form of shorthand is ⌐ and the second, *. It could not be argued that (56) is a haplography at the abstract *grapheme* level, referred to in the previous section, because (56) is not a case of writing one allograph, upper instead of lower case, for another, since the first form of "it" was an ideogram standing for the whole word. On the other hand, (57) is a suppressed haplography though one at the letter level, involving parts of letters. What would have been avoided by the haplography would have been writing the same shape, "a" , which was a part of the "g", twice in succession, as a consequence of which the downward vertical stroke of the "g" would have been omitted. Here the error is not one of accessing the wrong orthographic representation from the lexicon but of detecting a motor anticipation slip before it occurred.

One further example of a slip being suppressed so that an omission of a letter did not in fact occur is shown in (58).

(58)   . . . displ*cing* . . . (displacing)

In writing the "a" I mistook it for "c" and would have continued with "-ing", but suppressed this in time. The interest of this example is that it showed how visual monitoring of the writing might itself produce a slip. We shall see further examples of this in Section G, as well as how much monitoring may itself cause structural slips at the lexical level.

To conclude this section, the evidence of suppressed slips is that the much slower process of writing places within the reach of our reaction time the means to correct slips before they are made so that not only can these corrections be made more frequently in writing than in speech, but also much later stages in the processing of the skill. By the same token however the words which are being held in store prior to their being written will be more liable to short-term memory decay, as the following section illustrates.

C. Deterioration in Short-term Memory

A possible explanation of structural slips of the tongue is that they are due to deterioration of a word held in buffer storage before it comes to be articulated. However, the immediate correction of the error when it is identified, sometimes as in (45) and (46), before more than the first syllable has been articulated, makes this explanation unlikely. The experience of a speaker making such a slip is that he expected to say a particular word but found himself saying a different one. If there were a deterioration in buffer storage how would he know what the word he meant to say was? Similarly, a speaker who has made a structural slip which he did not detect, will sometimes deny that he made it, that is to say he will assert that he spoke the word alleged to have been forgotten. Of course, it might be claimed that the speaker rapidly regenerates the target word from its semantic specification. This would have to be extremely fast. Furthermore, the speaker's experience is more one of having just missed his phonological target but having been near it, rather than of the error word having been rejected because it had the wrong meaning, although of course it did in fact have the wrong meaning.

With structural slips of the pen, when the period during which words are held in buffer storage is longer, the case is sometimes different. Though I have not documented the claims made in the preceding paragraph concerning general experience, the evidence of some of my own structural slips of the pen, that were due to short-term forgetting, points out the contrast with slips due to errors in lexical access. The first examples I shall give are all of suppressed slips where sentences were composed, often in peripatetic fashion, preparatory to my sitting down and writing them out. In each of them a word similar in sound to the word I remembered originally accessing now substituted for that word. Though it might be argued that I could not know that I had correctly accessed a target word in the first place, the point of these examples is, firstly, that in no case was I, as in other slips of the tongue, able immediately to correct the error; instead there followed an attempt to recall the word originally accessed, which was like a very brief tip of the tongue experience; and secondly, that when the search was abandoned and another word substituted, i.e. regenerated, this, as in (59), (60) and (61), differed semantically from the target word that had been lost. On recommencing writing however in all the cases listed below, the original target word reappeared, that is to say, a word appeared that I "recognized" as being the word originally accessed. Perhaps the situation of explicitly attempting to recall a word blocks it and it is only when the situation of writing is reinstated, i.e. the full context in which the word originally appeared is replaced, that the word may be reaccessed. In the examples which follow, the error word, since it was not written, counts as a suppressed slip and is therefore italicized. When the search for the original is abandoned and a replacement substituted, this is indicated in bold print.

(59)   . . . that many problems of his *reading*, WRITING (meaning)
(60)   . . . processes of great generality and *flexity*, *flaxity*, FLEXIBILITY (complexity)

(61)   . . . though this *fault*, FEATURE (fact) has lead to neglect . . .†
(62)   . . . *revision*, ALLOCATION (division)
(63)   . . . *comprised, confined, con* . . .? (contrived)
(64)   . . . an *ordinary* (orderly) historical sequence.
(65)   . . . particularly with this *letter* (weather)
(66)   . . . due to their *face* (faith) in taxonomy . . .
(67)   . . . forced to fit into a conventional *mode* (mould)

Not all cases of short-term memory change were detected before they were written down. A few examples of ones actually committed in writing follow:

(68)   . . . all speech is incitive, unless we confine "incisive" (incitive) to that which aims . . .
(69)   It's a pity you can't be with us so that two mothers could be separated* (celebrated) together
(70)   . . . a certain minimum of technical confidence* (competence)
(71)   . . . but incidents in a sort of order* (certain order)

(68) is particularly clear cut in that, taking into account the speed of writing calculated in SP, we can say that about five seconds elapsed between taking the first occurrence of "incitive" from the buffer and writing the second, whereas in speech it would have been about one second. The other cases were identified as ones of short-term forgetting because they all involved a search for the original word, something which I have never known to occur with slips of the tongue.

In (71) a phrase is substituted for a word. There are a few other instances of this in my samples of slips of the pen, such as "a number" (another), but none are present amongst structural slips of the tongue; indeed one would expect none, if these slips are, as I hold, due to faults of lexical accessing rather than to short-term memory changes. Although some claims have been made for the inclusion of idiomatic phrases in the mental lexicon (Swinney and Cutler, 1979), these particular phrases are not of that kind.

D. Misspelling

Two kinds of misspelling can be distinguished – homophonic substitutions and "phonetic" spelling. The first kind I have included in the category of structural slips since one word which is a homophone is substituted for another. "Phonetic" spelling, that is, incorrect spelling which is nevertheless consistent with the sound of the word being spelled, has however not been included amongst structural slips since what are spelled are not words which are listed in the dictionary. I shall, however, argue that the two kinds of slip

---

† In this case the sentence had been written down but, wishing to reformulate it, I found myself repeating it with "fault" substituted for "fact". I then substituted "feature" before discovering by reference to the original what the word had been.

are related and that the latter are indeed slips which should be counted as lexical.

With these kinds of slips we pass to a later stage in the processing of writing, namely the retrieval from the graphological lexicon of forms to match those retrieved earlier from the phonological lexicon. Although these kinds of slips do not of course occur in speech, I will nevertheless discuss them for the sake of their theoretical bearing on the question of how we program words in writing.

1. *Homophone slips*

Structural slips which are homophones are not ones due to deterioration whilst being held in a buffer store, as far as their phonological form is concerned, because this is preserved intact. Their semantic classification changes of course just as it does in other structural slips. What strikingly differentiates homophone substitutions from the structural slips considered so far is the failure to observe syntactic constraints. This is manifested in three ways. Firstly, form class is not preserved. Whereas less than 5% of the structural slips of the tongue word pairs differed in form class, two thirds of open-class and all closed-class homophone word pairs differed in their output. Second, even where form class was preserved, grammatical morphemes were not. Though, as stated on p. 152, only 5% of structural slips of the tongue differed as between error and target word in grammatical morphemes, there was no evidence of this constraint amongst homophone substitutions. The following examples are illustrative.

(72)   . . . referents . . . (reference)
(73)   . . . he has done wrong in societies (society's) eyes
(74)   . . . how the patient see's (sees) his own conflict

In (72) a singular is substituted for a plural form, in (73) a plural for a possessive and in (74) an inappropriate possessive is applied to a verb form.

Thirdly, there is frequent failure amongst homophones of lexical segmentation in deriving the correct spelling of phonologically specified forms. Examples are of substitutions of words for multiword non-constituent expressions such as "your" (you're) and "there" (they're). Other examples are

(75)   This is not as small appoint* (a point) to make as . . .
(76)   . . . if the lie is not too greater (great a) one to tell.

(75) and (76) are of extra interest because they cut across the boundary of an immediate constitutent.

2. *Phonetic spelling*

We have already given as examples of phonetic spelling, "needent" (needn't) and "ridgid" (rigid). Others are "predjudiced", "incourage", "chrematorium", "imagenation", "excelerated", "reforence", "divice", "absalute", "idear" and "secondery". It might, however, be objected that these are not words and therefore these spelling slips of the pen should logically be allocated to the phoneme/letter rather than lexical level. "Non-words" play a large part in experimental research, and theories (cf., for example, Forster, 1976) concerning the organization of the mental lexicon are rather heavily invested in them. The criterion for determining whether a form is a word or not is whether it is listed in a dictionary. But of course many orthographic and phonological variants of words exist according to the region or class from which the speaker comes, what his native language is in the case of foreign speakers, whether he is a child or not, or to particular idiosyncrasies of his speech such as inability to pronounce his r's. We can identify these, when they are rendered phonologically or orthographically, in speech and in reading, and can produce them as well. They are therefore included in our mental lexicon or, perhaps more likely, we possess rules for receiving and producing them, albeit often in a highly simplified and stereotyped form. Such rules in the form of phoneme-to-grapheme correspondence rules are certainly used in transcriptions of accent used by novelists and playwrights and it is to these rules also that psycholinguists (e.g. Morton, 1980) have appealed in accounting for phonetic spelling. A difference however is that unlike the simplified and stereotyped rules usually employed to depict, say, Cockney or Scottish accents, phonetic spelling sometimes reveals a degree of sensitivity that may well be greater than any we could, unless we were trained linguists, achieve by conscious analysis. Examples of phonetic spelling that have not, because of our rules for allocating slips to categories, been classified as such but may in fact be cases of it are, as I have already argued, stem variants such as (13), (14), (16) and (17), and structural slips that are quasi-homophones such as (76) and

(77)   . . . that part of our minds wherein rests are (our) ideals

It is possible that certain other stem variants and structural slips may have a similar origin though this time in deviant phonology. Examples of this, including one already presented, are

(12)   Many experiments are still been (being) carried out . . .
(78)   . . . as useful as are intelligent (intelligence) tests . . .
(79)   . . . it can be an (and) quite often is . . .
(80)   . . . I do hope William's pasts his (passed his) test.

The interpretation of (80) is that the error, "pasts his" is a phonetic transcription of [pa:stsiz] where [s] is substituted for [h]. It is also of interest in that the morpheme "-d" is rendered in accordance with morphophonemic rules.

Not all phonetic spelling slips represent the operation of phoneme-to-grapheme rules as these are understood in studies of spelling. Some in their spelling are like what from the spelling point of view are described as irregular words. We have already come across one example of this in the suppressed slip, (53). Others are

(81)   Having expressed our meaning wri-* (rightly)

(82) . . . copywright (copyright)
(83) . . . before he support (supports) a contension (contention)
(84) . . . and the scientist kn* (now) has to be . . .
(85) . . . Edinborough (Edinburgh)
(86) . . . *Thimes* (Times)

Even if we extend the notion of homophone slips to include morphemes which are parts of words, as in (81), (82), (83) and (85), this still leaves (53), (84) and (86), the last being a slip of verbal thinking that misguided a search in the telephone directory. In these cases analogy seems to be at work through words like "rephrase", "know", and "Thames" or "thyme", as indeed may also be the case with regular phonetic spelling (cf. "ridge" and "ridgid", "dear" and "idear", "organization" and "organism").

3. *Translating phonological to graphological representation*

In discussions of deep dyslexia (Marshall and Newcombe, 1973; Coltheart, Patterson and Marshall, 1980) two routes from the orthographic to the phonological representations are frequently posited: the route via the lexicon and that via grapheme-to-phoneme correspondence rules. Homophone slips suggest use of the former and phonetic misspelling slips, that of correspondence rules, though proceeding from phonemes to graphemes. As pointed out in the previous section, the existence of such correspondence rules can scarcely be doubted, though there is not to the author's knowledge any detailed study of how these rules work. But can phonetic misspellings be fully accounted for in terms of these rules?

It is not possible to give anything more than a very tentative answer to this question because the data are fragmentary, phonetic misspellings and homophone slips being rather rare. But we found, as indicated in the last section, a number of cases where irregular spelling is used and phones like [n], [r], [t] and [f] are rendered by "kn", "wr", "th", "ph". It does not seem likely that such spelling, or the use of "-sion" as opposed to "-shun" for spelling [ʃvn], as in "conten*sion*", would ever be used in rendering provincial accents or idiosyncratic pronunciation. Rather it is as though the writer making slips like these is aware of the fact that the phonemes in question are occasionally spelled by such letters that causes him to make these mistakes. In other words, his attitude, which is to spell correctly according to conventions of spelling, is different from that when his aim is to copy the sound of words. Similarly, as we saw in the last section, some of his misspellings may be influenced by analogy with the spelling of other similar words.

Can we then attribute phonetic misspellings as well as homophone slips to the lexical route? The problem that presents itself here is what is meant by the lexical route. Models of language production and of reading hold, as shown in Section A, that words are accessed from the lexicon. Since the lexicon consists only of word stems, it follows that words in a phonetically fully specified clause must now be decomposed into base morphemes plus grammatical and perhaps derivational morphemes. This would mean that the program would have to regress to an earlier form. However since, as we have suggested, earlier forms of this program are still held in buffer storage in order to monitor for errors at the particular level for which they are responsible, it might simply be that a translation is made at the level of these earlier forms. Therefore there would be a transition from phonological base forms to graphological base forms with the syntactic structure regenerating bound morphemes, but now in abstract graphological rather than phonological form.

The trouble, however, with any theory that postulates reaccessing words from the graphological lexicon is that it does not account for the fact that the translation from the phonological to the graphological representation seems, in the case of phonetic misspelling slips, to proceed directly from the phonetic representation of a word in which the original syntactic distinctions are not observed. Thus, as shown in the two previous subsections, we have errors in lexical segmentation involving closed-class words, failure to preserve grammatical morphemes, and omissions or changes of complete bound morphemes, in everyone of which errors only phonetic shape is preserved. This means a failure to carry out the decomposition of the phonetically or articulatorily coded program into base forms and grammatical morphemes. It follows therefore that there can be a direct transition from a phonetically specified form to a graphological form. The latter may possibly be at the abstract graphemic level but it is already morphemically encoded. This implies that there can be graphological representations of words in long-term memory that can be accessed directly and not through the "lexicon", conceived as a list only of the base forms of words.

The question then arises as to why writing is nevertheless normally free from errors of this kind. One reason clearly is that not many homophones exist in our language and that most of them are infrequent in occurrence, the obvious exceptions being closed-class words like "their/there" etc. A second reason is that the syntactic and semantic representations of the program are normally still held in buffer storage and can monitor or control the translation from the phonological to the graphological, if reference is made to them. The extent of other demands upon our processing capacity can however sometimes result in the failure of such reference.

What remains is to account for phonetic misspelling errors. Can they also be explained in terms of an association between spoken and written forms? Some light may be thrown on this question by considering malapropisms, which is the subject of the next section.

E. Access Malapropisms

So far I have written as though there was only one kind of structural error that was due to a fault in lexical access. However in the process of collecting my own slips I have become aware that sometimes it is possible intentionally to produce a wrong word that is structurally similar to the right one, although normally I do not so. Such errors which seem to be due to temporary faults in memory cannot be called *slips*, because slips are defined as unintentional errors. I call these kinds of errors *access malapropisms*. They are different from the original malapropisms committed by the character of that name in Sheridan's play because those, which I call *storage malapropisms*,† were clearly errors of long-term memory storage. Access malapropisms, which are often though not invariably in their use accompanied by a feeling of uneasiness indicating a lower degree of confidence in their correctness, are formally identified by the speaker or writer recognizing that he has used the wrong word when given the correct one.

In the following examples, (87)–(90), the last of which was a blend, are errors in speech, (91) in typing and (92) and (93) in writing.

(87) I didn't realize they might be in cohorts together (cahoots)
(88) She rings me up and I try to jockey her along (jolly)
(89) He aupaired the meeting (compèred)
(90) Dumbstruck (Dumbfounded + thunderstruck)
(91) . . . some of the extra accommodation thereby released, which is in access (excess) of the amount envisaged
(92) Inset* Insert (Indent)
(93) . . . of two parts, an inducing part and a part on which the illusion has been induced. In conformity with this, evidence has been induced (adduced) . . .

The last example, which is an error of my own, is clearly a repetition slip at the lexical level. However, it seems itself to have induced an access malapropism since use of the word was intentional and, though I was uneasy about it, it was some time before the correct form could be accessed.

As for spelling, some of the cases of phonetic spelling already quoted were in fact access malapromisms of my own. These were "Edinborough", "excelerated" and "chrematorium". Normally, having very little difficulty with spelling, these are words I otherwise spell correctly. One cannot of course tell simply by inspection whether another's phonetic misspelling is a slip or an access malapropism, though it might be thought that homophone errors at least would be slips. However, even here one can be temporarily unsighted as occurred, for example, when I wrote "there" for "they're" and for a moment had surprising difficulty in telling which was right, or whether I should have written "their".

---

† The word "malapropism", has also been used by some researchers (e.g. Fay and Cutler, 1977) to refer to structural slips, that is to say, ones which were unintended. Given the origin of the word, I think this usage is unfortunate. Consider Mrs Malaprop's views about how young girls should be educated

"... above all ... she should be mistress of orthodoxy, that she might not misspell, and mispronounce words so shamefully as girls usually do; and likewise that she might reprehend the true meaning of what she is saying."

If unintentional errors of "orthodoxy" are to continue to be called malapropisms, it would be better to characterize them as *unintentional malapropisms*.

There is one clue which may suggest that access malapropisms are more frequent in writing than in speech. This is the frequency with which structural errors are detected when they are made. As shown in SP, where details of the method of judging immediate detection of errors are given, between 83% and 90% of open-class structural errors in, respectively, the Daily Life and Conference S-samples,[†] were corrected. In contrast to this, the proportion of such errors in the Group W-sample that were identified at the time they were made was only 20.8%. The significance of this lies in the fact that access malapropisms are, by definition, cases where the wrong word was spoken or written deliberately. One would not therefore expect them to be immediately corrected. Evidence such as this is consistent with the view that access malapropisms are more common in writing than in speech.

As for phonetic misspelling there is of course no parallel in speech for a comparison of frequency of correction to be made. However, implicit in the notion of access malapropisms in spelling is the idea that some spelling errors are more obvious, i.e. more easily edited out, than others. It is noteworthy that with one exception there are no cases of phonetic misspellings in which a grammatical morpheme is spelled as it is pronounced, such as "robz" (robs), "reachuz" (reaches) or "backt" (backed). When there is a phonetic misspelling involving a grammatical morpheme, the morpheme is omitted. This results in another word. Even the one exception, (80), where a phonetic spelling of a morpheme appears to have occurred, also resulted in a word. The prediction that would follow from these observations is that phonetic misspelling of grammatical morphemes that resulted in substitutions producing non-words would be far more quickly identified than those not involving grammatical morphemes. Therefore, depending upon which model one favoured, one could either say that errors involving phonetic misspelling of grammatical morphemes would be easily identified and edited out before being produced or that they would be less likely to be produced in the first place.

F.   Contextual Causes of Structural Slips

1.   Structural slips of closed-class words
We have not so far accounted for the large number of closed-class words that figure amongst structural slips in writing. It seems unlikely that many such slips are due to errors in lexical access. Perhaps substitution slips of closed-class words that preserve form class (p. 152) are due to errors in access. The error words would also, in the case of pronouns, articles and demonstratives,

---

[†] Noteboom (1980) in his analysis of corrections in the Meringer (1908) collection reports a much lower incidence of corrections than mine. I question whether one can reliably judge which of the slips reported in Meringer's books were corrected. In many cases Meringer reproduces both the slip and its correction. When he does not, but simply records the slip, sometimes simply giving only the error and target words, he may add the note "korr." or "nicht korr.", standing for "corrected" and "not corrected" but, with a substantial number, including some committed by himself, it is not stated whether the error was corrected or not. I do not think it is justified to assume in the latter case that none of these errors were uncorrected.

generally be structurally similar to the target words. However, slips of this kind are even rarer in writing than in speech, and, as we saw on p. 153, over 80% of structural slips of closed-class words *failed* to preserve form class between error and target word. As for short-term forgetting, no cases due to this, as judged by difficulty in recalling the target word when an error was identified, were observed. Homophones were necessarily limited to a few cases such as "there"/"their", "are"/"our", and "to" and "too" confused with each other or with "two". Homophone slips are of course by definition not structural slips of the phonological variety. However, there is no reason why phonological structural slips should not occur when the phonological item is converted into a graphological one. Certain pairings such as "where"/ "were", "with"/"which" and "that"/"than" are relatively frequent and they may indeed be cases of near-homophones or near-phonetic misspelling, which are favoured, just as we saw in the last section modifications of grammatical morphemes are, by a bias on the part of errors to lexicality.

There is an objection that may be made against my identification of closed-class word structural slips which must now be considered. This is that in many of these (e.g. it/if; on/or; be/by; do/to) only a single phoneme or letter is changed. Most researchers on slips (e.g. Shattuck (1975) and Fay and Cutler (1977) with regard to speech; Lecours (1966), Chedru and Geschwind (1972), Nauclér (1980) and Wing and Baddeley (1980) with regard to writing) do not count cases in which a single phoneme or letter is changed as word-substitutions but as slips at the phoneme/letter level. Yet if, in the case of writing, these were simply letter substitution slips, we would not expect words very frequently to result by chance from such substitutions. Table IV, which is based on the complete Wing and Baddeley sample (Wing and Baddeley, 1980, Appendix) and my Group W-sample, shows however that out of 74 cases of single letter substitutions, only 22 (29.7%) were non-words. About 90% of the words were closed-class words, most of them being two-letter words plus nine mutual substitutions of "that" and "than".

TABLE IV

Relative numbers of one-letter substitution slips converting closed-class target words into (a) closed-class words and (b) open-class words and (c) non-words.

Number of letters in target word	(a) Number of closed-class error words	(b) Number of open-class words	(c) Number of non-words
2	36	0	3
3	1	4	4
4	10	1	8
5	0	0	5
6	0	0	6
Total	47	5	22

2. *Anagrammatic word-formation*

If then we accept that closed-class word structural slips are not mere accidents resulting from substitutions at the letter level, may they not also be counted as cases of near-homophones or near-phonetic misspelling with a bias towards lexicality, such as was suggested earlier? There is however an alternative account that can be given of them and this is that they may be due to contextual influences. This is shown most clearly in the case of a special type of letter anticipation slip, namely, one where letters are omitted spanning the gap between two or even three words.

In the systematically collected samples there were 268 letter omission slips in all. 80.2% of these were of letters within a word, 18.7% between adjacent words† and 1.1%, of which (94) is an example, spanning three words.

> (94)   . . . seleva* (select the relevant) . . .

If we now ask what causes these jumps from one word to the next in writing, part of the answer is suggested by two features of these slips. These are (i) that they are frequently haplographies or involve jumping from a letter in one word to the same letter in the next word and omitting the intervening letters, or (ii) that they form new words as in anagrams from selected letters in two or three adjacent words, the letters of these new words being in the same order as in the adjoining words from which they are taken. If we add to my four systematically collected samples, between-word letter anticipation slips from the Wing and Baddeley W-sample, we have 106 cases in all. 31.1% of these are of the first kind (haplographies and telescoping between common letters), 52.8% of the second (new words), and 63.2% are of either.

We have already come across examples of haplographies amongst suppressed slips. (95) is an example from between-words letter anticipation slips.

> (95)   Forbiddencies (forbidden tendencies)

In (95) the same or a closely similar element "-den" or "-ten" is repeated three times and two of them are omitted. As for jumping from one occurrence of an element or string of elements in one word to another such occurrence in the next word, (55) and (94) are two examples of this.

With regard to the formation of new words, we have seen one example, (54) from suppressed slips. Other examples are

> (96)   seem* (see them)
> (97)   is* (in as)
> (98)   This* (The historical)
> (99)   whether* (where the father)
> (100) next* (now exists)
> (101) dew* (device we)
> (102) in order* (other words)

† The few cases where the space between two adjacent words was omitted as in "farm" (far more) were not included in this analysis.

Generally the order of letters in the source words is preserved in the error words, (102) being a rare exception. As can be seen from the examples given, the new words anagrammatically formed from the two or three words held in the program, include open-class words. However most of these new words (75%) were closed-class words.

It is possible that some omissions of single words, which again were very largely closed-class words, were also due to anagrammatic word formation operating between neighbouring words. This, for example, is what happened in (103) which was one of my own slips,

(103)   . . . has* (he has) . . .

After writing the "h" of "he" I found my pen against my will writing "as" so as to produce the succeeding word. One cannot, of course, tell whether this has happened in the case of others simply by inspection of their script, but clearly the possibility exists, sometimes causing the first of two words, as in (104) apparently to have been omitted, and sometimes, as in (105) the second.

(104)   . . . that is (it is) possible . . .
(105)   . . . this (this is) in experiment . . .

Fifteen word omission cases were of this kind, of which all but one word were closed-class words.

The question next arises whether the frequency, with which between-word letter anticipation slips form new words, can be expected by chance. It is, as pointed out before, difficult to judge this question when the slips are made by a number of different writers. I have therefore taken all the letter-anticipation slips of my own that spanned two words which together amounted to seven or fewer letters. There were 28 of these, of which 18 (64.3%) formed new words. The question is, what is the proportion of words and non-words that could be expected by chance? In calculating these, certain constraints were imposed. These were (i) that the sequence should start with the first letter of the first word, (ii) that the letters that were preserved should be in the same order as they were in the words they came from, (iii) that the omissions should be of intervening letters (cases which simply omitted the space between the two words were not included) and (iv) that only one break in the sequence of the 7 or fewer letters should be permitted.† Working on this basis, the total number of words that could be expected by chance was 71 (16.3%) out of a total of 434 sequences. The null hypothesis can thus be rejected ($\chi^2 = 35.82, P < 0.001$).

It must however be admitted that my own slips were particularly liable to this anagrammatic word production effect. Out of a total of 36 such slips formed from 7 or fewer letters committed by writers in my systematically collected samples, 18 (50%) were words. This was however still consider-

---

† These constraints, except for the third, were imposed because they largely characterized both my own slips and those of others. Only two exceptions to them (of which (100) is one) occurred and these were of course not included in the sample.

ably larger than the proportion that could be expected by chance which, at
17%, differed little from the chance expectation in the sample of my own
slips.

Between-words letter anticipation slips do not exhaust the possible
influences of the context in causing structural slips. Examples of slips which
may be due to the occurrences of a letter in the immediately preceding or
following words are the following:

(106)   I see no need for this is (in) intelligence
(107)   . . . from am* (an) experiment . . .
(108)   . . . and this* (thus) in the . . .
(109)   . . . most successful in (is) in the consideration . . .

Although there were more cases of structural slips where only one letter was
changed and the source of that letter was in the immediately preceding or
following word than otherwise, the number of cases was too small for the
null hypothesis to be tested.

3. *Theoretical issues posed by between-words letter anticipation slips*

Between-words letter anticipation slips raise two issues of theoretical
importance to our understanding of the production of writing. The first is
whether words which are produced anagrammatically in the way we have
just described may not be due to phoneme rather than, as I have described it,
letter anticipation. The second is that of the number of words held in buffer
storage when the translation from phonological to graphological representation takes place and the means by which a later word may affect the
transcription of an earlier one.

(i) Letter versus *phoneme between-words anticipation* Between-word
phoneme anticipation slips also occur in speech and may take the form of
haplophonies, as in (110) and (111).

(110)   I'll see you, tomorag* (tomorrow, Morag)
(111)   . . . Lorge* . . . (Lord George Brown)

Further, the span for phoneme omission slips in speech – 85.2% within
words, 12.3% spanning two and 2.4% spanning three words in the Meringer
S-sample – is closely similar to that obtaining in my four W-samples and, just
as in writing, none of these exceeded a span of three words. This contrasts
with ordinary phoneme *substitution* slips which are due to anticipation (i.e.
excluding anticipations manifested in the *omission* of intervening
phonemes). These show much larger spans; 25%, 47.1%, 16.8%, 6.1% and
4.9% for anticipations spanning 1, 2, 3, 4 and 5–7 words, respectively.

Can the slips we have been considering then be due to anticipation of the
phonologically rather than of the graphologically coded program? Three
types of evidence are relevant. First, it was argued on p. 159 above that
anticipation slips which involve substitutions occur very rarely in writing as
compared with speech because of more time being available for preparing

the program. By the same argument, it might be claimed that there should be very few anticipation slips involving omissions due to the phonological program. However, the difference in spans between the two kinds of phoneme anticipation slips and the similarity of the span for omissions in the two types of language production suggest that different mechanisms are at work for the two types of anticipation. For instance, anticipation slips involving substitutions might be due to errors in the assembling of the program whereas those involving omissions might be due to scanning the program ahead as the phonetic representation was being translated into a motor representation of a string of commands.

The second type of evidence is that although haplophonies occur in between-words phoneme anticipation slips, the formation of new words as a result of them is very rare. I have not been able to find more than three cases of this in the Meringer S-samples. Since most of the new words formed out of old ones in writing slips were short closed-class words, and closed-class words rarely figure amongst structural slips of the tongue, it may be this feature that is the main characteristic distinguishing anticipation in the two word-production situations.

A third source of evidence for determining the coding in which between-words anticipation effects occur is the relationship between the phonetic or graphic shape of the new word and those of the words from which it derives. Because of the close correlation between the phonetic and graphic shape noted in Part III, this type of evidence is generally ambiguous. However examples like the following suggest phonological anticipation.

(112)   make* (may characterise)
(113)   simple* (similar perceptual)
(114)   . . . Freudiand & (Freudian &) behavioural approaches . . .
(115)   Normand + Jill (Norman + Jill)

(114) and (115) are of particular theoretical interest. Both of them are haplographies of the repeated element "-an" and dittographies of the morpheme "and". They cannot be due to visual or motor coding since what is held in the program is an ampersand in the one case and a plus sign in the other. On the other hand, they cannot be attributed to phonetic coding because the [d] of "and" would in normal speech have been elided. It is unlikely that the phonetic representation that we make use of in our writing would be that characterizing the slowness and clarity we would use for addressing someone expected to have difficulty in understanding. By the logic of our argument in Section D, we have to accept that the phonological program in the case of (114) and (115) was at the more abstract phonemic level and that translation to the graphological form can sometimes occur at that rather than at the phonetic level, unless of course we accept the notion of abstract articulatory coding.

But although examples (112) to (115) suggest between-words phone or phoneme anticipations, there are many more cases of between-word anticipation slips that cannot be attributed to anticipations of phonemes than those that unambiguously can be. Examples that have already been quoted are (54) and (101). Others are

(116)   . . . the extent to which were* (we) are influenced . . .
(117)   . . . done it* (in) the first place . . .
(118)   . . . has not occurred before of* (or) frequently before.
(119)   Ready* (/re:d/) Harry Kaye's article

Similarly, there are cases of jumps between identical letters in adjacent words which cannot be attributed to phoneme anticipations, such as

(120)   . . . kneve* (knee) level . . .
(121)   . . . to sou* (sort) out . . .

It follows therefore that these slips and probably others that by their form could have been either phonological or graphological, must have occurred after the phonological-to-graphological conversion had taken place. Structural similarity in such cases would be graphological rather than phonological. This agrees with our finding shown in Table III of a closer match in terms of letters rather than phonemes for closed-class words.

(ii) How do between-words anticipation effects occur? The existence of structural slips due to anticipation of letters rather than phonemes indicates that conversion of the phonological forms of words into their graphological forms is done ahead of the word being written, though the span of these anticipation slips suggest that this programming is normally limited to one word ahead. Another source of evidence for this is provided by part-letter anticipation slips. I briefly described part-letter omissions and repetitions in Part II (p. 163), but have said very little concerning part-letter anticipation slips, which are all cases of haplography or telescoping between common letter strokes and of which (57), a suppressed slip, was an example. These slips, both in Ellis's (1979) and the Author's 2nd W-sample, are amongst the commonest, forming about a quarter of all slips at the letter and part-letter level in the author's 2nd W-sample.† Since this chapter is mainly concerned with slips at the lexical level, I have not said much about slips at the phoneme/letter level. However there is a feature of these slips which is of relevance here. Out of 81 such slips, 71 (86.6%) occur between neighbouring letters (including ones between the last letter of the one word and the first letter of the next) and 12 (14.6%) occur between adjacent words. These latter cases of telescoping between common letter strokes operate sometimes between the initial letters of adjacent words, as in (122).

(122) B*(Pure Behaviourism)

---

† Very few of these slips were noted in my first sample. This was the first systematic sample of any slips that I collected and it is possible that I was not at that time fully aware of them since they are easily missed. Further, monitoring for these kinds of slips requires a degree of vigilance that may make slips at a higher level less likely to occur.

When the capital "P" I was writing changed into a capital "B", I could not determine why I had done this. It was not until I crossed out the "B" and started again that I found the cause in the first letter of the next word. I must have been aware that I was going to write "Pure Behaviourism" but did not see the connection when I made the mistake and tried to find out why – the connection itself appears to have operated below the level of consciousness. Another example, this time of a suppressed slip, is (123).

(123)   J *(Tell Jill)

The impulse to curve the vertical downstroke was suppressed before the new intention, which was contrary to the original intention, was carried out. It may be of significance that (122) and (123) were of letters which, being upper case, were written separately. The next example, which again spans four letters was written in lower case. However since they were printed, they were again separate from one another.

(124)   would b*(would have been)

(124) is not a one-word omission slip because I was conscious of writing an "h" which changed before I could stop it by an inward curve into a "b".

In the last two examples I have referred to my awareness of what was happening in the process of writing, an awareness which enabled me to suppress the slip in (123), but was not quick enough for the one in (124). Similarly, in the case of between-words letter (as opposed to part-letter) anticipation slips, we saw, in (54) and (55), two other examples of suppression operating in time to avoid the slip. One is also sometimes aware of processes which appear to be responsible for a slip. It is often for example the case that in blends a speaker will report uncertainty concerning which form to produce (see also Garrett, 1980, p. 211). Similar considerations apply to between-words letter anticipation slips. Sometimes one may be aware of thinking of a word following the word one is in the act of producing. The following are examples of this:

(125)   exernam* (external examiners)
(126)   So I D* (So I don't)
(127)   To measures* (measure these)
(128)   kind *(kind of biassing)

(125) and (126) are typing slips. In the first, a telescoping between two occurrences of a common letter, I was thinking of the next word, "examiners" as I was coming to the end of the previous one. The second was due to my thinking ahead of the act of raising the carriage of the typewriter to type the apostrophe in "don't", anticipation of which lead to the premature raising of the carriage as a consequence of which an upper case 'D' was typed. Similarly, (127) and (128) are examples of thinking of the next word as the previous word was being completed. (127) is another example of telescoping between occurrences of a common letter, but (128), a part-letter anticipation between two words, does not depend upon a

common stroke, but simply the downward continuation of a vertical, which was suppressed before completion.

It is however by no means always the case that between-words letter anticipation slips are mediated by conscious awareness of a later word. Similar to haplographies and telescoping slips is the kind of error when a copy-typist, as a result of the same word or phrase appearing on successive lines, jumps, without realizing it, from one line to another and so misses out the intervening words. This is not necessarily a case of the typist losing his or her place when starting a new line because it also occurs when the word in common occurs somewhere in the middle of each line. It has indeed been shown in studies of reading (e.g. Rayner, 1975 a and b) that, in addition to the word being fixated in reading, information concerning word shape is obtained from words up to about $3°$ visual angle to the right of the fixation point, a distance which is large enough to account for the copy-typists jump from one word to another. By the same token, if we postulate an internal representation of words, graphically coded as strings of letters and held in a buffer store, then the scanning of these letters, which leads to the setting up of strings of motor commands, may also cover a larger area than a single letter and, given the left/right direction of the scan, jump from one to another occurrence of a given form.

It may be that a form similar or identical to one at present being fixated will have its threshold for perception lowered as a result of this similarity. This would not however account for the tendency for between-words letter anticipation slips to be favoured in cases where a new word is formed anagrammatically from parts of two adjacent word. On the other hand, errors in reading generally substitute one word for another rather than a non-word and these errors are anagrammatic in the sense that some letters from the correct word are present in the error word. I have collected many instances of these, including cases where in glancing through a newspaper a word, often from a headline, will catch the attention but when examined more closely is found not to have been there but to have been composed out of letters present in neighbouring words. However, unlike between-words letter anticipation slips, they do not preserve the order of the letters in the source words. Consecutive reading in a left to right direction rather than one's eye simply being caught by a set of words in a particular heading is what would be required to bring about this effect, but studies of errors in reading (e.g. Morton, 1964) do not report errors of this kind. This may be because in studies of reading the output is spoken aloud. As pointed out before, anagrammatic word-production slips, which mainly produce closed-class words of the wrong form class, rarely occur in speech, where form class is much better preserved.

G. Misinterpreting Visual Feedback

It was stated in Section A that even when the program was finally realized in writing, the writer was exposed to yet another source of slips. These derived from what was already written on the page or from what he was himself in the act of writing, as (58), a suppressed slip, showed. Some examples of these are the following.

(129)   . . . predominantly
         . . . rather thant (than)
(130)   environment
        1   2 0 (3)

In (129) the last word in the line above appears to have affected the last word in the next line, though in writing "thant", since the error was not corrected, I cannot have been aware of any such influence. Presumably this illustrates the influence of information received in parafoveal vision. In (130) the digits were written below the word in order to count the number of syllables in it. This digit "0", which substituted for "3", was presumably influenced by the letter, "O", printed above it. A more bizarre example is

(131)   12.3.45 (12.3.74)

(131) contained a suppressed slip in that writing the "5" was suppressed. To what was the slip in writing a date due? The only logically coherent reason that may be suggested is that the sequence, 1, 2, 3 leads to 4 and 5, "4" possibly being mediated by an anticipation of the "4" in the year . . . 74". The slip was clearly not due to phonological coding, which would have been "twelve, three . . .". This exemplifies a frequent finding in slips research, namely, that for all the awareness that may exist about what one is about to write, the causes of it, such as what is in the visual environment, are frequently not at all conscious and have to be inferred. (129) and (130) are examples of slips due to other information being picked up in parafoveal vision in the case of (129), and foveal vision in the case of (130). It is possible, however, that in (131) the very act of writing and the feedback from it, which we regard as necessary for the purposes of monitoring output, created the circumstances for the slip, a low level habit, that of counting, taking over from the intended output. The suppressed slip, (58), was another example of this. How this process may cause structural slips is suggested by (132).

(132)   . . . the (these) . . .
(133)   . . . speech (speed) . . .

(132), a typing slip, was a case of telescoping by jumping from one occurrence of a letter to a later occurrence, in this case a within-word letter anticipation slip. I took the "e" as the signal to continue to the next word. A touch typist would have avoided that particular source of error! In (133) I was consciously writing the word, "speed". However, the loop in the lower part of "d" was not closed, as in *speed*. When I came to the return vertical downstroke I found my pen adding an additional curve to produce *speech* . This was in the course of writing the present chapter, where the word "speech", was of course frequently in my mind. It appears to be another example of a lower level association taking over from conscious intention as a result of visual feedback.

H. Summing Up

Two issues were raised at the beginning of this part; to what extent structural similarity was based upon phonological or graphological similarity between error and target word, and whether it could be shown that errors in lexical access from the phonological lexicon were an infrequent cause of structural slips in writing as compared to speech. In this section, I will consider the extent to which the various sources of structural slips described above can answer these two questions.

1. *Phonological or graphological similarity?*
It is frequently claimed of slips that the regularities they show give an indication of the mechanisms underlying them. As pointed out earlier, the categories in which slips are classified are, as far as my own approach is concerned, in effect hypotheses or options for hypotheses concerning their genesis. In SP, I categorized structural slips of the pen as "sound pattern" slips. As we have seen, however, the matter is much more complex. This is basically because of the difficulty of differentiating between phonological and graphological similarity. The evidence presented in this section is that errors of access, whether intentional, as in access malapropisms, or unintentional; errors due to short-term memory deterioration; and homophone and phonetic misspelling errors, are ones due to phonological similarity. As for errors due to contextual contamination, though some may be due to phonological similarity, most are likely to be the result of graphological similarity, and all errors due to visual feedback are, of course, ones of graphological similarity. We cannot however estimate the relative frequency of errors due to the two kinds of similarity because of the difficulty in identifying in many cases what the particular source of the error was. In this I have had to rely on the testimony of writers, and particularly of course on my own slips. Furthermore, not all sources of these errors are equally represented. It is for example only in the last year that I have become conscious of the role that visual feedback may play in causing structural slips. It is not however very likely that one will ever, by these kinds of observations of processes occurring whilst one is writing, be able to collect material of any statistical significance. The function of observations such as these must be to suggest theories which may eventually be subject to experimental test and perhaps also warn experimentalists of the complexity of the processes concerning which they erect hypotheses for experimental testing.

2. *Is access to the phonological lexicon easier in writing than in speaking?*
Although we have identified a number of other factors besides errors in

lexical access, we do not, as far as open-class word structural slips are concerned, have enough evidence about the frequency of the different sources of error to suggest an answer to this question. There is, however, one other type of evidence that is relevant. This is the relative frequency of preservation of form class amongst open-class word structural slips. Assuming that all structural slips of the tongue of open-class words are due to errors of lexical access, form class is evidently preserved to the extent of 97% of all cases. The proportion amongst slips of the pen is at 72.2% still fairly high. But we cannot take this as suggesting that a substantial proportion of these slips are due to errors of lexical access since form class also appears to be preserved amongst errors due to deterioration in short-term memory. Furthermore, as we saw, there is a possibility that a larger proportion of these errors in writing as compared with speech are access malapropisms. So here also we must refer the question to experiment.

The function of observational studies such as these, which are part qualitative and, in so far as distributional evidence can be obtained, part quantitative, is, as has long been accepted, the suggestion of theories which can then be tested by experimental methods. It is also often suggested that when matters reach that stage, observation has fulfilled its purpose and is no longer required. My experience of researching slips is, however, that it is a process of continual discovery due both to the observation of new phenomena, such as, for example, suppressed slips, and the learning of how to observe them. They are not easy to record in full flight, as it were, without disrupting the flow of speech or writing and this is a skill, like any other, that needs practising. The gaining of a skill needs knowledge of results. This may in part be provided by criteria of internal consistency. But an important part is of course experimental validation. On the other hand, when a particular experimental technique is developed, such as the use of reaction time as a measure in lexical decision tasks, or the artificial induction of spoonerisms (Baars, Motley and MacKay, 1975), it often develops into an industry in its own right. But ultimately it too needs to be validated by reference to the real-life skills, observed in their actuality and not just in conventionalized form, that it is designed to explain.

Acknowledgements

I would like to thank Anne Koppel, Julia Grant and Malcom Hibberd for their help in new analyses of data for this chapter and Julie Fitzgerald for assistance in the phoneme and letter similarity count upon which Table III was based. I would also like to thank the editor, Brian Butterworth, for much help, advice and criticism throughout the writing of this chapter. Finally, I would like to thank the Leverhulme Trust for the Leverhulme Emeritus Fellowship which supported me in the research and writing of this chapter.

References

Aitchison, J. and Todd, P. (1981). Slips of the mind and slips of the pen. *In* "Language and Cognitive Styles; Patterns in Neurolinguistic and Psycholinguistic Development", (R. N. St Clair and W. von Raffler-Engel, eds). Swets and Zeitlinger B. V., Lisse.

Baars, B. J. (1980). On eliciting predictable speech errors in the laboratory. *In* "Errors in Linguistic Performance", (V. A. Fromkin, ed.) Academic Press, New York and London.

Baars, B. J., Motley, M. J. and MacKay, D. G. (1975). Output editing for lexical status in artificially elicited slips of the tongue. *Journal of Verbal Learning and Verbal Behavior*, **14**, 382–391.

Baars, B. J. and Motley, M. T. (1976). Spoonerisms as sequencer conflicts: Evidence from artificially elicited errors. *American Journal of Psychology*, **89**, 467–484.

Basso, A., Taborelli, A. and Vignolo, L. A. (1978). Dissociated disorders of speaking and writing in aphasia. *Journal of Neurology, Neurosurgery and Psychiatry*, **41**, 556–563.

Beattie, G. W. and Bradbury, R. J. (1979). An experimental investigation of the modifiability of the temporal structure of spontaneous speech. *Journal of Psycholinguistic Research*, **8**, 225–248.

Boomer, D. S. and Laver, J. D. M. (1968). Slips of the tongue. *British Journal of Disorders of Communication*, **3**, 1–12.

Butterworth, B. (1980). Some constraints on models of language production. *In* "Language Production", (B. Butterworth ed.) Vol. I, Academic Press, London and New York.

Chedru, F. and Geschwind, N. (1972). Writing disturbance in acute confusional states. *Neuropsychologia*, **10**, 343–353.

Chomsky, N. (1957). "Syntactic Structures". Mouton, The Hague.

Cole, R. A. and Jakimik, J. (1978). Understanding speech: How words are heard. *In* "Strategies of Information Processing", (G. Underwood, ed.) Academic Press, London and New York.

Coltheart, M. (1980). Deep Dyslexia: A review of the Syndrome. *In* "Deep Dyslexia", (M. Coltheart, K. Patterson and J. C. Marshall, eds). Routledge and Kegan Paul, London.

Coltheart, M., Patterson, K. and Marshall, J. C. (eds) (1980). "Deep Dyslexia". Routledge and Kegan Paul, London.

Dell, G. S. and Reich, P. A. (1980). Toward unified model of slips of the tongue. *In* "Errors in Linguistic Performance", (V. A. Fromkin, ed.) Academic Press, New York and London.

Dell. G. S. and Reich, P. A. (1981). Stages in sentence production. *Journal of Verbal Learning and Verbal Behaviour*, **20**, 611–629.

Duncan, S. Jr. and Fiske, D. W. (1977). "Face-to-face Interaction: Research, methods and Theory". Hillsdale, N. J.: Lawrence Erlbaum Associates.

Ellis, A. W. (1979). Slips of the pen. *Visible Language*, **13**, 265–282.

Ellis, A. W. (1982). Spelling and writing (and reading and speaking). *In* "Normality and Pathology in Cognitive Functions", (A. W. Ellis, ed.) Academic Press, London and New York.

Fay, D. A. and Cutler, A. (1977). Malapropisms and the structure of the mental lexicon. *Linguistic Inquiry*, **8**, 505–520.

Fodor, J., Bever, T. and Garrett, M. (1974). "The Psychology of Language", McGraw-Hill, New York.

Forster, K. I. (1976). Accessing the mental lexicon. *In* "New Approaches to Language Mechanisms", (R. J. Wales and E. Walker, eds). North-Holland, Amsterdam.

Fries, C. C. (1952). "*The Structure of English: An Introduction to the Construction of English Sentences*". Harcourt Brace. Jovanouich, New York and London.

Frith, U. (1978). From print to meaning and from print to sound or how to read without knowing how to spell. *Visible Language*, 12, 43–54.

Frith, U. (1979). Reading by eye and writing by ear. *In* "Processing of Visible Language", (P. A. Kolers, M. Wrolstad and H. Bouma, eds). Plenum Press, New York.

Frith, U. (1980). Unexpected spelling problems. *In* "Cognitive Processes in Spelling". (U. Frith, ed.) Academic Press, London and New York.

Fromkin, V. A. (1968). Speculations of performance models. *Journal of Linguistics*, 4, 47–68.

Fromkin, V. A. (1971). The non-anomalous nature of anomalous utterances. *Language*, 47, 1, 27–52.

Fromkin, V. A. (1973). "Speech Errors as Linguistic Evidence". Mouton, The Hague.

Fromkin, V. A. (ed.) (1980). "Errors in Linguistic Performance". Academic Press, London and New York.

Fry, D. B. (1969). The linguistic evidence of speech error. *BRNO Studies in English*, 8, 69–74.

Garrett, M. F. (1975). The analysis of sentence production. *In* "Psychology of Learning and Motivation", (G. Bower, ed.) Vol. 9, Academic Press, New York and London.

Garrett, M. F. (1980). Levels of processing in sentence production. *In* "Language Production", (B. Butterworth ed.) Vol. 1. Academic Press, London and New York.

Gibson, E. J. and Guinet, L. (1971). Perception of inflections in brief visual presentations of words. *Journal of Verbal Learning and Verbal Behaviour*, 10, 182–189.

Goldman-Eisler, F. (1968). "Psycholinguistics: Experiments in Spontaneous Speech". Academic Press, London and New York.

Hier, D. B. and Mohr, J. P. (1977). Incongruous oral and written naming: Evidence for a subdivision of the syndrome of Wernicke's aphasia. *Brain and Language*, 4, 115–126.

Hill, A. A. (1972). A theory of speech errors. *In* "Studies Offered to Einar Haugen", (E. S. Firchow *et al.*, eds). Mouton, The Hague.

Hockett, C. F. (1967). Where the tongue slips, there slip I. "To Honour Roman Jakobson, 2.910–36. (*Janua linguarum, series major*, 32), Mouton, The Hague.

Hotopf, W. H. N. (1968). Unintentional errors in speech and writing as clues to the processes underlying word production. Paper given to the Annual General Meeting of the British Psychological Society in Sheffield.

Hotopf, W. H. N. (1980a). Slips of the pen. *In* "Cognitive Processes in Spelling", (U. Frith, ed.) Academic Press, London and New York.

Hotopf, W. H. N. (1980b). Semantic similarity as a factor in whole word slips of the tongue. *In* "Errors in Linguistic Performance". (V. A. Fromkin, ed.) Academic Press, London and New York.

Kučera, H. and Francis, W. N. (1967). "Computational Analysis of Present-day American English". Brown University Press, Providence, Rhode Island.

Lashley, K. S. (1951). The problem of serial order in behavior. *In* "Cerebral Mechanisms in Behavior", (L. A. Jeffress, ed.) Wiley, New York.

Laver, J. D. N. (1969). The detection and correction of slips of the tongue, *In* "Work in Progress", **3**. Dept. of Phonetics and Linguistics, Edinburgh University.

Laver, J. D. M. (1970). The production of speech. *In* "New Horizons in Linguistics", (J. Lyons, ed.) Penguin, London.

Laver, J. D. M. (1980). Monitoring systems in the neurolinguistic control of speech production. *In* "Errors in Linguistic Performance", (V. A. Fromkin, ed.) Academic Press, London and New York.

Lecours, A. R. (1966). Serial order in writing – a study of misspelled words in 'developmental dysgraphia'. *Neuropsychologia*, **4**, 221–241.

Lenneberg, E. H. (1967). "Biological Foundations of Language". Wiley, New York.

Lhermitte, F. and Derouesné, J. (1974). Paraphasies et jargonaphasie dans le language oral avec conservation du language écrit. *Revue Neurologique*, **130**, 21–38.

Lieberman, P. (1967). "Intonation, Perception and Language". M.I.T. Press, Cambridge, Massachusetts.

MacKay, D. G. (1969). Forward and backward masking in motor systems. *Kybernetic*, **6**, 57–64.

MacKay, D. G. (1970). Spoonerisms: The structure of errors in the serial order of speech. *Neuropsychologia*, **8**, 323–350.

Maclay, H. and Osgood, C. E. (1959). Hesitation phenomena in spontaneous English speech. *Word*, **15**, 19–44.

MacNeilage, P. F. (1964). Typing errors as clues to serial ordering mechanisms in language behavior. *Language and Speech*, **7**, 144–159.

McNeill, D. (1979). "The Conceptual Basis of Language". Lawrence Erlbaum Associates, Hillsdale, New Jersey.

Marshall, J. C. and Newcombe, F. (1973). Patterns of paralexia, *Journal of Psycholinguistic Research*, **2**, 175–199.

Meringer, R. (1908). "Aus dem Leben der Sprache". Behrs Verlag, Berlin.

Meringer, R. and Mayer, K. (1895). "Versprechen und Verlesen, eine psychologisch linguistische Studie". Goschensche Verlagsbuchhandlung, Vienna.

Miller, G. A., Galanter, E. and Pribram, K. H. (1960). "Plans and the Structure of Behavior". Holt, New York.

Morton, J. (1964). A model for continuous language behaviour. *Language and Speech*, **7**, 40–70.

Morton, J. (1980). The logogen model and orthographic structure. *In* "Cognitive Processes in Spelling". (U. Frith, ed.) Academic Press, London and New York.

Motley, M. T. (1980). Verification of 'Freudian slips' and semantic prearticulatory editing via laboratory-induced spoonerisms. *In* "Errors in Linguistic Performance", (V. A. Fromkin, ed.) Academic Press, New York.

Motley, M. T. and Baars, B. J. (1976). Laboratory induction of verbal slips. *Communication Quarterly*, **24**, 28–34.

Murrell, G. A. and Morton, J. (1974). Word recognition and morphemic structure. *Journal of Experimental Psychology*, **102**, 963–968.

Nauclér, K. (1980). "Perspectives on Misspellings". CWK Gleerup.

Newman, S. E. and Nicholson, L. R. (1976). Speed of oral and written responding. *Bulletin of the Psychonomic Society*, **7**, 202–204.

Nooteboom, S. G. (1969). The tongue slips into patterns. *In* "Nomen: Leyden Studies in Linguistics and Phonetics", (A. G. Sciarone, *et al.*, eds). Mouton, The Hague.

Nooteboom, S. G. (1980). Speaking of unspeaking. *In* "Errors in Linguistic Performance", (V. A. Fromkin, ed.) Academic Press, New York and London.

Oshika, B. T., Zue, V. W., Weeks, R. V., Nue, H. and Aurbach, J. (1975). The role of phonological rules in speech understanding research. *I.E.E.E. Transactions of Acoustics, Speech and Signal Processing*, **ASSP-23**, 104–112.

Potter, J. M. (1980). What was the matter with Dr. Spooner? *In* "Errors in Linguistic Performance", (V. A. Fromkin, ed.) Academic Press, New York and London.

Rayner, K. (1975a). Parafoveal identification during a fixation in reading, *Acta Psychologica*, **39**, 271–282.

Rayner, K. (1975b). The perceptual span and peripheral cues in reading. *Cognitive Psychology*, **7**, 65–81.

Ross, J. R. (1975). Parallels in phonological and semantactic organization. *In* "The Role of Speech in Language". (O. F. Kavanagh and J. E. Cutting, eds). M.I.T. Press.

Rumelhart, D. E. (1975). Notes on a schema for stories. *In* "Representation and Understanding", (D. G. Bobrow and A. Collins eds). Academic Press, New York and London.

Ryan, J. (1969). Grouping and short-term memory: Different means and patterns of grouping. *Quarterly Journal of Experimental Psychology*, **21**, 137–147.

Shaffer, L. H. (1976). Intention and performance. *Psychological Review*, **83**, 375–393.

Shattuck, S. R. (1975). Speech errors and sentence production. Unpublished doctoral dissertation. M.I.T.

Simonini, R. C. (1956). Phonemic and analogic lapses in radio and television speech. *American Speech*, **31**, 252–263.

Snodgrass, J. G. and Jarvella, R. J. (1972). Some linguistic determinants of word classification times. *Psychonomic Science*, **27**, 220–222.

Swinney, D. A. and Cutler, A. (1979). The access and processing of idiomatic expressions. *Journal of Verbal Learning and Verbal Behaviour*, **18**, 523–534.

Taft, M. and Forster, K. I. (1975). Lexical storage and retrieval of prefixed words. *Journal of Verbal Learning and Verbal Behaviour*, **14**, 638–647.

Taft, M. and Forster, K. I. (1976). Lexical storage and retrieval of polymorphic and polysyllabic words. *Journal of Verbal Learning and Verbal Behaviour*, **15**, 607–620.

Wells, R. (1951). Predicting slips of the tongue. *Yale Scientific Magazine*, December, 9–12.

Wickelgren, W. A. (1954). Size of rehearsal group and short-term memory. *Journal of Experimental Psychology*, **68**, 413–419.

Wing, A. M. and Baddeley, A. D. (1980). Spelling errors in handwriting: a corpus and a distributional analysis. *In* 'Cognitive Processes in Spelling", (U. Frith, ed.). Academic Press, London and New York.

III

Commonalities and Differences
between Production and Perception

5

Perceptual Equivalence and Motor Equivalence in Speech

P. Howell
N. Harvey   *University College London*

I. Introduction

Workers in speech perception have argued that equivalence in perception between different acoustic cues is achieved by using knowledge that they are consequences of the same articulatory gesture (Liberman and Studdert-Kennedy, 1978; Studdert-Kennedy, 1980). On the other hand, those working in production have proposed that variability in the way a particular sound is produced is possible because perceptual knowledge is used to guide production (Nooteboom, 1970; Ladefoged *et al.*, 1972). In each case, equivalence of diverse patterns in one domain has been "explained" by appealing to a possibly non-existent invariance in the other domain. Perception cannot work by extracting production invariants if production works by using perceptual invariants. If there are perceptual invariants for use in production, then they should be used in perception. If there are production invariants for use in perception, then they should be used in production.

This buck-passing between production and perception has only been possible because few theorists have attempted to solve the problems of both areas within the same general theory. Equivalence in both perceptual and motor domains can only be satisfactorily explained by:

(1) Treating these areas independently but allowing them both the possibility of accessing common central representations.

(2) Solving problems of equivalence *within* one of these areas and referring problems of equivalence in the other area to that solution.

After outlining what the perceptual and production problems are, we shall discuss those few theories that have been developed to provide joint solutions to them along one of these two lines.

LANGUAGE PRODUCTION VOL. 2
ISBN 0-12-147502-6

II. Problems of Equivalence

To say that two different things are variations of one thing requires that they can be classified in the same way at some level. The level of constancy used to discuss variation in speech is usually that of the phoneme. If there was only a single articulatory specification or one signal corresponding to each phoneme, there would be little difficulty in classifying them. However, variation in both the articulation and signal do occur and present problems for both the perception and production theorist.

At least three types of variation may be distinguished. First of all, since the articulation corresponding to a particular phoneme depends on the adjacent phonemes, the signal for a phoneme usually varies with the context it occurs in.

Variation in the signal may arise from other than articulatory causes. Such variation arises in consequence of the medium of transmission and, to the extent that different speakers articulate sounds in the same way, because of the difference in the dimensions of the articulators of different speakers.

The final type of variation we will consider arises because speakers often produce the same signal in different ways. Speakers make compensatory changes in the positioning of their articulators so as to produce a constant signal.

Generally speaking, those theorists interested in explaining the process of speech perception have to account for how different signals can nevertheless be identified as the same phoneme. This is so whether the variations in the signal are or are not associated with variations in the signal. The problem of concern to the production theorist is how can many different articulations be regarded as a consequence of the same phonetic intent. This phenomenon has to be accounted for whether the articulations are or are not associated with variation in the signal. Before we consider how theorists have attempted to account for these phenomena, we will give examples of each of these kinds of variation in some detail.

A. Production of the Same Signal in Different Ways

There have been several reports that a given speaker can produce a particular sound in different ways. Typically in this type of study, the criteria for the identity of signals are acoustic, usually the resonant frequencies of the vocal tract (the formants designated $F1$, $F2$, $F3$ etc.). The signals are not completely identical but only so with respect to the lower formant frequencies. This qualification probably does not matter much because the intelligibility of the speech sounds that have been examined is determined mainly by the low-order formants.

Riordan (1977) has reported one example of this type of variability by showing that the vowels /i/, /y/, and /u/ may be produced either with lip-rounding or by lowering the larynx. Both of these manoeuvres increase the effective length of the vocal tract. Her acoustic analyses show that despite the two different ways of articulating these vowels, speakers can produce the same signal with respect to the first three formants.

Several authors have demonstrated that subjects can rapidly adapt their means of production of a vowel sound to conditions of mandibular constraint (e.g. Lindblom *et al.*, 1979). If speakers are prevented from moving their jaw by requiring them to hold a bite block between their teeth, they are still able to produce sounds which normally have a jaw position different to the constrained position. Acoustic analyses show that vowels produced with or without a bite block have the same first two or three formant frequency values.

The examples discussed so far have been concerned with vowels because it is easier to study the compensatory articulatory changes with them than with consonants. However, some less formal examples with consonants are also available. We will illustrate this point by considering some aspects of velar functioning. A schematic diagram of the vocal tract indicating the position of the velum is presented in Fig. 1.

The velum normally needs to be closed during the production of non-nasal consonants. However, clinically-based observations show that some speakers with cleft palates can produce perfectly acceptable non-nasal consonants. This is so despite speakers with cleft palates being unable to shut off their nasal cavity from their oral cavity, and some airflow through the nose always occurs. Such speakers must be able to compensate for the open velar port by modifying their articulations. Such compensations as these may not be restricted to speakers with such disabilities since cineradiographic studies

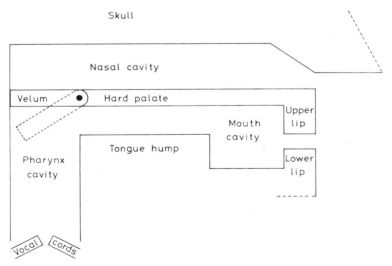

FIG. 1. A schematic diagram of the articulators indicating the position of the velum (lateral view).

on normal speakers have revealed that some of them have an open velum during consonant production too (Bjork, 1961).

So far we have considered consonant production when the velar port is open. There is also some indication that nasal consonants can be produced when coupling of the nasal cavity is impossible. For example, Wise (1948) had to have wadding plug his nasal cavities to stop haemorrhaging after he had sustained an automobile accident. Wise was a trained phonetician and he noticed that, after a few days, he was able to produce nasal consonants indistinguishable from his normally produced nasals. His phonetician colleagues who visited him were also surprised at his ability to produce such good nasals. Wise speculates that the nasal resonances may in fact be nasopharyngeal resonances. In fact this speculation is almost certainly wrong, as attested to by the experiments of Hattori *et al.* (1958) on nasalized vowels. It seems likely that Wise was making compensatory articulations to produce signals similar to those he would normally have produced for the nasals.

B. Articulators in the Same Position with the Signal Varying

We have already noted that this type of variation arises when the medium of transmission is changed or when considering the speech of different speakers. The medium of transmission can be changed by introducing gases of different densities into the vocal tract or by transmission to a listener over a man-made transmission device (e.g. a telephone).

One gas which is different in density from air is helium. The effect on intelligibility of speaking in a helium atmosphere has been studied because of its practical importance. Deep-sea divers must breathe oxy-helium mixtures yet still need to be in spoken communication with operatives on the water surface. Hence it is important to ascertain what effect on intelligibility the oxy-helium atmosphere has.

Helium changes the characteristics of the acoustic signal because the formant frequencies of the vocal tract are determined by the velocity of sound within them. This velocity is faster in less dense helium than in normal air. The vocal fold abduction/adduction which gives the pitch (Fo) of speech sounds is unaffected by the atmosphere. The net result is that the formants and inter-formant spacing are increased but the pitch of the sound is unchanged (Beil, 1962). Despite these distortions on the speech signal, helium speech is still quite intelligible.

Another example of this type of variation is provided by transmission of a signal through a telephone system. Once again this has been studied because of its practical importance. Transmitting the signal is an expensive business and telephone companies do not want to transmit frequencies which do not add anything to the intelligibility of the message. Although certain frequencies are lost from the signal, intelligibility is not seriously impaired.

Though we include intra-speaker variation as a further instance of variation in the speech signal without corresponding changes in the positioning of the articulators we cannot definitely say whether all speakers articulate a phoneme in exactly the same way. Even if it were the case that speakers produce sounds by positioning the articulators in corresponding positions, acoustic variability would be observed in the signal because of the variability in vocal tract size and in vocal fold length and thickness.

To illustrate how the formant frequencies vary when the dimensions of the vocal tract change, consider the schwa vowel (/ə/). This vowel is usually modelled by the formulae for an open tube with constant cross-sectional area. The first resonant frequency of such a tube is:

$$F1 = c/2L$$

where c = velocity of sound in air.
L = length of tube.
The higher resonant frequencies are given by:

$$Fn = (2n - 1) F1$$

where n is a positive integer.
The inverse relationship with L indicates that the formant frequencies will increase with shortening of the vocal tract and since the higher formant frequencies are a function of $F1$, the separation between the formants increases too.

This example illustrates why the formant frequencies of /ə/ are not constant across speakers. Similar considerations apply to all the other vowels as illustrated by the production data of, for example, Potter and Steinberg (1950). Plotting their measurements of $F1$ against $F2$ for vowels produced by different speakers reveals that the different vowels overlap to a considerable extent. Thus the vowels are confusable with respect to these parameters. A point worth noting is that the vowels do not overlap in a single speaker's speech so there is no confusion if the listener can identify the speaker.

C. Variation in Both Articulator Positioning and the Signal

All covariation between articulation and the resulting signal can be considered as instances of coarticulation. Coarticulation has been defined as ". . . the influence of one speech segment upon another; that is, the influence of a phonetic context upon a given segment" (Daniloff and Hammarberg, 1973, p. 239).

Though in Section II.A we pointed out that different articulatory positions can have the same acoustic output, this is generally not the case. Usually, different articulatory positions have signals with different acoustic characteristics associated with them. Hence, when a speaker is articulating a string of phonemes, he has to move his articulators through a variety of articulatory configurations, each of which will have a different signal associated with it. Since excitation of the vocal tract is applied continuously over adjacent phonemes, the signal changes as the intermediary positions are passed through. Though all workers have accepted that articulation and the signal for a phoneme vary with context, early workers denied that the control instructions to move the articulators vary. They claimed that mechanical effects and overlapping of commands can explain all of the observed variation in the speech signal.

For example, since the articulators vary in their masses and in the number and properties of the muscles attached to them, they also differ in their inertial properties. Because of these differences in the inertial properties, articulatory variability might be observed because some articulators are heavier than others so they take longer to get in and out of position. When speakers speak at different rates, the same commands could still be issued to the articulators but these would need to be interleaved to a greater or lesser extent.

In the early theories of speech production, these two principles – inertia and overlap of commands – were thought sufficient to explain all coarticulatory phenomena. Such an account is appealing because it offers a simple account of speech production. Moreover the claim that constant commands are issued to the articulators takes on an additional importance because it would then be possible for this invariant to be used in perceiving speech (see Section III.B.1).

However, the evidence renders such a position untenable. On the one hand, all instances of coarticulation cannot be explained in terms of inertia and overlap. We distinguish what we call phoneme sequencing from other instances of coarticulation. A good case can be made that phoneme sequencing can be accounted for by the inertial properties of the articulators and overlapping of the control instructions but this position cannot be sustained for other instances of coarticulation.

We shall first review evidence showing that all coarticulation cannot be accounted for in terms of inertia. This still leaves the possibility that whatever articulatory specifications are made they are overlapped in a fairly simple way when speech is spoken at different rates. So we shall then review findings that demonstrate speech undergoes complex restructuring when it is spoken at different rates. Thus the second principle accounting for the lack of articulatory-phonetic invariance is also shown to be inappropriate.

Consider first the acoustic variation that occurs when an articulator has to be positioned differently for the production of adjacent segments (phoneme sequencing). The type of variability that arises here can be illustrated by considering the "locus" theory of stop consonant production which was developed to explain the acoustic variation observed with each of the stop consonants when they are spoken in different vowel contexts (Delattre *et al.*, 1955). The main assumption in the theory is that the speaker moves his articulators from the position specified for one phoneme to that of the next.†
The acoustic signal varies as the vocal tract changes shape provided that the

---

† The assumption of independence or lack of it is concerned with mechanisms within the individual and not those concerning evolutionary development.

vocal tract stays sufficiently open for the signal to be transmitted. For utterances starting from a given articulatory position, signal variability arises because the articulators have to pass through different intermediary positions to reach the different target positions. For example, the articulatory gesture for /d/ starts with closure in the vocal tract at the alveolar ridge irrespective of the following vowel. At closure no sound emerges. As the tongue is released it follows a trajectory towards the vowel configuration. The resulting formant movements are illustrated schematically in Fig. 2. Since it is reasonable to suppose that when an articulator has different positions specified on adjacent segments the movement is limited by the inertia of the articulators, this variability in the signal is not inconsistent with fixed commands being issued for each of the phonemes. However, such an account does not appear to explain all coarticulation. As one example of coarticulation which is difficult to reconcile with the assumption that the same commands are issued to the articulators whatever context the phoneme occurs in, consider the syllable /stru/ (Daniloff and Moll, 1968). In this syllable, the lips round at the phoneme /s/ and remain rounded in anticipation of the vowel which does not occur until three phonemes later. This lip rounding affects the acoustic output too. The differences in the phoneme /s/ in the syllables /si/ and /su/ can be detected on close listening. The /s/ in /su/ is produced with lip rounding as in /stru/ while that in /si/ is not. In this example, coarticulation occurs over three phonemes and has been observed over as many as seven phonemes. It seems unreasonable to argue that inertial effects could operate over time intervals of this length.

Investigations of speech spoken at different rates show that speakers restructure their articulations in a complex way. If speakers issue the same commands whatever rate the speech is spoken at, then articulators would undershoot their targets at fast rates (Lindblom, 1963). Undershoot of the tongue occurs for vowels (Lindblom, 1963) and undershoot of the velum for consonants (Kent *et al.*, 1974). However, speakers change the velocity of the lips (Gay and Hirose, 1973; Gay *et al.*, 1974) and mandible (Abbs, 1973) to minimize such undershoot. Thus increased speaking rate does not just lead to an overlapping of the same commands. The commands are changed in a variety of different ways so that the whole command sequence is restructured at different rates.

III. Proposed Solutions to Problems of Equivalence

We have discussed three types of phenomena – those concerning variation only in the way the signal is produced, those concerning variation in the signal alone and those concerning variation in both. We have pointed out that, in general, theories of perception have been concerned with the second and third of these and theories of production with the first and third of them. Typically, though, theories restricted to one explanatory domain have made

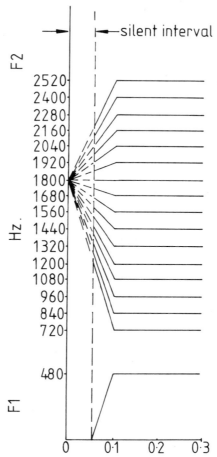

FIG. 2. Schematic spectrograms indicating the expected formant frequencies of the consonant /d/ before different vowels predicted from the locus theory of stop consonant production (Delattre *et al.*, 1955). The point where the *F*2 transitions intersect is the locus frequency of the stop consonant. The formant transitions are not observed in real spectrograms until the vocal tract is sufficiently open to transmit the signal (represented by the solid lines).

assumptions that are difficult to reconcile with both the theories and phenomena in the other domain. It is no use explaining perceptual equivalence by appealing to production constancies that will not explain motor equivalence or to account for motor equivalence by referring to perceptual constancies that do not fit with perceptual data.

General theories of speech processing (i.e. those concerned with both perception and production) have tackled problems of equivalence in one of two ways. First, we shall consider those theories that regard perception and production as independent processes, each of which may take advantage of some central representation common to them both. Second we shall discuss theories where problems of equivalence for one process (e.g. production) are solved within its own explanatory domain, and problems for the other (e.g. perception) are dealt with by referring them to that solution.

A. Perception and Production as Independent Processes

Invariant relations for particular phonemes may be in the speech signal as a consequence of how it is produced. These relations may then be retrieved during perception without any reference to their means of production.

1. Template models

It has been proposed that there are unique patterns (templates) associated with each of the phonemes. Perception then takes place by matching input directly to a set of these templates, production by activating a set of them which then specify all aspects of output. Wickelgren's (1969) context-sensitive allophone theory is an example of this type of model. He argued that although the acoustic properties of a phoneme vary with context (see Section II.C), there are only about 10^6 permissible interfaces between phoneme segments. There might be a template for every context a phoneme occurs in. Wickelgren considers that this is not an unreasonably large number of representations to be held in memory and input could be matched against the representations or they could be strung together to produce a message in the manner just outlined. Although Wickelgren (1969) originally formulated his theory as a model for production, he has recently argued that templates may also be involved in (apparently independent) perceptual processing. As a theory of production, it provides a satisfactory account of how phonemes could be sequenced. However, it fails to explain the other types of variation outlined in Section II.C (those associated with other types of coarticulation and with differences in speech rate). These problems could be circumvented by proposing more and more templates but such a solution would render the theory even less parsimonious. Extending the theory to perception only serves to increase these problems for still more templates would be required to provide a satisfactory account of the sources of variation outlined in Section II.B (e.g. that arising from differences in the size and shape of different speakers' vocal tracts).

2. Feature models

According to feature models, the invariant relations between linguistic segments and the speech signal are represented as sets of features. These features may be used to specify control parameters for production and be extracted from the signal during perception. The perceptual advantages of this more abstract mode of representation over that provided by templates has been discussed by a number of authors (e.g. Neisser, 1967).

Stevens (1972, 1981), Stevens and Blumstein (1975) and Stevens and Perkell (1977) have argued that features are not specific to speech. Speech did not appear spontaneously independent of other systems but evolved to take advantage of certain properties of the productive and perceptual systems. In his production theory, for example, Stevens (1972) argues that there are certain quantal regions of the vocal tract within which articulatory variation produces little or no effect on acoustic output. Use of these areas enables constant and predictable signals to be emitted with relative ease. For example, Stevens (1972) calculated that the vowel /i/ shows small changes in acoustic output with changes in the point of tongue constriction. Stevens went on to show that the other point vowels (/u/ and /a/) are acoustically stable too. Recently, Stevens (1981) has argued that the particular sensitivities of the auditory system have been taken into account during the evolution of speech perception. Thus, sounds that the auditory system responds to in a similar manner tend to have the same phonological function.

There are several objections which can be raised concerning Steven's theory of speech production. First, though there may be acoustically stable regions in a speaker's vocal tract, we saw in Section II.C that a speaker does not always use the articulatory configurations which would allow him to exploit them (Riordan, 1977; Lindblom et al., 1979). Second, although vocal tract surgery would remove the stable regions of the vocal tract, patients do regain intelligible speech after such operations (Fourcin, 1974). Finally, the theory does not provide a rationale for how distinctions cued by the rate of articulatory movement (e.g. /ba – wa/) could arise. The same acoustically stable regions might be used at the start and end of the utterance but an additional factor would be required to account for the evolution of such rate-cued distinctions.

The two lines of evidence that can be regarded as support for Stevens' perceptual model concern categorical perception. This term refers to phenomena first observed in the identification and discrimination of speech sounds. If listeners are asked to identify speech stimuli along certain continua (e.g. voice onset time, VOT), their categorizations change sharply from one category to another. A range of stimuli are clearly heard as one phoneme and then there is an abrupt change to hearing the phoneme in the adjacent category. Furthermore, two stimuli given the same phoneme label in identification experiments are discriminated at chance level but two stimuli with the same physical difference given different phoneme labels are discriminated well. Within category discrimination is at chance level but there is a discrimination peak at the same position on the continuum as the point of abrupt changeover in the identification function. These characteristics of categorical perception are illustrated in Fig. 3. Stevens' view is consistent with experiments showing categorical perception of non-speech continua by humans and with the perception of speech continua by non-

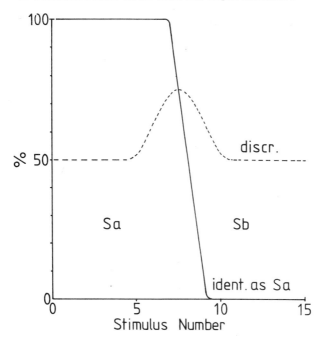

FIG. 3. Idealized results for a categorically perceived continuum, the three features to note are: (a) the sharp identification function; (b) chance discrimination performance within phoneme categories; (c) a peak in the discrimination function at the point of changeover in the identification function.

humans. He interprets these findings as showing that there are regions on some continua in which the mammalian auditory system is highly sensitive.

Do these reports of categorical perception really provide evidence for auditory features? There are reasons to doubt some of the results. For example, Cutting and Rosner (1974) found that non-speech sounds varying in rise time were identified (as sounding like a plucked or a bowed string) and discriminated in the way that is held to be evidence for categorical perception. Rosen and Howell (1981) failed to find the mid-continuum peak in the discrimination function that Cutting and Rosner did. Instead subjects were best at discriminating sounds at the pluck end of the continuum and became gradually worse as stimuli were drawn from nearer the "bow" end. On rerunning the experiment with Cutting and Rosner's original stimuli, the mid-continuum discrimination peak appeared. Measurements of Cutting and Rosner's stimuli, however, showed them to be non-uniformly spaced along the rise time continuum (i.e. there was a relatively broad spacing of stimuli in the centre of the continuum) which was responsible for the original results. Despite doubt that these particular non-speech stimuli show categorical perception, categorical perception has been reported with two relative onset time continua (Miller *et al.*, 1976; Pisoni, 1977). However, it appears to be restricted to non-speech dimensions of this type. Moreover, Summerfield (1982) has questioned whether perception of such non-speech continua is analogous to their supposed VOT analogues. His experiments show that while speech VOT continua show shifts in their category boundaries as a result of shifts in their first formant onset frequencies, non-speech VOT analogues do not show similar shifts when their analogous "first formant" onset frequencies are shifted.

In fact there are other fundamental reasons to be dissatisfied with the suggestion that these categorical perception effects provide evidence for auditory features. The phenomena may in no way reflect the natural auditory sensitivities that, according to Stevens, were exploited during the evolution of speech. Were it the case that they did so, then they would be invariant and phoneme boundaries would be immutable. Unfortunately for the theory, they are not. They vary across languages (Abramson and Lisker, 1970) and speaking rates (Summerfield and Haggard, 1972), and are subject to range/frequency effects. These effects, familiar to psychophysicists, demonstrate that the context within which a stimulus occurs influences the decision about the category to which it belongs. For example, if a listener is presented with a tone at some particular frequency it may be judged as "low" when it is paired with relatively high frequency sounds but as "high" when paired with relatively low frequency ones (range effect). Also subjects tend to place equal numbers of stimuli in each category and so adjacent stimuli that are presented relatively frequently tend to be allocated a relatively wide range of categories (frequency effect). Although Eimas and Miller (1978) and Strange and Broen (1980) have asserted that range/frequency effects do not occur in the judgment of stop consonants, Rosen (1979) has reported both range and frequency effects in the perception of stop consonants varying in place of articulation while Brady and Darwin (1978) have reported a range effect in the perception of VOT continua. Range and frequency effects provide further demonstrations that category boundaries are not fixed.

The evidence from animals does not provide unequivocal support for the notion of natural auditory sensitivities. First, Kuhl and Miller (1975) did not demonstrate discrimination peaks, but only sharp categorization functions which corresponded with those found for English-speaking humans. Second, animals show range/frequency effects on speech continua like the humans (Waters and Wilson, 1976). This finding indicates that if the animals are perceiving like humans, it is not because of either's sensitivity to the auditory contrast.

B. Non-independence of Perception and Production

The theories we have just discussed treat perception and production independently. The perceptual process does not use information about or employ mechanisms connected with the production process and neither does production take perception into account. We have seen that there are a number of problems with theories that have taken this approach.

An alternative view is that the problems of equivalence can be solved within one of these areas and that the problems in the other area can be referred to that solution. Nooteboom (1970), for example, has suggested that auditory targets provide the constant reference necessary to account for motor equivalence in production. The most detailed theories, however, argue in the opposite direction. Problems of motor equivalence are solved within the production system and problems of perceptual equivalence are referred to that solution. We shall consider two theories of this type – motor theory and action theory.

1. *Motor theory*

According to motor theory (Liberman *et al.*, 1967) there is a constant one-to-one mapping between phonemes and sets of categories of myomotor commands responsible for their production. Output variability could arise because different inertial effects occur at the periphery when these commands are executed in different sequences and at different rates as described in Section II.C. Because the constant set of commands associated with a particular phoneme is retrieved during perception the problems of both perceptual equivalence and categorical perception can be explained. A speech sound can be identified as an instance of a particular phoneme by reference to the constant myomotor commands responsible for production of that phoneme in all contexts. Perception of speech may be categorical because the hearer only has available what he can produce and production occurs by reference to constant categories of myomotor commands.

Motor theory attempted to explain something about which very little was known (i.e. speech perception) in terms of something else about which even less was known (i.e. speech production). The problems associated with it are legion. They may be conveniently summarized in terms of the three types of variation we outlined above. First, the assumption of constancy in production is untenable. We saw in Section II.A that articulatory positioning may vary even when the output signal is constant. Also it is difficult to account for how the articulatory reorganization required to produce adequate output after vocal tract surgery takes place if the old inappropriate commands provide the only basis on which it can occur (Fourcin, 1974). Second, the perceiver may be able to understand without being able to emulate what he is hearing (Section II.B). A perceiver cannot produce in air a sound that corresponds to speech transmitted in helium and yet the helium speech may be understood without experience of speaking in that medium. Similarly, it is possible to understand individuals of a different age and sex or with some pathological condition even though it is not possible to speak using their vocal tracts. Even individuals who are congenitally unable to speak can perceive speech (Fourcin, 1975). Third, when variation in the speech signal and its means of production do occur together (Section II.C), they do not appear to do so in the manner required by motor theory. In order for motor commands to be used for perception, the commands responsible for a particular segment must be constant despite variation in segmental and suprasegmental context. Any variation in the output signal must arise because of influence at the periphery. However, it is very difficult to support the claim that all the variability within the speech of a single individual is caused by articulatory inertia or command overlap. Hence the muscle commands giving rise to such movement must be reorganized. For instance, an inertia account of all anticipatory coarticulation is, as we mentioned above, very difficult to sustain. Various other accounts of it are more credible – it may serve to make execution easier for the speaker (Henke, 1966; Perkell, 1980) or even be planned to provide the listener with advance cues about forthcoming segments (MacNeilage, 1972; Daniloff and Hammarberg, 1973). That all variability in articulator positioning is not caused by inertia is reinforced by EMG measurements. They have shown that muscle activity does not stay the same as context changes. EMG activity associated with stop consonant and vowel production varies with preceding and following segmental context (Fromkin, 1966; Lubker, 1968; MacNeilage and De Clerk, 1969).

The final piece of evidence we will present concerning the covariation between speech production and speech perception has been conducted on French–English bilinguals (Caramazza et al., 1973). We mentioned above that VOT varies in different languages (Abramson and Lisker, 1970). If speakers are truly bilingual they should produce different VOTs in different languages. Perception by reference to how the speech was produced should lead to different perceptual boundaries in the two languages. Caramazza et al. (1973) found two distributions of VOT in the speech of French–English bilinguals which corresponded to the respective boundaries of French or English unilingual speakers. The unilingual speakers had different perceptual boundaries but the bilinguals had only one perceptual boundary whichever language context they were tested in. Moreover the perceptual boundary did not correspond to either unilingual boundary but was intermediate between them. Thus, though these speakers appear to have two sets of language commands, perception is not referred to either.

2. Action theory
Action theory is a general theory that has aroused much interest recently in all areas of motor control. Following Easton (1972), Turvey and his associates argue that muscles are inherently organized into systems (co-ordinative structures) that reduce the number of individual muscles that have to be controlled during performance (Turvey, 1977; Turvey, et al., 1978). Coordinative structures may be expressed as mapping rules that relate activity in different muscles. Thus, for example, the activity (P) of one muscle may be related to that (Q) of another according to the rule $P = KQ$, where K is a parameter. After a particular coordinative structure is specified as output, tuning to different execution contexts (e.g. jaw constraint) is

carried out automatically. This tuning varies the activity of different muscles within the specified invariant relationship. Thus, if the activity P is affected by external constraints, Q automatically assumes the value that is necessary to keep the invariant ratio, K. Automatic tuning at the periphery is possible because specification of a coordinative structure physically yokes muscles together so that they are organized as "a vibratory system – that is, a system with an intrinsic goal which it attains from any starting point by virtue of its dynamic configuration".

Action theory can be directly applied to both the production (Fowler *et al.*, 1980) and perception (Tuller and Fowler, 1980) of speech. Perception is not referred to invariant motor commands but the coordinated movement of the articulators as reflected in the speech signal. It then becomes, like motor theory, a production-based model designed to account for both perceptual and motor equivalence. However, relative to motor theory, the production side of the model is filled out in greater detail and so some discussion of this aspect of it is appropriate here. The requirement to produce a particular linguistic segment results in specification of the coordinative structures subserving it. This specification may involve setting various modulable parameters within each coordinative structure. The effect of this would be to alter the invariant relationship between the activity of the muscle groups involved in performance. Thus in the above example, the activity (P) of one muscle group would be related to that (Q) of the other muscle group by a new value of the parameter K. Automatic tuning would still be carried out during execution but would be directed to reaching this new value of K. Thus the speaker controls the parameters of the equations of constraint between muscle groups rather than controlling the muscles directly as assumed by motor theory.

One function of parameter setting is to allow variation in the way a particular segment is produced. Another function is to distinguish different segments that activate the same coordinative structures. During speech planning, fine-grained coordinative structures, corresponding to relatively short segments, are functionally embedded within coarser grained ones, corresponding to larger segments. This nesting is a top-down process whereby "the more coarse-grained levels are established by altering the relationships among smaller coordinative structures". The constraints on possible movements that are specified by coordinative structures correspond not only to linguistic segments but also to (fairly abstract) acoustic patterns. Thus, during the perceptual extraction of linguistic segments from acoustic patterns, knowledge about execution constraints may be used to delimit the class of possible input patterns.

Action theory is rich but not powerful. It provides a number of possible mechanisms for accounting for variation in speech production but does not specify when one is appropriate and not another. Consider, for instance, variation in the means of production of a constant signal (Section II.A). This could occur because of differences in the way coordinative structures are functionally embedded during speech planning. Alternatively, it could occur because of the operation of the peripheral tuning mechanisms during execution. Certain types of covariation in the signal and its means of production (Section II.C) can be explained in terms of speech planning or speech execution – phoneme sequencing is a case in point.

Anticipatory coarticulation across a number of phonemes is, on the other hand, unlkely to be due to compensation during execution. It must therefore show evidence of a coarse-grained coordinative structure stretching across the intervening phonemes. Is it reasonable to talk of a segment of such a size being controlled as an open-loop vibratory system? If it is and if it is correct to assume that gestures are only spread when they do not change the phonetic identity of intervening segments, then there must be a check during planning to determine whether or not such a change would occur. Such a check would require reference to perception because languages vary in the articulatory gestures that are distinctive.

When considering perception it is not clear how the theory deals with the type of variation discussed in Section II.C. If perception *requires* reference to the invariants used in production, how can we perceive a signal that we cannot produce (because we do not have the appropriate vocal tract)? One possible answer is that higher-order invariants that are appropriate to many speakers can be extracted from the various lower-order invariants appropriate to our own vocal tract at different stages of growth (Shankweiler, *et al.*, 1979). However, this would not provide an obvious explanation for the perception of speech emanating from abnormal vocal tracts or of speech that no one could produce (i.e. speech distorted by helium transmission or other means). If the weaker suggestion (not favoured by the action theorists themselves) is that perception does not require, but can be *influenced* by, reference to the invariants used in production, the problem becomes one of demonstrating that influence. A number of phenomena may be regarded as doing so. First, no sound is emitted when the vocal tract is completely occluded and use of this articulatory information in perception may explain why silence can be perceived as a stop consonant (Bailey and Summerfield, 1980). Second, both bursts and formant transitions occur during the production of stop consonants and this may explain why such markedly different acoustic cues result in the same percept and can be traded off against one another (Fitch *et al.*, 1980). Third, CV syllables are produced in such a way that extra cues to the vowel are present which are absent when the vowel is produced alone and use of this articulatory information may explain why identification of vowels is better in consonant contexts than in isolation (Shankweiler *et al.*, 1976). While this effect like the previous two, is consistent with the use of articulatory knowledge during perception, it would be rash to take it as positive support. In fact, Howell (1981) has found that not only a consonantal context that provides no information about the vowel but also a non-speech context (a 1 kHz tone) improve vowel identification over that obtained with no context.

Since action theory shares the assumption that perception is not independent of production, the study on bilinguals by Caramazza *et al.*, (1973) poses problems for action theory too. In addition, the specific proposals that muscles operate as coordinated structures and that perception uses knowledge of their operation do not fit with some perceptual data. The data come from a developmental study of VOT perception. VOT involves several changes in the acoustic signal as well as the onset of voicing. For example, transitions of the first formant are seen clearly in spectrograms of voiced stops but are less clear or even absent for the voiceless stops. First formant transitions might be an additional cue to the voiced–voiceless distinction. Simon and Fourcin (1978) found that English children are not able to make use of this cue until the age of 5 years old. This work raises problems about whether knowledge of the operation of coordinative structures is used during perception since it indicates that perception develops with knowledge of the language. Knowledge of coordinating structures cannot, however, be acquired bit-by-bit.

In sum, the extent and means of incorporation of articulatory information into the speech perception process is still an issue for debate.

IV. The State of Play: Summary and Assessment

We have observed that there are three classes of phenomena when a speaker decides to produce a particular segment:
  (1)   There is articulatory variability for the same acoustic output.
  (2)   The same articulation can give rise to different acoustic outputs.
  (3)   The articulation and acoustic output vary when the speaker is producing the same segment.
We have posed two problems to be solved: how does a listener determine that different acoustic patterns are perceptually equivalent and what is the basis of motor equivalence?

The theories we have discussed commended themselves to us because they do not simply use production invariants to "explain" perception or perceptual invariants to "explain" production but offer some explanation of the phenomena in the unexplained domain too. In this final section, we want to summarize general issues raised by the different theoretical approaches and point to some problems that we consider have received insufficient attention.

We will first consider a general issue which has been raised with respect to the perceptual theories we have discussed. Motor theory and action theory require a mechanism which is specialized for the perception of speech sounds, the former by reference to constant motor commands, the latter through knowledge of what movements the articulators can make. This issue has been a matter of debate for some years. At present the need for such a specialized mechanism has been called into question by the two experimental findings Stevens uses to support his theory – categorical perception by humans on non-speech continua and categorical perception of speech by animals. Recollect that categorical perception refers to the phenomena observed in the identification *and* discrimination of some speech sounds and illustrated in Fig. 3 and which were originally thought to be peculiar to speech. Several questions remain to be solved concerning the findings on categorical perception that call into question the status of a specialized speech decoder.

First, since the only demonstrations of categorical perception with non-speech are restricted to relative-onset time continua, should they be regarded as oddities? In contrast to non-speech continua, it is widely considered that categorical perception is commonly found with speech sounds. Though categorical perception may not be exclusive to speech it may be more typical. Hence the findings on non-speech need not be damaging for the hypothesis of a specialized processing mechanism for speech. Summerfield's demonstration that categorically-perceived non-speech continua are not sensitive to the same type of variation as their supposed speech analogues might suggest that categorical perception on such non-speech continua is fortuitous. Further demonstrations of categorical perception on non-speech continua or delimiting the circumstances under which it occurs for speech would clarify whether speech is or is not perceived by a specialized mechanism. With respect to categorical perception on speech continua it is surprising that demonstrations are restricted to a limited number of speech cues (formant transition cued series in particular).

The claim that non-speech continua are categorically perceived by humans and demonstrations of categorical perception on speech continua by animals raises many questions. For example, there is the general question of why phoneme boundaries are not fixed. Why do chinchillas show phoneme boundaries at the same value as English speakers on VOT continua when phoneme boundaries in different languages occur at different values of VOT? If listeners are sensitive to specific auditory values how can speech be perceived when the auditory properties change as a function of rate and stress? The omission of discrimination tests with animals further limits the claim that animals perceive speech categorically. The sharp categorization function in itself is not sufficient to claim "categorical perception".

The questions we have posed concerning these recent demonstrations of categorical perception do not imply that we consider there is firm evidence for a specialized speech processor. Aside from the phenomena of categorical perception, much of the evidence for a specialized speech decoder is of a negative nature. For example, it is only by ruling out other explanations that workers have supported the claim that the superior identification of vowels in consonant necessitates articulatory knowledge being used during perception.

We have presented the study of Caramazza *et al.* (1973) as a demonstration that perception does not depend on production. This is an important study from our perspective because such studies demonstrate which of the two approaches to the questions of perceptual and motor equivalence is preferable. Other approaches to the question of the independence or interdependence of the two domains are needed but those we examined are fraught with more serious difficulties than the bilingual work. For example this question might be approached from a developmental viewpoint. Menyuk and Anderson (1969) demonstrated that children can identify minimal word pairs like light-white or white-write better than they can speak them. This study would appear to indicate that perception develops before production and presumably independently of production. However, Strange and Broen (1980) demonstrate that the findings made depend largely on how perception and production are assessed. If these methodological issues can be resolved such studies would offer a promising way of testing whether perception develops in concert with production.

In the area of speech production, action theory offers some promise. Besides addressing the problems we have posed these theorists are also trying to tackle the question of how the brain can control the vast number of muscles involved in each articulation. The deficiency of this approach is that to date there is little experimental support or tests trying to discriminate between action theory and other theories. It is clear that many questions about speech perception, speech production and their inter-relation remain.

Acknowledgement

Both authors are supported by grant G 979/647/N from the M.R.C. The co-operation of Stuart Rosen and Michael Ashby is gratefully acknowledged.

References

Abbs, J. H. (1973). The influence of the gamma motor system on jaw movements during speech: A theoretical framework and some preliminary observations. *Journal of Speech and Hearing Research*, **16**, 175–200.

Abramson, A. S. and Lisker, L. (1970). Discriminability along the voicing continuum: Cross language tests. *Proceedings of the 6th International Congress Phonetic Sciences, Prague, 1970*, pp. 569–573.

Bailey, P. J. and Summerfield, Q. (1980). Information in speech: Observations of [s] – Stop Clusters. *Journal of Experimental Psychology: Human Perception and Performance* **6**, 536–563.

Beil, R. G. (1962). Frequency analysis of vowels produced in a helium-rich atmosphere. *Journal of the Acoustical Society of America*, **34**, 347–349.

Bjork, L. (1961). Velopharyngeal function in connected speech. *Acta Radiologica Supplement* No. 202.

Brady, S. A. and Darwin, C. J. (1978). Range effect in the perception of voicing. *Journal of the Acoustical Society of America*, **63**, 1556–1558.

Caramazza, A., Yeni-Komshian, G. H., Zurif, E. B. and Carbone, E. (1973). The acquisition of a new phonological contrast: The case of stop consonants in French–English bilinguals. *Journal of the Acoustical Society of America*, **54**, 421–428.

Cutting, J. E. and Rosner, B. S. (1974). Categories and boundaries in speech and music. *Perception and Psychophysics*, **16**, 564–570.

Daniloff, R. G. and Hammarberg, R. E. (1973). On defining coarticulation. *Journal of Phonetics*, **1**, 239–248.

Daniloff, R. and Moll, K. (1968). Coarticulation of lip rounding. *Journal of Speech and Hearing Research*, **11**, 707–721.

Delattre, P. C., Liberman, A. M. and Cooper, F. S. (1955). Acoustic loci and transitional cues for consonants. *Journal of the Acoustical Society of America*, **27**, 769–773.

Easton, T. A. (1972). On the normal use of reflexes. *American Scientist*, **60**, 591–599.

Eimas, P. D. and Miller, J. L. (1978). Effects of selective adaptation on the perception of speech and visual patterns: Evidence for feature detectors. *In* "Perception and Experience", (R. D. Walk and H. L. Pick, eds). Plenum, New York.

Fitch, H. L., Halwes, T., Erickson, D. M., and Liberman, A. M. (1980). Perceptual equivalence of two acoustic cues for stop-consonant manner. *Perception and Psychophysics*, **27**, 343–350.

Fourcin, A. J. (1974). Laryngographic examination of vocal fold vibration. *In* "Ventilatory and Phonatory Control Systems", (B. Wyke, ed.) Oxford University Press, Oxford.

Fourcin, A. J. (1975). Speech perception in the absence of speech productive ability. *In* "Language, Cognitive Deficits, and Retardation", (N. O'Connor, ed.) Butterworths, London.

Fowler, C. A., Rubin, P., Remez, R. E. and Turvey, M. T. (1980). Implications for speech production of a general theory of action. *In* "Language Production", (B. Butterworth, ed.), Vol. 1. Academic Press, London and New York.

Fromkin, V. A. (1966). Neuromuscular specification of linguistic units. *Language and Speech*, **9**, 170–199.

Gay, T. and Hirose, H. (1973). Effect of speaking rate on labial consonant production. *Phonetica*, **27**, 44–56.

Gay, T., Ushijima, T., Hirose, H. and Cooper, F. S. (1974). Effect of speaking rate on labial consonant-vowel articulation. *Journal of Phonetics*, **2**, 47–63.

Hattori, S., Yamamoto, K. and Fujimura, O. (1958). Nasalization of vowels in relation to nasals. *Journal of the Acoustical Society of America*, **30**, 267–274.

Henke, W. L. (1966). Dynamic articulatory model of speech production using computer simulation. Doctoral dissertation, M.I.T.

Howell, P. (1981). Identification of vowels in and out of context. *Journal of the Acoustical Society of America*, **70**, 1256–1260.

Kent, R. D., Carney, P. J. and Severeid, L. R. (1974). Velar coarticulation and timing: Evaluation of a model for binary control. *Journal of Speech and Hearing Research*, **17**, 470–488.

Kuhl, P. K. and Miller, J. D. (1975). Speech perception by the chinchilla: Voiced-voiceless distinction in alveolar plosive consonants. *Science*, **190**, 69–72.

Ladefoged, P., DeClerk, J. L., Papcun, G. and Lindau, M. (1972). An auditory-motor theory of speech production. *Working papers in Phonetics*, No. 22, 48–75. U.C.L.A. Linguistics Department, Los Angeles.

Lehiste, I. (1970). "Suprasegmentals". MIT Press, Cambridge, Massachusetts.

Liberman, A. M., Cooper, F. S., Shankweiler, D. P. and Studdert-Kennedy, M. (1967). Perception of the speech code. *Psychological Review*, **74**, 431–461.

Liberman, A. M. and Studdert-Kennedy, M. (1978). Phonetic perception. *In* "Handbook of Sensory Physiology", (R. Held, H. Leibowitz and H.-L. Teuber, eds). Vol. VIII. Springer-Verlag, Heidelberg.

Lindblom, B. Spectrographic study of vowel reduction. (1963). *Journal of the Acoustical Society of America*, **35**, 1773–1781.

Lindblom, B. E. F., Lubker, J. and Gay, T. (1978). Formant frequencies of some fixed-mandible vowels and a model of speech motor programming by predictive simulation. *Journal of Phonetics*, **7**, 147–162.

Lubker, J. F. (1968). An electromyographic-cinefluorographic study of velar function during normal speech production. *The Cleft Palate Journal*, **5**, 1–17.

MacNeilage, P. F. (1972). Speech physiology. *In* "Speech and Cortical Functioning", (J. H. Gilbert, ed.) pp. 1–72. Academic Press, New York and London.

MacNeilage, P. F. and De Clerk, J. L. (1969). On the motor control of coarticulation in CVC monosyllables. *Journal of the Acoustical Society of America*, **45**, 1217–1233.

Menyuk, P. and Anderson, S. (1969). Children's identification and reproduction of /w/, /r/, and /l/. *Journal of Speech and Hearing Research*, **12**, 39–52.

Miller, J. D., Wier, C. C., Pastore, R. E., Kelly, W. J. and Dooling, R. J. (1976). Discrimination and labelling of noise-buzz sequences with varying noise lead times: An example of categorical perception. *Journal of the Acoustical Society of America*, **60**, 410–417.

Neisser, V. (1967). "Cognitive Psychology". Appleton, New York.

Nooteboom, S. G. (1970). The target theory of speech production. *I.P.O. Annual Progress Report*, No. 5, 51–53. Institute for Perception Research, Eindhoven: Holland.

Perkell, J. S. (1980). Phonetic features and the physiology of speech production. *In* "Language Production", (B. Butterworth, ed.), Vol. 1, pp. 337–372. Academic Press, London and New York.

Pisoni, D. B. (1977). Identification and discrimination of the relative onset time of two component tones: Implications for voicing perception in stops. *Journal of the Acoustical Society of America*, **61**, 1352–1361.

Potter, R. K. and Steinberg, J. C. (1950). Towards the specification of speech. *Journal of the Acoustical Society of America*, **22**, 807–820.

Riordan, C. J. (1977). Control of vocal-tract length in speech. *Journal of the Acoustical Society of America*, **62**, 998–1002.

Rosen, S. M. (1979). Range and frequency effects in consonant categorization. *Journal of Phonetics*, **7**, 393–402.

Rosen, S. M. (1979). Range effects as obstacles in the search for natural sensitivities. *In* "The Cognitive Representation of Speech", (T. Myers, J. Laver and J. Anderson, eds). North-Holland, Amsterdam.

Rosen, S. M. and Howell, P. (1981). Plucks and bows are not categorically perceived. *Perception & Psychophysics*, **30**, 156–168.

Shankweiler, D., Strange, W. and Verbrugge, R. R. (1979). Speech and the problem of perceptual constancy. *In* "Perceiving, Acting, and Knowing", (R. Shaw and J. Bransford, eds). Erlbaum, Hillsdale, New Jersey.

Simon, C. and Fourcin, A. J. (1978). Cross-language study of speech-pattern learning. *Journal of the Acoustical Society of America*, **63**, 925–935.

Stevens, K. N. (1972). The quantal nature of speech: Evidence from articulatory-acoustic data. *In* "Human Communication. A Unified View", (P. B. Denes and E. E. David, eds). McGraw-Hill, New York.

Stevens, K. N. (1981). Constraints imposed by the auditory system on the properties of speech sounds: Data from phonology, acoustics and psychoacoustics. *In* "The Cognitive Representation of Speech", (T. Myers, J. Laver and J. Anderson, eds). North-Holland, Amsterdam.

Stevens, K. N. and Blumstein, S. E. (1975). Quantal aspects of consonant production and perception: A study of retroflex stop consonants. *Journal of Phonetics*, **3**, 215–233.

Stevens, K. N. and Perkell, J. S. (1977). Speech physiology and phonetic features. *In* "Dynamic Aspects of Speech Production", (M. Sawashima and F. S. Cooper, eds). University of Tokyo Press, Tokyo.

Strange, W. and Broen, P. A. (1980). Perception and production of approximant consonants by three-year-olds. *In* "Child phonology: Perception Production and Deviation", (G. Yemi-Komshian, J. F. Kavanagh and C. A. Ferguson, eds). Vol. 2. Academic Press, New York and London.

Studdert-Kennedy, M. (1980). Speech perception. *In* "Proceedings of the Ninth International Congress of Phonetic Sciences". Institute of Phonetics, University of Copenhagen.

Summerfield, Q. (1982). Differences between spectral dependence in auditory and phonetic temporal processing: Relevance to the perception of voicing in initial stops. *Journal of the Acoustical Society of America*, **72**, 51–61.

Summerfield, A. Q. and Haggard, M. P. (1972). Speech rate effects in perception of voicing. *Speech Syn Percept*, No. 6, Progress Report, Psychological Laboratory, University of Cambridge, 1–12.

Tuller, B. and Fowler, C. A. (1980). Some articulatory correlates of perceptual isochrony. *Perception and Psychophysics*, **27**, 277–283.

Turvey, M. T. (1977). Preliminaries to a theory of action with reference to vision. *In* "Perceiving, Acting, and Knowing: Toward an Ecological Psychology", (R. Shaw and J. Bransford, eds). Erlbaum: Hillsdale, New Jersey.

Turvey, M. T. Shaw, R. and Mace, W. (1978). Issues in the theory of action: Degrees of freedom, co-ordinative structures and coalitions. *In* "Attention and Performance", (J. Requin, ed.) Vol. VII.

Waters, R. S. and Wilson, W. A. (1976). Speech perception by rhesus monkeys: The voicing distinction in synthesized labial and velar stop consonants. *Perception and Psychophysics*, **19**, 285–289.

Wickelgren, W. A. (1969). Context-sensitive coding, associative memory, and serial order in (speech) behaviour. *Psychological Review*, **4**, 118–128.

Wise, C. M. (1948). ɪz neɪzəl rɛzənənts æktʃʊəlɪ neɪzoʊ-fərɪŋgəl rɛzənənts? mɛːtrə fənɛiˈk, 4–5.

6

Aphasia: Information-processing in Language Production and Reception

W. E. Cooper   *Harvard University*
E. B. Zurif   *Boston University School of Medicine*

I. Introduction

Aphasia – a specific disruption to language skills consequent to brain damage – is a devastating experience for those who endure it. Yet, however ruefully viewed, aphasia also provides a unique vantage point from which to study brain–language relations. There is, to be sure, considerable inter-individual variation in the manner in which language is affected, but of central interest here is the fact that much, if not most, of this variation can be accounted for by the general site of lesion; and indeed, work over the past century has led to a reliable typology of the patterns of linguistic deficit that turns solely on the location of the damage. In this chapter, we will explore the extent to which these different patterns of deficits can be interpreted – both for comprehension and production – as a disruption to one or another of the putative component processes that normally interact to yield the faculty of language. This account will be assembled in relation to distinctions among levels of linguistic information – standardly, the distinctions among phonology (including here the acoustic and phonetic characteristics subsumed by this level), syntax, and semantics.

Within this general framework, we will seek to show (1) that aligning processing distinctions with linguistic information types will enable one to reconstruct some of the consequences of brain injury upon language processing, specifically, upon the processing of features of sentence form; and (2) that the nature of the processing losses uncovered in the light of these distinctions will increase the understanding of normal linguistic activity (for a detailed discussion of this point, see also Saffran, Schwartz and Marin (1980) in Volume I).

As a first step in forming this account, we will briefly sketch the clinical features of a number of aphasic syndromes pertinent to our analyses, includ-

LANGUAGE PRODUCTION VOL. 2
ISBN 0-12-147502-6

ing Broca's aphasia and two forms of fluent aphasia – Wernicke's and anomic aphasia. We will then deal primarily with sentence comprehension, reviewing, for each of the syndromes separately, studies revealing less "public" comprehension limitations that in some respects parallel those of the clinically observable productive disorders. In this context, we will explore possible interdependencies of the processes underlying both comprehension and production, being concerned with the extent to which these two sets of processes might similarly reflect the structural constraints of language. We will also in this section attempt to account for these overarching linguistic deficits in terms of distinct stages of processing, and in the case of Broca's aphasia – for which there exist more detailed analyses – in terms of a partially elaborated model that implicates the organization of lexical retrieval mechanisms as an aid to syntactic processing.

In light of our discussion of comprehension and its relation to production in aphasia, and in response to some of the issues raised therein, we will turn to more detailed studies of speech production, and in particular, to studies of the prosodic characteristics of aphasic utterances that have not yet been treated in other reviews. These recent studies focus on the acoustic attributes of speech timing and fundamental frequency (Fo), attempting to infer from the measurement of these acoustic variables the aphasic patients' capacity to plan utterances over phrasal and clausal domains. Here, too, we will attempt to delineate aphasic disruptions in terms of separable information processing stages and in terms of the information-flow routes among them.

A final introductory remark: Our analyses will not represent an attempt to develop brain–language relations in physiological terms. In short, our analyses will not be mechanistic at the level of neurological structure and function. We will, however, assume that the manner in which language breaks down after focal damage does point in a non-trivial way to the manner in which it is organized in the brain, however complicated the relation might be between the neuroanatomical locus of the damage and the neurological organization of the disordered computational unit.

II. Some Clinical Phenomena

Clinically, the speech output of aphasic patients can usually be characterized as belonging to one of two patterns – fluent or nonfluent, each pattern in turn typically being correlated with a particular lesion site. Consider patients with Broca's aphasia, a "non-fluent" syndrome associated with damage to the anterior portion of the left hemisphere just in front of or involving the primary motor strip for the muscles involved in speech (Geschwind, 1970; Levine and Sweet, 1979). Such patients show a reduced output that is awkwardly articulated and effortful. The output is also restricted to simple syntactic forms, and it is telegraphic – or agrammatic – in the sense that grammatical morphemes, both bound and free, are usually omitted, with a corresponding reliance on nouns and, to a lesser extent, on verbs, these latter items usually appearing in uninflected or in nominalized form. Equally noteworthy is the general clinical impression that, in conversational settings, Broca's aphasics generally seem to show relatively spared comprehension abilities (Goodglass and Kaplan, 1972).

The syndrome of Broca's aphasia is made the more striking for its contrast with the patterns of speech and comprehension exhibited by patients with Wernicke's aphasia, a syndrome usually resulting from a lesion in the posterior portion of the first temporal gyrus of the left hemisphere – a region adjacent to primary auditory cortex (Geschwind, 1970). The output of Wernicke's aphasic patients is motorically facile, and, to the clinical ear, it seems to retain intact syntactic frames and the normal melodic patterns of speech. However, their speech is also remarkably empty of content and features sound errors (literal or phonemic paraphasias), errors of word usage (semantic paraphasias), and sometimes even neologistic, or nonsense, elements. Yet another critical feature of this syndrome is that comprehension is notably impaired (Goodglass and Kaplan, 1972).

The speech of anomic aphasics – a second, somewhat less common form of "fluent" posterior aphasia – is also relatively empty of content words. Yet, in contrast to the Wernicke's patients (and indeed, to all other types of aphasic patients who also have word-finding difficulties to a greater or lesser extent), the word-finding problem in anomic aphasia seems to be a relatively *isolated* one, without neologisms and semantic and phonetic paraphasias. Also, unlike Wernicke's aphasia, comprehension in the anomic aphasia syndrome is relatively intact (Goodglass and Kaplan, 1972). Admittedly, some patients initially presenting as Wernicke's aphasics evolve into anomic aphasics in the course of their recovery. However, the syndromes are nonetheless distinct and also usually marked by contrasting lesion sites: the lesion responsible for anomic aphasia is somewhat more variably located than that for Wernicke's aphasia, but is generally observed in the tempero-parietal area and may extend to the angular gyrus (Tonkonogy and Goodglass, 1980).

While acknowledging the grammatical limitations of the various aphasias in a general way, traditional clinically-based expositions of these syndromes have tended to elaborate upon the distinctions among them in terms of a distinction between sensory systems and motor systems (e.g. Marie, 1906; Weisenberg and McBride, 1935). Descriptions of this sort, even today (Levine and Sweet, 1979), emphasize the fact that the lesions underlying Broca's and Wernicke's aphasia are, respectively, adjacent to or involve primary motor and auditory cortex. To be sure, Broca's aphasics most often do have a problem with the motor implementation of speech, and Wernicke's patients do have profound auditory comprehension problems. Even so, it has become increasingly clear – witness the developing abandonment of the labels "expressive" and "receptive" aphasia – that describing the deficits in sensory-motor terms provides a too narrow and somewhat misleading view. That is, although the neurological capacity for speaking and listening obviously incorporates and is shaped by channel-specific characteristics, the brain seems also to honour processing distinctions that reflect "higher-order" linguistic constraints, subserving *both* comprehension and production. And certainly, in reflection of this view, the ways in which sensory-motor systems break down under conditions of left-sided brain damage do not predict the ways in which focal brain damage also selectively affects language capacity and the processes implementing this capacity (Marin and Gordon, 1980; Zurif, 1980).

III. Comprehension Deficits and Their Relation to Production Deficits in Broca's Aphasia

A. Parallels Between Comprehension and Production

Without dwelling at length on individual contributions – which at any rate have been reported in detail elsewhere (Caramazza and Berndt, 1978; Schwartz, Saffran and Marin, 1980; Zurif and Blumstein, 1978; Zurif and Caramazza, 1976) – it may be fairly stated that recent studies are in agreement in concluding that, to the extent that Broca's aphasics show *relatively* intact comprehension, it is largely based on their ability to utilize semantic and pragmatic cues independent of sentence structure. They understand a sentence primarily by sampling from it in terms of what each of the major lexical items – that is, the nouns and verbs – refers to and by combining these referential meanings in terms of what makes factual sense. In effect, this evidence provides a picture of an impairment in the recovery of appropriate grammatical strutures – an impairment that is not readily apparent to clinical observation and is made public only in those situations (usually experimental) where semantic and pragmatic constraints fail to predict the structural relations among words.

More particularly, the Broca's inability to assign syntactic analyses to sentences has been traced, at least in part, to a problem in their use of function words. The data from a number of different experiments strongly suggest that Broca's aphasics have no knowledge of the *structural* roles played by grammatical morphemes and that they are thereby unable to use these items as markers of phrasal constituents – that is, as syntactic place holders (Gardner, Denes and Zurif, 1975; Kolk, 1978; Ulatowska and Baker, 1975; von Stockert and Bader, 1976; Zurif, Caramazza and Myerson, 1972; Zurif *et al.*, 1976). Just as they speak agrammatically, so too can they be characterized as agrammatic comprehenders; the deficit, in other words, appearing to be central to the language faculty.

B. Processing Accounts of the Grammatical Limitation

With this evidence in mind, a number of investigators have lately attempted to account for the grammatical limitation – particularly the problem with function words – in terms of specific levels of processing. In this respect, one account turns on the fact that, in English, function words are generally unstressed, and guided by this fact, this account locates the comprehension problem at the point of assigning phonetic representations to the acoustic input. In effect, the claim made is that Broca's aphasic patients selectively attend to stressed (content) words and not to unstressed (function) words (Brown, 1979; Kellar, 1978).

This description, however, should not be viewed as having explanatory force in the sense of implicating the acoustic level of processing. That is, it is not likely to be the case that the brain damage underlying Broca's aphasia forecloses grammatical analysis by "blocking off" the analysis of the unstressed function words on a purely acoustic basis (Kean, 1980). Relevant to this point is experimental evidence which suggests that function words place an extra burden on the Broca's processing capacities quite apart from acoustic considerations – namely, Swinney, Zurif, and Cutler (1980), have observed that, although both Broca's aphasics and neurologically intact subjects responded faster in a monitoring task to stressed than to unstressed words appearing in sentences, only the Broca's showed an effect of vocabulary class by responding to content words faster than to function words *regardless of stress*.

This is not to claim that the level at which the sound structure of a sentence is represented is not implicated in the Broca's aphasic's agrammatism. Indeed, Kean (1980) has persuasively argued that the contrast between content and function words – a contrast required for any analysis of agrammatism – can be formally described only at the phonological level of representation. Rather, our claim is that this phonological distinction is not likely to be computationally relevant at the stage at which the acoustic input is phonetically recoded.

At what point, then, will this distinction be exploited in the processing chain? In light of recent work initiated by Bradley and Garrett (1980; also Bradley, 1979), one current bet is that it applies at the stage of lexical access. Specifically, making use of a number of lexical decision tasks, Bradley and Garrett (1980) provide evidence to suggest that, in the neurologically intact, there exist separate routes for the lexical access of these two phonological classes of words. The route by which content words are accessed appears to be frequency sensitive – the more frequently a word appears in the language, the more rapidly it is classified. By contrast, the route by which function words are accessed appears not to be subject to such an effect. These initial findings may lead to a partial characterization of parsing in normals. Namely, the separate recognition device for function words might reasonably be supposed to provide an important basis for syntactic inference – a basis for imposing form class designations on content words – establishing, for example, that a word is an article leads to the inference that the adjacent content word is a noun or an adjective but not a verb.

Supporting this notion, and of central concern here, is the finding that agrammatic Broca's aphasics do *not* exploit the processing distinction between these two vocabulary classes (Bradley, 1979; Bradley, Garrett and Zurif, 1980). Instead, they seem to treat the function words as they do content words, showing a frequency effect for both. It does not appear, therefore, that the grammatical problem in Broca's aphasia amounts to a simple dropping out of function words or to a blocking off of these items at an acoustic level. After all, the function words were processed by the patients and recognized as belonging to the language. Rather, the problem seems tied to a disruption of the specialized mechanism that accesses function words for their structure-building relevance.

To extend this line of reasoning, it may be suggested, in view of the finding that Broca's correctly identify function words as words in their language, that these items are normally doubly "registered" or "contacted" – once via their specially accessed route and in addition, via the frequency-sensitive route that contacts also the content words (Bradley, Garrett and Zurif, 1980). The question, therefore, arises as to whether we can assign a semantic function to the frequency-sensitive route, in complementary fashion to the parsing function word route.

Preliminary evidence from a study using articles as a test case is consistent with this possibility. Although the Broca's aphasics cannot integrate articles structurally (Zurif *et al.*, 1972), they nonetheless appear to appreciate the semantic value of articles in situations in which these elements critically signal partitions in the environment and in which on-line demands are minimized (see also Friederici, 1980). In the Zurif, Garrett and Bradley study currently being run, a patient is instructed to point to a single geometric figure from an array of three, the critical instances being those in which the article used in the instruction is inappropriately definite with respect to the array, as, for example, when the patient is faced with *two* round shapes and one square and is instructed to point to *the* round one. Although the patients seem not to process the article when the instructions are delivered orally at a normal speaking rate (Goodenough, Zurif and Weintraub, 1977), they show clear evidence of recognizing an anomalous use of the article when the instructions are delivered in written form and when they are given unlimited time to read the sentences. That they do so in these delimited circumstances suggests that, quite apart from any syntactic capacity, they can connect the article with some such semantic/pragmatic notion as "ready identifiability". Stated more generally, they appear to be able to involve articles in the assignment of reference, even if not in the assignment of structure.

C. Relations Between Comprehension and Production Reconsidered

The convergence of the Broca's telegraphic output and their inability to use function words as syntactic placeholders during sentence understanding suggests that the processes of production and comprehension are similarly constrained by left-anterior brain damage in their implementation of linguistic structure. In light of the lexical decision experiments just mentioned, we may now speculate further on this issue. It seems that the disruption common to production and comprehension in Broca's aphasia can be located at that point at which the function-content word distinction is normally exploited, in which case it seems reasonable to suppose that this aspect of the organization of the lexical inventory normally serves as a resource both for production and comprehension.

To this point we have speculated on a connection between production and comprehension within the confines of a functional decomposition of language that highlights the contrast between sentence form and meaning in terms of the partition between content and function words. Indeed, thus far our entire reconstruction of the comprehension and production deficits in Broca's aphasia has focused only on those processes implicating the grammatical morphemes. But the fact remains that syntactic information is also associated with the content word vocabulary (e.g. that certain verbs take complements whereas others do not, *believe* vs. *hit*, etc). And it is certainly possible that disruption to the special function word route may be only one reflection of a larger inability to gain syntactic information, whether carried by function *or content* words.

It is noteworthy with respect to this last possibility that the omission of function words is only one of several diagnostic features of the Broca's aphasics' output. The utterances produced by these patients are also significantly impoverished in the sense that constructions more complex than simple active declaratives such as verbal complement constructions are very rarely, if ever, observed, even in elicited production situations such as in sentence completion tasks. And, as Caplan (pers. commun.) has pointed out, this restriction in production could as well be due to an inability to use the structural information in verbs as to an inability to use function words as a syntactic vehicle.

Considerations of a similar nature arise also in relation to comprehension. As already mentioned, Broca's aphasic patients are clearly able to gain understanding on the basis of semantic and pragmatic constraints. But what is at issue here, and what is less certain, is their ability to use *order* information to establish meaning relations. The question, specifically, is whether the patients can apply a strategy operating independently of a deterministic structural decoding capacity – a "perceptual" strategy that relies on a sequential regularity in the language whereby many surface arrangements of the form noun phrase–verb–noun phrase (NP–V–NP) can be taken to signify the semantic structure agent–action–object (Bever, 1970; Frazier, 1978).

While a number of studies (Blumstein *et al.* 1979; Caplan *et al.*, in press; Rubin, 1978) have indicated that Broca's aphasics can apply such a strategy, a recent analysis has raised the possibility that their ability in this respect is illusory, and that, when faced with NP–V–NP sequences, their capacity to assign semantic roles appropriately to the two NP's is based entirely on "semantic" cues (Schwartz *et al.*, 1978). The evidence – at best marginal and therefore only suggestive, as the investigators themselves acknowledge (Schwartz *et al.*, 1978 and pers. commun.) – is based on an intuition as to whether or not verbs are biased towards one or another of their arguments. Thus, in the few relevant instances tested, Broca's aphasics were more likely to assign semantic roles correctly for sentences like, "Bob applauds Tom", in which the action "inheres" in the agent, than for sentences like, "Bob chases Tom", in which the action may be viewed as encoding some form of relation between the agent and object, but having no special link with either. In effect, then, the data suggest that Broca's are relatively disrupted in their ability to use order information, at least in linguistic contexts, such that when verbs are "neutral" with respect to their arguments, they are more likely than otherwise to make comprehension mistakes.

If there is some such problem in dealing with order information, should we take it as an indication that the syntactic disruption in Broca's aphasia implicates content as well as function words? Not necessarily. The problem could still be characterized in terms of a breakdown to the putative specialized function word route. That is, if the successful operation of the function word access and parsing system is crucial in most instances to the isolation of the phrasal constituents to be ordered, then clearly in those instances, its disruption would foreclose the use of any NP–V–NP strategy employing order information. But again, there are no strong data to rule out the possibility that the syntactic information carried by the content words (particularly by verbs and derived forms) is also unavailable to Broca's aphasics, and that this, too, is contributing to the parsing and order problems.

The possibility – again, still largely untested – that Broca's are unable to use word order cues raises yet another question: namely, if the order of the verb's arguments are of no significance to the Broca's aphasics in comprehension, how are we to view their ability to string and order words together appropriately (albeit telegraphically) in production? Does their output consist of nothing other than a series of labels – planned one at a time and sequenced according to some semantic strategy (e.g. start with an animate element), or ordered according to pragmatic constraints (e.g. put the topic first)? Or, are they indeed able to encode relational meanings in their output? In which case, can we so easily dismiss those reports – indeed, the majority of reports – that claim that Broca's aphasics *are* able to extract structural relations from word order in comprehension?

Fortunately, the results of a recent analysis of Fo during speech production in Broca's aphasia bear on these questions (Danly, de Villiers and Cooper, 1979; Danly and Shapiro, 1981). In normal speech, Fo declines over the course of major constituents, indicating, thereby, that such constituents in some way enter as units during the course of planning speech (Cooper and Sorensen, 1981); see also p. 239 of this chapter). Surprisingly, and to forecast the substance of a later section of this chapter, this general form of declination was also observed for Broca's aphasics, even though in some cases the words comprising an utterance were separated from each other by pauses lasting five or more seconds. This finding suggests that Broca's aphasics are not reduced to programming their intended message one word at a time but rather are capable of formulating supralexical meanings, at least in the sense that the messages sent to innervate the vocal apparatus are comprised of units that extend beyond the single word and presumably, therefore, of some relational structure. This argument will be pursued – and refined – in greater detail in a later section. Yet, even this cursory description should suggest that the patients are *not* reduced to collocating single labels in the absence of *all* mediating linguistic structures.

Just what these remaining structures are, or conversely, just how to characterize the syntactic problem – both for comprehension and production – of course remains unanswered by these data. As already remarked, the problem, essentially, is one of determining whether the Broca's inability to process aspects of sentence form implicates the content as well as the function word vocabulary. Or, to place the issue in a larger context: Does normal sentence analysis require a syntactic decision for every lexical item, or do function words play a pivotal role in syntactic analysis as suggested by the experimental demonstration of a special access route for these items?

IV. Comprehension Deficits and Their Relation to Production Deficits in the Fluent Aphasias

A. Wernicke's Aphasia

As a general point, the Wernicke's aphasic's unravelled sentence processing capacity has not yet been as successfully reconstructed in terms of a functional decomposition of language as has that of the Broca's aphasic. The problem is that, compared to the Broca's aphasic, the Wernicke's lexical knowledge appears not to be so spared, nor his syntax so disrupted. In effect, the pattern of sparing and loss in Wernicke's aphasia less palpably reflects distinctions among linguistic information types. Yet, some beginnings in characterizing the lexical semantic problem and in disentangling this disorder from the syntactic deficits have been made, and these efforts are briefly reviewed in what follows (see also Caramazza and Berndt, 1978).

Investigators attempting to account for vocabulary disruption in Wernicke's aphasia have, in part, striven to implicate the mapping procedures that relate input and output to the conceptual representations in which word meanings are embedded – as if, in production, the semantic representation for a word would be found intact if only the mechanisms by which it is activated or retrieved for speech were spared (Bisiach, 1966; North, 1971); or equivalently for comprehension, that a word's meaning would be understood if only the acoustic input could be properly coded for the purpose of addressing the semantic lexicon (e.g. Luria, 1970). Thus, studies of naming and word-finding problems in Wernicke's aphasia have pointed to the patients' less-than-normal ability to integrate the sensory qualities of objects to be named (North, 1971). In a similar vein, studies of word comprehension in Wernicke's aphasia have attempted to implicate a ". . . disturbance of auditory analysis which leads to the loss of phonemic hearing, and, as a secondary result, to the disturbance of all functions which are dependent upon this physiological (sic) function" (Luria, 1970).

Yet, although disruptions at these initial "processing" stages likely exist, recent findings suggest that they cannot – either alone or in any straight-forward fashion – account for the Wernicke's lexical comprehension and production problem, nor, for that matter, do they predict what is spared of his vocabulary (Gardner, 1973; Goodglass and Baker, 1976; Grober et al., 1980; Grossman, 1978; Whitehouse et al., 1978). A number of studies indicate that the Wernicke's performance at the acoustic/phonetic level does not reliably predict his performance at the level of word comprehension (Blumstein et al., 1977; Naeser, 1974), and in a like spirit, that his problem in integrating the sensory information inherent in an object to be named cannot be divorced from a disruption to the manner in which functional and perceptual information is structured at the semantic level (Caramazza et al. 1978).

In a more positive vein, a number of recent investigations point to a connection between, on the one hand, the ability of aphasics (considering Broca's and Wernicke's together) to find and to understand words, and on the other hand, their ability to trace conceptual relations among words (Caramazza et al., 1978; Goodglass and Baker, 1976; Whitehouse et al., 1978; Zurif et al., 1974). The suggestion here is that the conceptual elements or semantic features into which words may be factored – and which may serve as a basis for tracing relations among words – might be importantly involved in the process of using and understanding words in aphasia. This notion is supported also by the Wernicke's semantic paraphasias and off-target word comprehension responses – supported in the sense that, for the patient to presumably intend one lexical item and to perceive or produce instead another semantically related one, there must be some level in the chains of comprehension and production at which the representations of the items overlap in terms of their semantic features.

But, however internally consistent this line of reasoning might be, it is not at all clear that it should serve as an account of the processes involved in the normal access of lexical forms and meaning, the reason being that it does not make contact with what presently seems a functionally defensible analysis of normal language use. Specifically, a recent argument against semantic decomposition as a fact of real-time processing suggests that there is no reasonable analysis of normal function such that a constituent can be isolated which implements a semantic feature analysis of lexical meaning (Fodor et al., 1980; see also Caplan, 1980).

If this view is correct (and it must be emphasized that the data are sufficiently scanty as to blunt any point), it would appear that the semantic feature "explanation" offered above serves solely to reconstruct the basis upon which *only aphasic* vocabulary skills operate – pointing, as it were, to a backup system that is error prone and palpably less efficient than that utilized by normals. We have assumed that aphasia does not create new information processing systems, but rather disrupts those that existed pre-morbidly. Clearly, this view was supported in our analysis of sentence processing in Broca's aphasia in which we reconstructed the patients' inability to processes features of sentence form in terms of a disruption to a particular component specified within a functionally defensible account for normal processing. But what of our analysis of vocabulary skills in Wernicke's aphasia, where we have argued that the process mediating between the phonological shape of a word and its meaning is one that is not normally used? Does this violate the assumption? We think not; the inferential processes by which aphasics appear to gain word meanings are clearly processes that are also available to normals, and indeed, appear to be used, not for on-line comprehension, but rather in situations that draw upon long-term memory (Gentner, 1975). Accordingly, our analyses of vocabulary skills in aphasia are still understandable within the context of a functional decomposition of the language faculty, and further, they exemplify how a system present in normals for one purpose is inefficiently used by aphasics for another.

However imperfectly Wernicke's aphasics attain the form and meaning of lexical items, the fact remains that they are not completely unable to connect verbal labels to their referents. Their lexical knowledge is, in fact, sufficiently spared for them to more than occasionally infer the content of a verbal message. And it is in the context of such partial sparing that we can analyse the extent to which syntactically indicated meaning relations influence the Wernicke's comprehension, the rationale being that, even if the words in an utterance can only be partially processed, or even if only some of them can be processed, a spared ability to impose some syntactic analysis on the input should enhance understanding.

But is syntactic processing spared to Wernicke's aphasics? Not entirely, it seems. Several studies employing a sentence–picture matching paradigm are in agreement in concluding that, although Wernicke's can use order information in the service of assigning meaning to sentences, they do not have the normal capacity to algorithmically compute full structural descriptions – either for complex sentences featuring discontinuous constituents (Caramazza and Zurif, 1976; Blumstein *et al.*, 1979) or for simpler sentences in which structural relations are signalled morphologically (Heeschen, 1980). In effect, they seem restricted to the use of a minimum distance principle which relies on a sequential regularity of English, whereby in many instances the noun closest to and preceding a verb can be taken as signifying the agent of the action specified by the verb. As an example (from Blumstein *et al.*, 1979), faced with two pictures, one of a young girl bandaging herself and one of a waitress bandaging herself, Wernicke's routinely pointed to the correct depiction of the sentence, "The girl watched the waitress bandage herself." In contrast, they were far less successful in pointing to the picture corresponding to, "The girl, watching the waitress, bandaged herself." The first-mentioned of these two sentences maintains the noun–verb sequence, waitress being mapped as agent, bandage as action; the last-mentioned sentence does not, a clause intervening between the agent, on the one hand, and the action and reflexive pronoun, on the other.

This restriction on syntactic capacity seems to extend also by the Wernicke's output. That is, notwithstanding the fact that clinicians have in the past claimed that Wernicke's speech contains complex constructions (e.g. Goodglass and Kaplan, 1972), a recent careful charting of their output shows that they are far less likely to depart from simple declarative utterances than are normals (Gleason *et al.*, 1980). Further, we cannot at present dismiss the possibility that, insofar as Wernicke's aphasics do occasionally produce embedded constituents and relative clauses, these may be simply meaningless, over-learned automatisms, as opposed to outputs planned over well-formed (and semantically informed) syntactic representations. Thus, although some subordinate clause constructions were observed in a recent study of Wernicke's aphasics' output, these were most often found to be semantically unrelated to the matrix clause (Delis *et al.*, 1979).

One line of current research pertinent to the issue of grammatical capacity in Wernicke's aphasia turns on an analysis of pauses and neologistic elements in their speech. For example, having observed a disproportionate number of hesitations and long pauses preceding neologisms in the output of a jargon aphasic, Butterworth (1979) has suggested that the neologisms represent an adaptation to a failure of lexical search (see also Buckingham and Kertesz, 1974; Lecours and Rouillon, 1976; Buckingham, 1979) and are not simply inserted by the speaker because the normal constraints on word formation are disinhibited (e.g. Rochford, 1974; Pick, 1931). Of greater relevance to this chapter, Butterworth has reported that the hesitation pauses seem to be specific to the lexical search problem, and correspondingly, that pauses at clause boundaries appear normal in their occurrence.

Yet, it would be premature to interpret this last finding as indicative of a relatively intact syntactic-to-phonetic path of information flow, for there are other indications that such is not the case. As will be shown in a later section, while neologisms might reflect "local" disturbances of lexical access, there appears in addition to be a more general problem of utterance planning in Wernicke's aphasia. Specifically, recent analyses of Fo contours in sentence contexts have indicated that Wernicke's do not seem to take into account the overall length of their target utterance in programming their first Fo speaking, thus suggesting a deficit in long-range planning capability – a deficit that can be defined in terms of constituents larger than the single word.

However, we shall defer a detailed consideration of this work until the section on prosody in Wernicke's aphasia, and conclude at this point only that Wernicke's aphasics are impaired in their ability both to use syntax productively and to carry out semantic inference on the basis of syntactically indicated meaning relations – despite, in this latter instance, some ability to gain word meaning and a seemingly greater sensitivity than Broca's both to form class distinctions (Friederici, 1980) and to constituent order (Heeschen, 1980).

Finally, let us reconsider Luria's (1970) claim that the general deficit in speech comprehension for Wernicke's aphasics is attributable to an inability to perceive minimal phonemic distinctions that differentiate words (e.g. *dear* and *tear*), a so-called loss of "phonemic hearing". In this regard, a recent study of Baker *et al.* (1980) is noteworthy for its joint appraisal of phonological and semantic factors that contribute to aphasic deficits in phoneme discrimination. *Contra* Luria (1970), a study by Blumstein *et al.* (1977) showed that Wernicke's aphasics were not as impaired in discriminating phonemes as other aphasic groups who had scored higher than Wernicke's aphasics on a speech comprehension test. On the basis of this and other studies reviewed by Baker *et al.*, it appeared rather that the comprehension deficit in Wernicke's aphasics is primarily due to an inability to associate the phonemic representation of a word with its meaning. To test this hypothesis, Baker *et al.* conducted a series of experiments in which patients were required to exhibit increasing amounts of semantic processing of words presented auditorily and visually. The experiments included a same–different matching test in which both items were presented auditorily, a similar matching test in which one item was presented auditorily and one visually, and a multiple choice auditory–visual matching test. In the first test, discrimination could be performed without semantic processing; in the second, semantic processing would be necessary to relate the auditorily and visually presented members of each pair to be discriminated; in the third, a multiple choice test included both inappropriate semantic and phonological choices, allowing for the possibility of either type of error.

The results showed that Wernicke's aphasics committed more errors than Broca's aphasics in all three tests. However, the difference in performance between the two groups widened when semantic processing was required. Wernicke's aphasics do appear to exhibit a deficit in linking a word's sound with its meaning, and the interactive nature of this deficit was most clearly illustrated in the multiple choice discrimination test. The results showed that, as either the phonological or semantic discriminations increased in difficulty, Wernicke's ability to make word discriminations based on the other processing component also suffered. That is, phonologically difficult phoneme discriminations impeded semantically-based ones as well and vice-versa. By studying both phonological and semantic aspects of word discrimination jointly, Baker *et al.* were able to infer that the primary deficit in speech comprehension for Wernicke's aphasia lies not within the isolable aspects of phonological and semantic processing so much as with the interaction between the two.

B. Anomic Aphasia

Our discussion of Wernicke's aphasia should not be construed as a blanket indictment of the fluent v. non-fluent distinction as a means of bracketing different constituent linguistic processes. Rather, the relevant contrast in this respect seems to be one between Broca's aphasics and anomic aphasics who never presented with features of Wernicke's aphasia – that is, between those who have a disproportionately severe syntactic problem (in relation to the other aspects of their language functioning) and those who present with a relatively circumscribed "lexical" problem. Indeed, the validity of this contrast is underlined by the fact that, unlike the Broca's aphasics, anomic aphasics tested on lexical decision tasks show the normal dissociation between content and function word access (Bradley 1980). Thus, the failure to separately access function words (with the attendant, unfortunate consequences for parsing) seems tied to left-anterior agrammatism and not to brain damage in general. And, in this sense, we may be encouraged in our claim that different sites of brain damage are likely to selectively affect different "computational units".

V. Speech Prosody in Aphasia

Having presented an overview of the major deficits in aphasics' comprehension and production of language, we turn to a more detailed examination of difficulties in speech production, with particular emphasis on prosodic attributes of speech. In so doing, it will be possible to assesss characteristics of the information-flow routes among the syntactic, semantic, and phonological components of aphasic speech production.

Among prosodic attributes, the general property of *fluency* has been widely utilized as a means of distinguishing the speech of Broca's and Wernicke's aphasics, with Broca's of course exhibiting far less fluent output (e.g. Goodglass and Kaplan, 1972). In addition, measures of fluency have been employed as a means of quantifying the severity of speech deficit among individual patients (e.g. Wagenaar et al., 1975; Demeurisse et al., 1979; Kreindler, 1980).

Recently, attempts have been made to study component aspects of fluency in conjunction with other salient characteristics of aphasic speech. Such studies have been motivated in large measure by the finding that prosodic attributes have been useful in characterizing aspects of information-flow among the various processing operations mediating normal speech. For example, detailed analyses of pausing and word durations have provided information about aspects of lexical retrieval during speech production (e.g. Goldman-Eisler, 1968; Grosjean and Deschamps, 1975; Butterworth, 1980) as well as about the hierarchical nature of the speaker's syntactic representations (e.g. Lieberman, 1967; Grosjean, Grosjean, and Lane, 1979; Cooper and Paccia-Cooper, 1980). Acoustical measures of fundamental voice frequency (Fo) – corresponding to the rate of vocal fold vibration during voiced portions of speech – have yielded further insight about the speaker's structural representations of phrasal units as well as about the speaker's relatively long-range planning capabilities (e.g. Lea, 1973; O'Shaughnessy, 1976; Maeda, 1976; Cooper and Sorensen, 1981).

A schematic fundamental frequency contour for the utterance "If Harry leaves, John will be furious" is presented in Fig. 1, displaying some of the salient aspects of Fo to be examined in aphasic speech. These attributes include *declination, declination resetting, terminal fall,* and *continuation rise. Declination* refers to the notion that the Fo peaks on successive stressed syllables typically decline throughout a clause in declarative utterances (e.g. Bolinger, 1964; Lea, 1973; Maeda, 1976; O'Shaughnessy, 1976; Cooper and Sorensen, 1981). This characteristic is particularly apparent in utterances that do not contain emphatic or contrastive stress. *Declination resetting* refers to the notion that the declination function may be reset within an utterance, most typically at a major clause boundary (Lea, 1973; Cooper and Sorensen, 1981). In Fig. 2, declination resetting occurs at the clause boundary, such that the peak values in the second clause are systematically higher than would be predicted on the basis of a single declination function for the entire sentence. Research with oral reading in normals has shown that the essence of the declination function in this situation can be captured by an abstract mathematical formula that is approximately invariant across a number of features, including the sex of the speaker, speaking rate, and sentence structure (Cooper and Sorensen, 1981). In addition, such research has indicated that declination resetting may accompany major clause boundaries but seldom accompanies phrase boundaries within clauses unless such phrases are particularly long.

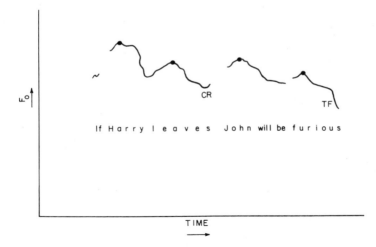

FIG 1. Schematic Fo plot of the sentence *If Harry leaves, John will be furious.* The Fo peaks for each stressed word are marked by points. Other salient features include the continuation rise (CR) at the end of the first clause and the terminal fall (TF) at the end of the utterance. The printed version of the sentence below the Fo plot coincides roughly with the temporal course of Fo.

The features of declination and declination resetting have been investigated for aphasia in order to determine whether such patients exhibit deficits in higher-order operations that influence Fo programming and, in addition, whether the domain of such programming is shorter-than-normal, as would be expected from informal clinical observations, especially in the case of non-fluent Broca's aphasics. As noted earlier, Broca's aphasics can often transmit semantic intentions via speech without being able to apply normal syntactic frames. This fact raises the question of whether such patients are capable of planning speech in units that accommodate the basic subject–predicate relations in their semantic intentions. According to the most stark possibility, Broca's aphasics might only formulate their speech one word at a time. By examining the prosodic attributes of speech containing more than one word, it is possible to determine if such a limitation exists for speech planning.

The syntactic domains over which Wernicke's aphasics can construct representations in on-line fashion have also not yet been determined, nor is it known whether or not these patients can use semantic variables to inform their syntactic computations. Given their fluent but empty speech and the variety of syntactic forms they can produce, it might be expected that, at the level of constructing an utterance, their performance is normal. But, as alluded to earlier, the problem is more complex. It is unclear whether, even at the level of phonetic realization, planning can proceed normally in the face of possible disruptions at a semantic level. For example, do semantic paraphasias and neologistic elements in Wernicke's speech merely represent "local" disruptions – problems with accessing particular lexical items? Or, are these elements to be viewed as reflecting a more general type of problem with utterance-planning, extending beyond the single-word domain? In their spontaneous speech, Wernicke's aphasics produce syntactic frames including both main and subordinate clauses, but, as indicated earlier, the subordinate clause may be semantically unrelated to the matrix clause (Delis et al., 1979). Thus, the fluent syntactic constructions observed in the speech of these patients may merely have the status of prefabricated routines, as opposed to constructions planned over well-formed syntactic representations, and examining the prosodic attributes of Wernicke's speech should enable one to determine whether limitations constrain their speech planning to shorter-than-normal domains.

In addition to declination and its resetting, two other aspects of Fo contours may also provide information about aphasics' domain of speech planning. A *terminal fall* in Fo denotes a large peak-to-valley drop at the end of an utterance, typically accompanying the last syllable, as shown in Fig. 1. While falling patterns of Fo appear at many locations in an utterance, the terminal fall in normal speech is typically larger in magnitude and quite consistent in character from one utterance to another.

The *continuation rise* is a special Fo attribute utilized to mark locations in continuation with a rise in Fo at the end of a word, as on the clause-final *leaves* in Fig. 1. Together, the absence of a large terminal fall and the presence of continuation rises at the ends of non-final words signify that the speaker wishes to continue speaking, and an examination of these features in aphasia has helped to provide information about patients' speech planning capabilities.

In subsequent discussion, acoustical studies of these Fo characteristics and pausing will be reviewed with an emphasis on examining the relationship between these characteristics and salient non-prosodic abnormalities of aphasic speech. Before considering such studies, however, we wish to highlight the importance of utilizing acoustical measures in this work over impressions derived by the unaided ear. Studies of both pausing and fundamental frequency have indicated that the human ear is often a poor judge of acoustic reality (e.g. Lieberman, 1965; Martin, 1970; Breckenridge, 1977), and acoustical measures, representing direct consequences of the speaker's vocal tract, provide a more direct means of inferring aspects of the speaker's internal processing operations. Currently available computerized techniques for acoustic analysis provide a precise and highly efficient means of examining the prosodic characteristics of both normal and aphasic speech, and researchers have recently begun to apply these techniques to the task of assessing processing operations in aphasia, with largely encouraging results.

VI. Broca's Aphasia

Because the speech of Broca's aphasics is so manifestly non-fluent, one might question whether such patients retain any of the rudiments of normal speech prosody. To examine this possibility, an acoustical analysis was conducted on two-word utterances spoken by moderate-to-severely disordered Broca's aphasics under two conditions, including a spontaneous interview and the oral reading of a select group of sentences (Danly *et al.*, 1979). In this and subsequently-described oral reading tests, the patients were instructed to avoid the use of contrastive or emphatic stress while reading the sentences. When the patient grossly misarticulated a content word or exhibited unusual stress, he was asked to repeat the sentence until a satisfactory utterance was produced. In the case of Broca's speech, agrammatic speech output was acceptable as data, and, in the case of Wernicke's speech, paraphasias and neologisms were acceptable as long as the output utterance contained the same number of content words as the target utterance. With these provisions, one could analyse the difference between target and typical output for these aphasic groups in order to determine isolated and interactive aspects of their computational deficits.

The utterances in this particular study of Broca's speech were analysed for three prosodic characteristics that would be indicative to normal speech for two-word utterances, as opposed to successive single-word utterances. These features include a terminal falling pattern of fundamental frequency on the second word from peak to valley, the declining of Fo peaks from the first word to the second, and an elongation of the second word. Of these attributes, the Broca's two-word utterances reliably exhibited both a terminal falling Fo contour and Fo declination. On the other hand, the duration of the first of the two words was longer than that of the second word, contrary to findings for normal adults and children (Branigan, 1976a,b; Danly and Shapiro, 1980; Stokes and Branigan, 1978). The same pattern of results was obtained in a comparison of the second and third words of three-word utterances spoken by Broca's aphasics in an oral reading test (Danly and Shapiro, 1980), suggesting that the lengthening of the first word in two-word utterances was not entirely attributable to a start-up effect in producing this word with heightened stress (cf. Goodglass *et al.* 1967). It seems, rather, that the difference in duration between the last word of the utterance and the next-to-last word is attributable to an abnormal shortening of the utterance-final word, accompanied by unusually low amplitude in many cases. Clinically, Broca's patients seem to "run out of gas" at the ends of even short utterances, and this impression might result from a physiological run-down accompanied by abnormally low subglottal pressure, yielding low speech amplitude. Exactly why the duration of the utterance-final word should be shortened in these patients remains unexplained, however.

One possibility is that Broca's speakers elongate *non*-final words in order to allow an extra fraction of time to plan upcoming material as well as to allow for proper execution of current motor programs. At the end of the utterance, the need for extra planning time is no longer present, yielding somewhat shorter durations for utterance-final words.

The fact that Broca's aphasics produce a larger terminal Fo fall on the last word of an utterance, despite producing a short word duration is consistent with the view that utterance-final lengthening in normal speech is probably not produced in order to allow time for a large terminal Fo fall (cf. Klatt, 1975; Lyberg, 1979). The dissociation between utterance-final duration and Fo effects for the Broca's aphasics is consistent with the finding that, in normal speech, there exists no strong correlation in individual utterances between the amount of utterance-final lengthening and the amount of terminal Fo fall at major syntactic boundaries (Cooper and Sorensen, 1977, 1981). It appears that, while the programming of timing and Fo information is considered jointly at some high-level stage of processing, the programming of specific durations and Fo values proceed largely independent of one another.

Aside from the findings for duration, the results of the Fo analyses reveal that Broca's aphasics do retain some of the basic attributes of normal speech prosody, even though these characteristics are typically camouflaged by their very slow rate of speech and numerous large inter-word pauses. To the clinical ear, the speech of Broca's aphasics would no doubt seem much improved, albeit still abnormal, if it was tape recorded and then represented after someone had excised some of the more lengthy pauses. In this study, relatively normal terminal Fo fall and declination were observed despite inter-word pauses that averaged more than one second and included pauses as long as seven seconds. No significant correlation was obtained between the length of these interword pauses and the magnitude or presence of the normal Fo attributes. †

To further examine the Fo characteristics of Broca's aphasics, oral reading tests were conducted using longer sentence strings, ranging from seven to fourteen words each (Danly and Shapiro, 1980). The sentences had originally been tested with normals to investigate the mathematical form of Fo declination as well as the slope of declination in short v. long utterances (Cooper and Sorensen, 1981). An example sentence pair bearing on this latter issue is presented below. The underlined words represent stressed words, common to both sentences, measured for peak Fo.

The *cat* was *asleep* in the *tree*.
The *cat* that Sally owned was asleep on the large branch in the *tree*.

In their study of normal speech, Cooper and Sorensen found that speakers produced higher Fo peaks on the first stressed word of an utterance in long v. short sentences, presumably in order to allow a greater range for Fo declination in long utterances. In a study of Broca's speech using the same sentence materials, however, Danly and Shapiro (1980) found that the aphasics failed to produce higher Fo peaks in longer strings, unlike a group of non-neurological hospitalized control patients. These results suggest that Broca's aphasics do not consider the general length of a sentence when programming Fo in oral reading. This inference is consistent with their very limited capability to produce multiple word sentences. In addition, such patients did not show the same gradual trend of declining Fo peaks throughout the course of such utterances. Rather, the Broca's aphasics seemed to produce declination over two or three word phrases, and to reset their declination function many times within the sentence (especially for longer sentences), suggesting that their programming of Fo is carried out over domains that are much shorter than normal. The resetting generally respected syntactic boundaries, however, rarely occurring within the confines of phrasal units. Thus, the Broca's seems to retain some degree of syntactic integrity in his speech, although in line with our earlier discussion of comprehension in

---

† It is tantalizing to speculate that the relative preservation of Fo control, in contrast to speech timing, is due, at least in part, to the possibility that the intact right hemisphere can program attributes associated with Fo contours in Broca's aphasia. This possibility is consistent with the general results of Melodic Intonation Therapy (Helm, 1979), in which severely disordered Broca's patients are trained to produce utterances by first learning to produce them with a highly exaggerated intonation contour. However, the imposition of such a contour may allow the speaker to chunk the utterance into manageable small units more easily, and it is possible that this factor accounts for the success of this type of therapy without the need to invoke right-hemisphere involvement. If it turns out, alternatively, that the effectiveness of such therapy is due to the ability of exaggerated intonation contours to engage the intact right hemisphere, this same right-hemisphere involvement might account for the fact that Fo contours are relatively intact in the speech of more moderately disordered Broca's patients (see also Cooper, 1981).

Broca's aphasia, it is also possible that this feature can be linked to intact semantic processing, a question for future study.

The patients partially compensated for their halting speech by typically ending words within each phrase with a sizable continuation rise in Fo. The continuation rises produced by such patients do appear to warrant the description "compensatory", inasmuch as their frequency of occurrence and magnitude are greater than normal yet are quite appropriate given the shorter-than-normal domains of production with lengthy interword pauses. The frequency of continuation rises was positively correlated with the severity of language disorder across the five patients tested. Whether or not the Broca's speaker intends to aid the listener by producing these continuation rises, such rises undoubtedly serve this function, possibly in addition to helping the speaker demarcate his own units of processing. The effective utilization of continuation rises at the ends of words in Broca's speech seems to represent one aspect of a general tendency for these patients to exhibit more sophisticated control over Fo during the middle and final portions of a word than at or near a word's beginning. A closer examination of the Fo contours is needed at various locations within words to investigate this possibility further, but, if substantiated, Broca's difficulty in controlling Fo at the *beginnings* of words may be attributed to their need to devote so much of their processing at this point to motor commands associated with producing a correct phonemic representation of the first phoneme of a word, a region of special difficulty in the speech of such patients (Goodglass *et al.*, 1967). This possibility rests on the assumption that, although the detailed programming of Fo and phonemic representations are largely independent, a general executive of limited processing capacity may simplify or abandon certain Fo programming operations when the demands on processing phonemic representations are at a premium.

The presence of large and frequent continuation rises also provides the first piece of convincing evidence in favour of the notion that Broca's speakers plan for an upcoming word before completely executing a current one. Originally, the presence of declination and terminal Fo fall were taken as evidence in favour of this view (Danly *et al.*, 1979; Danly and Shapiro, 1980), but a closer examination of these phenomena reveal problems with this interpretation. According to the notion that these patients program Fo over a span of at least two words, the speaker pre-plans an Fo contour for the two words prior to the uttering of either, complete with declining Fo peaks and terminal Fo fall. But, according to another alternative, the patient might not be endowed with such pre-planning capability, but rather produces a default Fo contour for the first word, and only after uttering this word might the patient program Fo for a subsequent word. According to this alternative, the speaker must simply recognize when he is about to utter the terminal word of an utterance, programming a low peak Fo and terminal falling pattern for this word. Such recognition could be delayed until just before the terminal word is spoken.

On the basis of declination and terminal Fo alone, it is difficult to distinguish between these two possible accounts. Both models predict, for example, that an analysis of single-word utterances would show Fo patterns similar to those of utterance-final words. Ideally, we would like to know exactly what the speaker pre-plans before the utterance has already been initiated and what the speaker plans thereafter, and an answer to this question must await research in which acoustical measures are combined with a task sensitive to the distinction between pre-planning and planning-cum-execution, such as reaction time to initiate speech (see Cooper and Ehrlich, 1981).

The continuation rises that appear at the ends of non-terminal words, do suggest however, that Broca's speakers *are* capable of planning for an upcoming word. While it remains a possibility that such planning does not take place until some portion of a current word has been produced, continuation rises would not be expected if these speakers did not begin to plan for an upcoming word until the current word was completely uttered. In effect, then, the presence of strong continuation rises at the ends of non-terminal words in Broca's speech can be taken as evidence that some planning capabilities do span a unit encompassing more than a single word. What remains to be determined is whether such planning can take place for the patients even before the first word of an utterance is spoken.

In studies now under way, particular attention is also being paid to the distinction between the target utterance and the patient's output. One question of major interest is whether substantial differences in the form of the target utterance will influence the prosodic attributes of Broca's patients, even in cases for which the utterances themselves contain the same words or other commonalities as a result of agrammatism. For cases in which differences in the target utterance produce such influences, one can infer that some aspects of an intended utterance are available to the speaker when programming prosodic effects but are then lost at a subsequent level of programming leading to speech output. In these and other target v. output studies, it is helpful to utilize an oral reading procedure, since the target utterances can be unambiguously defined. On the other hand, such studies run the risk of yielding results at least some of which are particular to the task of oral reading, not generalizable to spontaneous speech. In the earlier study of two-word utterances, the findings for spontaneous speech and oral reading for Broca's were quite similar, but only future work can determine whether such a congenial dovetailing of results is typical.

To conclude, the studies of Broca's speech indicate that a few rudimentary attributes of normal Fo patterns are preserved in short utterances despite lengthy interword pauses and laboured articulation. On the other hand, these aphasics do not exhibit utterance-final lengthening as in normal speech, and Broca's speech is marked by evidence of shorter-than-normal domains of prosodic programming. The results imply a deficit in speech planning, but the extent to which this deficit is incurred before the initiation of speech and/or after initiation remains unknown. Additionally, it remains to be determined whether the planning domain available to Broca's aphasics is more properly characterized in terms of syntactic or semantic/pragmatic representations, but these questions can be addressed in future work using the same testing procedures.

As for the traditional clinical view that Broca's asphasics exhibit dysprosody, it now appears that this description is more applicable to speech timing – including both the durations of segments and pauses – than to fundamental frequency. While segmental timing in even short two-word utterances shows abnormally short durations of the utterance-final word and long interword pauses, fundamental frequency analysis shows at least a few normal characteristics, including the declining of Fo peaks from the first word to the second and a terminal Fo fall from peak to valley in the utterance-final word. In addition, Broca's patients exhibit an ability to compensate in part for their shorter-than-normal domains of Fo declination by producing substantial continuation rises in Fo at the ends of utterance non-final words, signifying the intent to continue speaking. This highly adaptive employment of Fo suggests that these patients retain a rather sophisticated ability to program this prosodic attribute on the basis of higher-order considerations. Yet, because such control of Fo is not readily discerned by the clinical ear, when camouflaged by the very slow, halting rate of speech, so the impression of dysprosody is understandable. It is equally apparent, however, that the continued use of the term *dysprosody* is somewhat misleading insofar as it commonly connotes a primary deficit in the programming of Fo.

VII. Wernicke's Aphasia

In marked contrast to the utterances of Broca's aphasics, Wernicke's speech is quite fluent and gives the appearance of nearly normal prosody in clinical evaluation. Duchan *et al.* (1980), for example, remark that intonation contours of a jargon aphasic are generally appropriate, respecting syntactic boundaries and other structural aspects of sentences. Lecours and Rouillon (1976) have noted, however, that intonation is exaggerated in the speech of some Wernicke's aphasics, and a recent acoustical study of such patients supports this observation (Cooper, Danly and Hamby, 1979).

A careful analysis of Wernicke's speech reveals other systematic irregularities that provide information relevant to the conceptual view previously outlined. We shall consider two studies which combine acoustical measures of Wernicke's speech with some consideration of the unique characteristics of the disorder.

In one study, alluded to earlier, hesitation pauses in the spontaneous interview speech of a single patient were analyzed to determine whether any relation existed between the amount of pausing and the presence of immediately following neologisms or paraphasias (Butterworth, 1979). The results showed that the aphasic produced significantly longer pauses preceding neologisms than preceding paraphasias. In addition, the appearance of a hesitation was more likely preceding neologisms, with about half of the neologisms being preceded by a pause, compared with only about a fourth of the verbal paraphasias. As already mentioned, Butterworth hypothesized that the speaker's neologisms represent an adaptation to a failure of lexical search, which presumably takes place during at least part of the pause interval, the key assumption here being that hesitation pausing represents an interval of silence during which the speaker is engaged in word-finding activity, and correspondingly that neologistic forms are not simply inserted by the speaker because the normal constraints on word formation are disinhibited.

A detailed analysis of the pause durations revealed a systematic difference in the durations associated with "pure" neologisms – bearing no phonological relation to either the target word or to an adjacent word in the utterance – and neologisms which did bear some such phonological relation. The pause durations for the "pure" neologisms were about twice as long as average, suggesting that these neologisms were produced by a special device which generates a stereotypical nonsense form when lexical search is aborted. In addition, the pauses preceding phonologically related neologisms were about twice as long as pauses preceding verbal paraphasias. Butterworth's claim that neologisms are often produced by a special device is supported by evidence from other investigators who have reported that some individual patients' neologisms often have a sterotypical phonological form (e.g. Green, 1969; Lhermitte et al., 1973; Buckingham, 1974; Duchan et al., 1980 and references therein). Unlike Butterworth, however, Duchan et al. report informally an absence of long pauses before neologisms in the speech of one jargon aphasic, suggesting that this patient either does not require pausing for lexical search at the locations eventually occupied by neologisms (perhaps lexical search for the key word is planned ahead of time) or that neologisms for this speaker do not in fact represent a replacement for aborted lexical search.

The *locations* of neologisms within an utterance may eventually provide another peg of support for the view that these forms reflect a failure of lexical search. Green (1969) observed that neologisms generally appear in the predicate rather than the subject NP of Wernicke's speech. This finding suggests that the patient might adopt a strategy of withholding speech until the lexical and phonological representation of the subject NP is programmed, with the predicate being unspecified in large part before speech is initiated. According to this view, neologisms appear primarily within the predicate because the speaker incurs the most difficulty with lexical search in this region. Alternatively, the finding that neologisms appear more prevalently in the predicate may simply be due to the fact that more words generally appear in the predicate, rendering more individual opportunities for lexical search difficulty. Both Green (1969) and Butterworth (1979) report that the bulk of neologisms replace target nouns, but more nouns typically appear in the predicate of a sentence than in the subject, and future work must be conducted to unravel the alternative accounts of this predicate effect.

The relationship between pausing and neologisms observed by Butterworth and others also appears to distinguish the word-finding difficulty of Wernicke's aphasics from that of anomics. As noted by Buckingham (1979), anomic patients typically exhibit hesitation pauses in the absence of neologisms when they incur word-finding difficulty, whereas Wernicke's aphasics are more likely to exhibit neologisms immediately following hesitation pauses. One question which remains, however, is whether the neologisms prevalent in Wernicke's speech reflect the output of a special device utilized as part of a clever strategy for camouflaging difficulty with word-finding, as Butterworth suggests, or whether these neologisms represent a natural consequence of partial retrieval of lexical information, including a few semantic and phonological features that are combined to form a neologistic output (e.g. Marshall, 1979). The stereotypical form of many neologisms for an individual patient does seem to implicate a special generation device.

Recently, a general acoustical analysis of speech prosody in Wernicke's speech has been undertaken to determine whether such patients exhibit subtle but systematic prosodic deficits which typically go undetected during informal clinical observation (Cooper et al., 1979). Salient aspects of fundamental frequency contours in sentence contexts were examined, including the form of Fo declination and the first peak value of Fo in relatively long v. short sentences. As noted earlier, for normal subjects, the form of Fo declination for successive peaks in a single main-clause sentence can be captured by an abstract mathematical rule. Given the first and last peak values and their times of occurrence, the rule can adequately predict the Fo values of intermediate peaks in the utterance, largely invariant across a wide variety of variables such as speaker sex, speaking rate, sentence length, and others (Cooper and Sorensen, 1981). By examining the detailed form of declination for Wernicke's speech in the same sentence contexts, it was possible to determine whether their speech adhered to this mathematical formulation and whether their declination was perturbed in any way by the presence of paraphasias or neologisms.

In addition to this issue, the Fo values of the first peak in long v. short utterances were examined as in the study of Broca's speech to determine whether Wernicke's exhibit long range planning in their speech prosody. Recall that, in normal speech, the first peak in a longer single-clause sentence is higher in Fo than is the first peak in a shorter sentence.

The results of the study indicated that Wernicke's speech does exhibit systematic departures from the oral reading of normals. Of five patients tested, four regularly exhibited some form of Fo declination, but none of these patients adhered to the mathematical formulation of declination in a normal fashion. The patients generally started their first peak in Fo higher than normal for *both* long and short sentences. The peak values for this first peak did not differ significantly in the long v. short sentences, however, indicating another departure from normal speech. Like Broca's aphasics, Wernicke's patients do not seem to take into account the overall length of the target utterance in programming their first Fo peak, suggesting a deficit in long-range planning capability. Since their values for the first peak were higher than normal for all sentences, this possible failure did not lead to a restriction in the range of Fo declination in long sentences, however.

Perhaps the most interesting finding of this study was that the form of the aphasic's declination was relatively unperturbed by the presence of paraphasias or neologisms. This result was most apparent for a patient who produced literal paraphasias for approximately half of the key words spoken correctly. The similarity of the declination functions for correct and paraphrastic output for this and other patients suggests that the programming of Fo declination proceeds in a manner that is relatively independent of proper phoneme selection.

In addition to these findings, the acoustical analysis revealed other abnormalities in the oral reading of Wernicke's patients. Although the sentences used in the study involved simple syntactic structures and relatively high frequency words, the speech of the patients was, on average, almost twice as slow as normal, primarily due to an increase in hesitation pauses just prior to content words. This finding suggests that Wernicke's speakers are not really very "fluent" in a demanding reading situation and that their apparent fluency in spontaneous speech derives from their ability to cover up problems of lexical retrieval by producing neologisms and circumlocutions, as discussed earlier in relation to studies of pausing (e.g. Butterworth, 1979). In addition, Wernicke's speech displayed larger than normal peak-to-valley fluctuations in Fo, indicating that their fundamental frequency is often more contrastive than normal, supporting the observation of Lecours and Rouillon (1976).

In conclusion, while the speech of Wernicke's aphasics is far more fluent than that of Broca's, it does exhibit prosodic abnormalities. Regarding speech timing, hesitation pauses often precede neologisms, and it appears that these two features in conjunction represent difficulty in word-finding. The finding that neologisms are likely to follow hesitation pauses allows one to infer tht neologisms represent a default output when lexical search fails. It seems quite possible that these neologisms are generated by a special device and serve to camouflage the speaker's failure to retrieve target words.

The fundamental frequency of Wernicke's speech shows more of a tendency toward declination of peaks than does Broca's speech, although the precise programming of declination is not equivalent to normal speech. In addition, Wernicke's aphasics show the same deficit in long-term planning as Broca's for programming the first Fo peak of an utterance with respect to the overall length of the utterance. Despite these deficits, Wernicke's programming of Fo seems largely unperturbed by the presence of literal paraphasias and neologisms, suggesting that the operations involved in programming Fo are, for the most part, independent from those that select phonemes.

VIII. Conclusion

The study of aphasia has provided a means of examining some of the key processing stages in language production and comprehension, both from the standpoint of determining their individual characteristics and their interaction. Thus, from the available evidence on Broca's aphasia, it seems reasonable to propose – though clearly not with any strong assurance – that lack of a specialized processor for accessing function words is responsible for both their agrammatic speech output and their inability to decode closed class elements efficiently in comprehension. This latter deficit may in turn account for Broca's impairment in parsing sentences into well-formed constituents. Wernicke's aphasics, in contrast, appear to be more sensitive to form class distinctions, but are impaired in their ability to make semantic inferences on the basis of syntactically-determined meaning relations. As is doubtlessly apparent, the work upon which these claims are based has been motivated by, and embodies, a particular theoretical stance: namely, that language requires structural representations that are formally dissimilar to those involved in non-linguistic motor and perceptual tasks, and that these linguistic structures have a neurological independence at some level of organization – as revealed, however indirectly, by the phenomena of aphasia.

For the most part, neuroanatomical specification of the constituent processes comprising this linguistic capacity has been attempted via studies of aphasic comprehension. More recently, however, analyses of the independence of processing stages have also been carried out in relation to production. In particular, new studies combining acoustical measures of speech prosody with some of the more salient abnormalities of aphasic speech have begun to provide an intriguing testing ground. Thus, in some instances, as in the combined study of hesitation pauses and neologisms, the co-occurrence of prosodic and lexical abnormalities formed the basis of a case favouring the notion that neologisms represent the output of a special device when lexical search is aborted. In other cases, as in the study of declination and literal paraphasias, an inference regarding the independence of processing stages could be advanced on the basis of a lack of perturbation in declination by the occurrence of paraphrastic output. These examples suggest that the exploration of possible relations between prosodic and non-prosodic characteristics may improve our ability to specify both separable and interactive aspects of the processing stages that compute the major types of linguistic representation in normals and aphasics.

The comparison of normal and aphasic performance has shown some converging lines of inference. For example, the conclusion that a specialized processor is normally utilized to access function words for the purpose of structural analysis was supported by evidence from both normals and Broca's aphasics, as was the conclusion that the programming of segment durations and Fo values proceed for the most part independently. Such instances add a measure of weight to the claim that a joint consideration of normal and aphasic speech leads to a better understanding of processing operations that subserve both. At the same time, the pattern of disorder in aphasia also illustrates that the centrally-impaired language user can muster certain compensatory processes (e.g. Broca's producing large and frequent continuation rises in Fo at the ends of non-terminal words) and backup strategies (e.g. Wernicke's conceptual factoring of word meaning in terms of semantic elements as an aid to comprehension and the production of neologisms to possibly camouflage failed lexical search) that the normal language user seldom, if ever, finds the need to rely on. Our belief is that much of the compensatory aspects of aphasic performance represent the working of intact processing that is also available to normals, selectively revealed in aphasia as a consequence of disturbances to other processing sites. By assessing the patterns of preservation and impairment, it seems possible both to unveil otherwise hidden aspects of each processing stage and to determine the intact system's overall flow of information.

Acknowledgements

The writing of this chapter was supported by NIH Grants NS 11408, NS 15059, and NS 06209. The authors contributed equally to the preparation of each section, and the ordering of authorship was determined alphabetically. We are grateful to David Caplan and Alfonso Caramazza for detailed comments and suggestions on portions of an earlier version of this manuscript.

Some of the material contained in this chapter was presented at the 18th Annual Meeting of the Academy of Aphasia, October, 1980.

References

Baker, E., Blumstein, S. E. and Goodglass, H. (in press). Phonological versus semantic factors in auditory comprehension. *Neuropsychologia*.

Bever, T. G. (1970). The cognitive basis for linguistic structures. *In* "Cognition and the Development of Language", (J. R. Hayes, ed.) Wiley, New York.

Bisiach, E. (1966). Perceptual factors in the pathogenesis of anomia. *Cortex*, 2, 90–95.

Blumstein, S. E., Baker, E. and Goodglass, H. (1977). Phonological factors in auditory comprehension in aphasia. *Neuropsychologia*, 15, 19–30.

Blumstein, S. E., Cooper, W. E., Goodglass, H., Statlender, S. and Gottlieb, J. (1980). Production deficits in aphasia: A voice-onset time analysis. *Brain and Language*.

Blumstein, S. E., Cooper, W. E., Zurif, E. B. and Caramazza, A. (1977). The perception and production of voice-onset time in aphasia. *Neuropsychologia*, 15, 371–384.

Blumstein, S., Statlender, S., Goodglass, H. and Biber, C. (1979). Comprehension strategies determining reference in aphasia: A study of reflexivization. Paper presented at Academy of Aphasia, San Diego.

Bolinger, D. (1964). Intonation as a universal. *In* "Proceedings of Linguistics IX", pp. 833–844. Mouton, The Hague.

Bradley, D. C. (1979). Computational distinctions of vocabulary type. Ph.D. Thesis, MIT.

Bradley, D. C. and Garrett, M. (1980). The lexical component and sentence processing. Unpublished Manuscript, MIT.

Bradley, D. C., Garrett, M. and Zurif, E. B. (1980). Syntactic deficits in Broca's aphasia. *In* "Biological Studies of Mental Processes", (B. Caplan, ed.) pp. 269–286. MIT Press, Cambridge.

Branigan, G. (1976a). Sequences of single words on structural units. Paper presented at the Eighth Annual Child Language Research Forum, Stanford University.

Branigan, G. (1976b). Organizational constraints during the one-word period. Paper presented at the First Annual Boston University Conference on Language Development.

Breckenridge, J. (1977). Declination as a phonological process. *Bell Laboratories Technological Memo*, Murray Hill, N.J.

Brown, J. (1979). Comments on Arbib paper. Paper presented at University of Massachusetts Conference on Neural Models of Language.

Buckingham, H. W. Jr. (1974). A neurolinguistic description of neologistic jargon aphasia. Doctoral dissertation, University of Rochester.

Buckingham, H. W. Jr. (1979). Linguistic aspects of lexical retrieval disturbances in the posterior fluent aphasias. *In* "Studies in Neurolinguistics", (H. Whitaker and H. A. Whitaker, eds), Vol. 4. Academic Press, New York.

Buckingham, H. W. Jr. and Kertesz, A. (1974). A linguistic analysis of fluent aphasia. *Brain and Language*, 1, 43–62.

Butterworth, B. (1979). Hesitation and the production of verbal paraphasias and neologisms in jargon aphasia. *Brain and Language*, 8, 133–161.

Butterworth, B. (1980). Evidence from pauses. *In* "Language Production", (B. Butterworth, ed.) Vol. 1. Academic Press, London and New York.

Caplan, D. (1980). On the cerebral localization of linguistic functions. Unpublished manuscript, Department of Medicine (Neurology), University of Ottawa.

Caplan, D., Matthei, E. and Gigley, H. (in press). Comprehension of gerundive constructions by Broca's aphasics. *Brain and Language*.

Caramazza, A. and Berndt, R. S. (1978). Semantic and syntactic processes in aphasia: A review of the literature. *Psychological Bulletin*, 85, 898–918.

Caramazza, A., Brownell, H. and Berndt, R. S. (1978). Naming and conceptual deficits in aphasia. Paper presented at Academy of Aphasia, Chicago.

Caramazza, A. and Zurif, E. B. (1976). Dissociation of algorithmic and heuristic processes in language comprehension: Evidence from aphasia. *Brain and Language*, 3, 572–582.

Cooper, W. E. (1981). The analytic/holistic distinction applied to the speech of patients with hemispheric brain damage. *The Behavioral and Brain Sciences*, 4, 68–69.

Cooper, W. E., Danly, M. and Hamby, S. (1979). Fundamental frequency (Fo) attributes in the speech of Wernicke's aphasics. *In* "Speech Communication Papers Presented at the 97th Meeting of the Acoustical Society of America", (J. J. Wolf and D. H. Klatt, eds). Acoustical Society of America, New York.

Cooper, W. E. and Ehrlich, S. F. (1980). Planning speech: Studies in choice reaction time. *In* "Attention and Performance IX". (A. Baddeley and J. Long, eds). Lawrence Erlbaum Associates, Hillsdale, New Jersey.

Cooper, W. E. and Paccia-Cooper, J. (1980). *Syntax and Speech*. Harvard University Press, Cambridge, Massachusetts.

Cooper, W. E. and Sorensen, J. M. (1977). Fundamental frequency contours at syntactic boundaries. *Journal of the Acoustical Society of America*, **62**, 682–692.

Cooper, W. E. and Sorensen, J. M. (1981). "Fundamental Frequency in Sentence Production". Springer-Verlag, New York.

Danly, M., de Villiers, J. G. and Cooper, W. E. (1979). Control of speech prosody in Broca's aphasia. *In* "Speech Communication Papers Presented at the 97th Meeting of the Acoustical Society of America", (J. J. Wolf and D. H. Klatt, eds). Acoustical Society of America, New York.

Danly, M. and Shapiro, B. E. (in press). Fundamental frequency attributes in the speech of Broca's aphasics.

Delis, D., Foldi, N. S., Hamby, S., Gardner, H. and Zurif, E. B. (1979). A note on temporal relations between language and gestures. *Brain and Language*, **8**, 350–354.

Demeurisse, G., Demol, O., Robaye, E., Coekaerts, M.-J., de Beuckelaer, R. and Derouck, M. (1979). Quantitative evaluation of aphasia resulting from a cerebral vascular accident. *Neuropsychologia*, **17**, 55–65.

Duchan, J. F., Stengel, M. L. and Oliva, J. (1980). A dynamic phonological model derived from the intonational analysis of a jargon aphasic patient. *Brain and Language*, **9**, 289–297.

Fodor, J. A., Garrett, M. F., Walker, E. C. T. and Parkes, C. H. (1980). Against definitions. *Cognition*, **8**, 263–367.

Frazier, L. (1978). On comprehending sentences: Syntactic parsing strategies. Ph.D. Thesis, University of Connecticut.

Friederici, A. (1980). Structure and semantic processing in Broca's aphasia. Paper presented at Academy of Aphasia, Cape Cod, Massachusetts.

Gardner, H. (1973). The contribution of operativity to naming in aphasic patients. *Neuropsychologia*, **11**, 200–213.

Gardner, H., Denes, G. and Zurif, E. B. (1975). Critical reading at the sentence level in aphasics. *Cortex*, **11**, 60–72.

Gentner, D. (1975). Evidence for the psychological reality of semantic components: The verbs of possession. *In* "Explorations in Cognition", (D. A. Norman and D. E. Rumelhart, eds). W. H. Freeman & Co. San Francisco.

Geschwind, N. (1970). The organization of language in the brain. *Science*, **170**, 940–944.

Gleason, J. B., Goodglass, H., Obler, L., Hyde, M. and Weintraub, S. (1980). Narrative strategies of aphasic and normal-speaking subjects. *Journal of Speech and Hearing Research*, **23**, 370–382.

Goldman-Eisler, F. (1968). *Psycholinguistics*. Academic Press, London and New York.

Goodenough, C., Zurif, E. B. and Weintraub, S. (1977). Aphasics' attention to grammatical morphemes. *Language and Speech*, **20**, 11–19.

Goodglass, H. and Baker, E. (1976). Semantic field, naming, and auditory comprehension in aphasia. *Brain and Language*, **3**, 359–374.

Goodglass, H., Fodor, I. and Schulhoff, C. (1967). Prosodic factors in grammar—evidence from aphasia. *Journal of Speech and Hearing Research*, **10**, 5–20.

Goodglass, H. and Kaplan, E. (1972). "The Assessment of Aphasia and Related Disorders". Lea and Febiger, Philadelphia.

Green, E. (1969). Phonological and grammatical aspects of jargon in an aphasic patient. *Language and Speech*, **12**, 103–118.

Grober, E., Perceman, E., Kellar, L. and Brown, J. (1980). Lexical knowledge in anterior and posterior aphasics. *Brain and Language*, **10**, 318–330.

Grosjean, F. and Deschamps, A. (1975) Analyse contrastive des variables temporelles de l'anglais et du francais: Vitesse de parole et variables composants, phenomenes d'hesitation. *Phonetica*, **31**, 144–184.

Grosjean, F., Grosjean, L. and Lane, H. (1979). The patterns of silence: Performance structures in sentence production. *Cognitive Psychology*, **11**, 58–81.

Grossman, M. (1978). The game of the name: An examination of linguistic reference after brain damage. *Brain and Language*, **6**, 112–119.

Heeschen, C. (1980). Strategies of decoding actor–object-relations by aphasic patients. *Cortex*, **16**, 5–20.

Helm, N. A. (1979). Melodic intonation therapy (studien zur sprach therapie). "Patholinguistica", G. Peuser, Hrsg. Verlag, Munich.

Kean, M. L. (1977). The linguistic interpretation of aphasic syndromes. *Cognition*, **5**, 9–46.

Kean, M. L. (1980). Grammatical representations and the description of language processing. *In* "Biological Studies of Mental Processes". (D. Caplan, ed.) MIT Press, Cambridge, Massachusetts.

Kellar, L. (1978). Stress and syntax in aphasia. Paper presented at Academy of Aphasia, Chicago.

Klatt, D. H. (1975). Vowel lengthening is syntactically determined in a connected discourse. *Journal of Phonetics*, **3**, 129–140.

Kolk, H. H. L. (1978). Judgment on sentence structure in Broca's aphasia. *Neuropsychologia*, **16**, 617–625.

Kreindler, A., Mihailescu, L. and Fradis, A. (1980). Speech fluency in aphasics. *Brain and Language*, **9**, 199–205.

Lea, W. A. (1973). Segmental and suprasegmental influences on fundamental frequency contours. *In* "Consonant Types and Tone", (L. M. Hyman, ed.) pp. 15–70. USC Press, Los Angeles, California.

Lecours, A. R. and Rouillon, F. (1976). Neurolinguistic analysis of jargonaphasia and jargonagraphia. *In* "Studies in Neurolinguistics", (H. Whitaker and H. A. Whitaker, eds), Vol. 2. Academic Press, New York and London.

Levine, D. N. and Sweet, E. (1979). The neuropathologic basis of Broca's aphasia and its implications for the cerebral control of speech. Paper presented at the University of Massachusetts Conference on Neural Models of Language.

Lhermitte, F., Lecours, A. R., Ducarne, B. and Escourolle, R. (1973). Unexpected anatomical findings in a case of fluent jargon aphasia. *Cortex*, **9**, 433–446.

Lieberman, P. (1965). On the acoustic basis of the perception of intonation by linguists. *Word*, **21**, 40–54.

Lieberman, P. (1967). Intonation, perception and language. *Research Monograph No. 38*, MIT Press, Cambridge, Massachusetts.

Luria, A. R. (1970). "Traumatic Aphasia". Mouton, The Hague.

Luria, A. R. and Hutton, A. (1977). A modern assessment of the basic forms of aphasia. *Brain and Language*, **4**, 129–151.

Lyberg, B. (1979). Final lengthening–partly a consequence of restrictions on the speed of fundamental frequency change? *Journal of Phonetics*, **7**, 187–196.

McAllister, R. (1971). Predicting physical aspects of English stress. *Quarterly Progress and Status Report, Speech Transmission Laboratory*, **1**, 20–29. Royal Institute of Technology, Stockholm, Sweden.

Maeda, S. (1976). A characterization of American English intonation. Unpublished Ph.D. Thesis, MIT, Cambridge, Massachusetts.

Marie, P. (1906). La troisième circonvolution frontale gauche ne joue aucun role special dans la fonction du language. *Semaine Medicale*, **26**, 241–247.

Marin, O. and Gordon, N. (1980). Neuropsychological aspects of aphasia. *In* "Modern Neurology", (H. Tyler and D. Dawson eds). Vol. II. Wiley, New York.

Marshall, J. C. (1979). Disorders in the expression of language. *In* "Psycholinguistics", (J. Morton and J. C. Marshall), MIT. Press, Cambridge, Massachusetts.

Martin, J. G. (1970). On judging pauses in spontaneous speech. *Journal of Verbal Learning and Verbal Behavior*, **9**, 75–78.

Naeser, M. (1974). The relationship between phoneme discrimination, phonemic picture perception and language comprehension in aphasia. Paper presented at American Academy of Aphasia, Virginia.

North, E. (1971). Effects of stimulus redundancy on naming disorders in aphasia. Ph.D. Thesis, Boston University.

O'Shaughnessy, D. (1976). Modelling fundamental frequency and its relationship to syntax, semantics and phonetics. Ph.D. Thesis, MIT, Cambridge, Massachusetts.

Pick, A. (1931). "Aphasia". (Translated by Jason W. Brown. Charles Thomas, London 1973).

Rochford, G. (1974). Are jargon dysphasics dysphasic? *British Journal of Disorders of Communication*, **9**, 35–44.

Rubin, W. (1978). Unpublished manuscript, Aphasia Research Center, Boston University School of Medicine.

Saffran, E. M., Schwartz, M. F. and Marin, O. S. M. (1980). Evidence from aphasia: Isolating the components of a production model. *In* "Language Production", (B. Butterworth, ed.) Vol. 1, pp. 221–241. Academic Press, London and New York.

Schwartz, M., Saffran, E. and Marin, O. (1978). The nature of the comprehension deficits in agrammatic aphasia. Paper presented at International Neuropsychological Society, Minneapolis.

Schwartz, M. F., Saffran, E. M. and Marin, O. (1980). The word order problem in agrammatism: Comprehension. *Brain and Language*, **10**, 249–262.

Stokes, W. and Branigan, G. (1978). On the definition of two-word utterances: Or when does 1 + 1 = 2. Unpublished Manuscript, Boston University.

Swinney, D., Zurif, E. B. and Cutler, A. (1980). Interactive effects of stress and form class in the comprehension of Broca's aphasics. *Brain and Language*, **10**.

Tonkonogy, J. and Goodglass, H. (1980). Broca's aphasia, foot of F3 and Rolandic operculum. Unpublished Manuscript, Aphasia Research Center, Boston University School of Medicine.

Ulatowski, H. and Baker, W. (1975). Linguistic study of processing strategies in right- and left-brain damaged patients. Unpublished manuscript, University of Texas.

von Stockert, T. R. and Bader, L. (1976). Some relations of grammar and lexicon in aphasia. *Cortex*, **12**, 49–60.

Wagenaar, E., Snow, C. and Prins, R. (1975). Spontaneous speech of aphasic patients: A psycholinguistic analysis. *Brain and Language*, **2**, 281–303.

Weisenberg, T. H. and McBride, K. E. (1935). "Aphasia". Commonwealth Fund, New York.

Whitehouse, P., Caramazza, A. and Zurif, E. B. (1978). Naming in aphasia: Interacting effects of form and function. *Brain and Language*, **6**, 63–74.

Zurif, E. B. (1980). Language mechanisms: A neuropsychological perspective. *American Scientist*, **68**, 305–311.

Zurif, E. B. and Blumstein, S. E. (1978). Language and the Brain. *In* "Linguistic Theory and Psychological Reality", (M. Halle, J. Bresnan and G. A. Miller, eds). MIT Press, Cambridge, Massachusetts.

Zurif, E. B. and Caramazza, A. (1976). Psycholinguistic structures in aphasia: Studies in syntax and semantics. *In* "Studies in Neurolinguistics", (H. Whitaker and H. A. Whitaker, eds), Vol. 1. Academic Press, New York and London.

Zurif, E. B., Caramazza, A. and Myerson, R. (1972). Grammatical judgments of agrammatic aphasics. *Neuropsychologia*, **10**, 405–417.

Zurif, E. B., Caramazza, A., Myerson, R. and Galvin, J. (1974). Semantic feature representations in normal and aphasic language. *Brain and Language*, **1**, 167–187.

Zurif, E. B., Green, E., Caramazza, A. and Goodenough, C. (1976). Grammatical intuitions of aphasic patients: Sensitivity to functors. *Cortex*, **12**, 183–186.

7

Lexical Representation

B. Butterworth · *University College London*

I. Introduction

It is curious that, despite innumerable studies of word-recognition, "lexical decision", "lexical memory", "lexical access" and so on, very little attention has been paid by psychologists to basic questions as to how words are represented in the mind. In this essay, I shall raise some of these questions, and review some, but by no means all, of the evidence that bears on their answers.

To avoid confusion, and theoretical prejudice, let me start by introducing some terminological and typographical conventions. Words printed in italics, *cat*, designate in, as neutral as possible a manner, the word, independent of modality; slashes, e.g. /kæt/, designate an abstract phonemic representation of the sound of the word, independent of whether the sound is spoken or heard; the square brackets indicate the word sound with reference to either hearing or speech as indicated in the context, [kæt]. Capitals indicate orthographic form, and are intended as neutral as among cases, fonts, handwriting v. print etc., e.g. CAT. I shall use traditional categories in their traditionally understood meanings, unless specifically stated to the contrary. These categories include "morphemes", "inflexions", "derivations", "morphologically related". Where these terms prejudge issues, I shall employ the pretheoretical term "Lexical Representation" (LR) to stand for any entity at all that could be a candidate for the form of representation of words in the mind – it could, for example, be a morpheme, or a "lexeme" (Lyons, 1981); it could be modality-specific or modality-neutral. The nature of LRs is what is under consideration, and answers should not be prejudged by injudicious definitional fossilization. I also wish to introduce two further pretheoretical terms which are intended in the most neutral way

LANGUAGE PRODUCTION VOL. 2
ISBN 0-12-147502-6

possible: "base forms", by which I shall denote the simplest, or, where appropriate, the citation, form of a word (e.g. *sing*) and "compound forms", by which I shall denote what are traditionally described as "polymorphemic" words, for example, inflections and derivations of base forms (e.g. *sings, sang, singer*).

Intuitively, LRs are those linguistic elements that are permanently listed in the heads of speakers of a language, and which serve as terminal elements in grammatical constructions. Linguists have traditionally been concerned to characterize regularities in such a listing in order to minimize the number of items needed, and to capture speakers' knowledge about the relations among items listed. From a statement about such regularities one can set a lower theoretical bound to the number of items a speaker needs, but one cannot set an upper bound. For example, a rule which adds -*s* to form the third person singular *sings* from the base from *sing*, and to other appropriate verb forms, theoretically allows speakers to list only *sing* plus the general rule for adding -*s*. Psychologically, however, we are concerned, not with a theoretically minimal listing, but with the listing that speakers actually employ.

In addition to a simple listing of forms, base or compound, other information, associated with each form, is required by speakers. Miller (1978) has set out the following "minimal list" of the kinds of information the lexicon would contain for each lexical entry. It is minimal in the sense that every (literate) speaker of the language would have to have access to this information for each word in order to use it properly (Miller, 1978, pp. 62–63).

A. Pronunciation (and spelling for written languages)
    (i) Phonology (including stress features)
    (ii) Morphology (including inflected and derived forms)
B. Syntactic categorization
    (i) Major category (N, V, A, P . . .)
    (ii) Subcategory (syntactic contexts into which it can go)
C. Meaning
    (i) Definition (concept expressed; relation to other concepts)
    (ii) Selection restrictions (semantic contexts)
D. Pragmatic constraints
    (i) Situation (relation to general knowledge)
    (ii) Rhetoric (relation to discourse contexts)

Miller's idea of lexical entry links together a base form and all its compounds. Now it is possible, *a priori*, for each compound to have its own lexical entry. Indeed, inflected forms of, say, *sing*, will have different subcategorization contexts from the base form. So *singing* can appear in the context "was ___" but *sing* cannot; and derived forms, like *singer*, have a different major category – N as opposed to V. If identical characterizations under the headings A–D are required for two forms to appear under the same lexical entry, then almost any two words will need separate lexical entries: *sing* and *sings* are pronounced differently, and even *sing*(1) and *sing*(2) in *we sing* and *you sing* have different selection restrictions in that they can occur only with certain noun or pronoun types. If some criterion, looser than identity, is proposed for grouping under a single lexical entry, what is this criterion to be?

One possibility, following Zimmer (1964) and Aronoff (1976), would be to suggest that two forms A and B fall under the same lexical entry if the specifications under each of the heads for B can be predicted from A plus the appropriate lexical rules. So, in the case of a verb like *sing*, the forms of the various conjugations can be predicted, except for the past tense and the past participle – *sang* and *sung*; the meanings of these forms also seem straightforwardly predictable, as do the syntactic contexts appropriate for them; presumably, the pragmatic conditions in use are identical for all forms. One way of treating the unpredictable, exception forms, would be to list these explicitly in locations which for regular verbs would be filled in default by reference to the relevant rule. The speaker, then, would consult the lexical entry for *sing*, look up the location for, say, the third person present singular, find no explicit form, and deduce that it could be correctly computed from the base plus the rule for adding *-s*.

We still need a principle for grouping forms, explicit or not, under one lexical entry headed by a base form. Identity of pronunciation seems to be necessary but not sufficient. Identity of meaning appears inadequate since it would imply that forms like *teach* and *instruct*, perhaps, should share a lexical entry. Identity of pronunciation alone would imply that *palm* (hand) and *palm* (tree) share an entry: this entry would bifurcate in sections C and D, and the denominal verb will be derivable only from the first meaning (hand) (see below pp. 264–266 for a further discussion of this issue).

From a psychological perspective, one may ask what advantage a speaker (or a hearer) could derive from listing the various forms of *sing* under a single heading. One intuitively plausible reason would be that such an arrangement allows the speaker to see the relations holding among these forms – morphological, semantic and pragmatic. But other arrangements (to be discussed below) may also permit this with equal efficiency. A second reason, commonly advanced in the psychological literature (e.g. Forster, 1976) is that listing under a common heading, allows the speaker to leave blank locations for forms that can be predicted by rule, and this will minimize memory load. At the same time, as Bradley (1980) has pointed out, such a scheme will increase online computational load: every time the speaker needs the third person present singular of *sing*, he will have to locate the base form, *sing*, the relevant rule, and from these compute that *-s* is to be added and then add it. Given some processing assumptions, one might be able to predict that access to *sings* should therefore take longer than access to *sang* – which, on most accounts would have to be listed and therefore accessible directly without computation.

Miller also assumes, in A(i), that only one representation of the form is needed. This falls under the general heading "Pronunciation" though it is described as "phonological". Perhaps he is thinking of phonological features as articulatorily based (cp. Chomsky and Halle, 1968). It is not clear whether this representation is intended as specific to the speech modality, thereby requiring (nonlexical) procedures for converting auditory input into phonological features as precondition for recognizing the word: or whether nonlexical conversion is required for speaking too, implying a form of representation neutral as between speech and hearing.

This claim, though widely-held by linguists and psychologists, is by no means unequivocally supported by the data (e.g. Morton, 1981), and it remains open whether there might not be words we can recognize and understand, but cannot pronounce.

Certainly this seems to be so for children in the early stages of language development; whether this observation is to be explained in terms of separate sets of LRs for hearing and speaking, or in terms of the development of more peripheral skills, especially of pronunciation, has been a matter of some dispute (see Menn, this volume). At any event, this question should not be foreclosed prematurely.

We start then with four basic questions, to which psychological experimentation should be able to provide the answers. These questions are independent, though the answer to one may predispose investigators to certain answers to the others.

(a)   Is every word-form the speaker knows explicitly listed? I shall refer to this as the "Full Listing Hypothesis" (FLH).

(b)   What is the unit type for LRs? That is to say, do speakers list all words, or all morphemes, or words with internal morpheme boundaries marked in, or what?

(c)   Are LRs modality-neutral? Is there one format or code for listing words? Linguists suggest a modality-neutral phonemic representation, but it is possible that each word has several representations – one acoustic, one articulatory, one orthographic for reading, one motor-manual for writing and so on, and perhaps a phonemic one as well. I can best illustrate this claim by reference to hearing. The word, *sing*, will be associated with a specific acoustic template which is employed in analysing the acoustic input to the ears. This is to be distinguished from the modality-neutral claim that the acoustic input is translated into, say, a sequence of phonemes and it is this that is matched with the stored phoneme sequence /sɪŋ/.

(d)   How are LRs organized? Are there distinct sublists for different kinds of words, for example "function words" as compared with content words (as Bradley, 1980 has claimed). Is the list (or lists) organized by meaning, by sound or by frequency of use, or some combination of all three? Or in some quite different way?

The independence of these questions yields a quite unmanageable combinatorial explosion of potential characterizations of LRs. For example, it is *a priori*, possible for there to be modality specific lexicons, each of which is organized according to some different principle. Indeed, it would not be implausible to propose that the lexicon for hearing is arranged according to the principle of sound – i.e. words with similar sounds being located close together in a multidimensional sound space since access to this lexion is from an analysis of sounds, whereas the lexicon for speaking is arranged according to meaning, since it is from a prior specification of word meaning that the appropriate word is located. Moreover, it may turn out that the FLH applies, say, to the hearing lexicon, but not to the reading lexicon.

Unfortunately, the available evidence does not address the whole range of potential combinations of answers, and in many cases leaves even the simple questions unresolved.

II. The Full Listing Hypothesis

Linguistics have traditionally rejected the Full Listing Hypothesis (FLH), preferring an approach by which regularities in lexical representation are stated by rules, and only elements not so stated need a listing in the lexicon. Bloomfield (1933, p. 274) wrote:

> Any form that a speaker can utter without having heard it is regular in its immediate constitution and embodies regular functions of its constituents, and any form which a speaker can utter only after he has heard it from other speakers is irregular. Strictly speaking then every morpheme of a language is an irregularity, since the speaker can use it only after hearing it used . . . The lexicon is really an appendix of the grammar, a list of basic irregularities. This is all the more evident if meanings are taken, since the meaning of each morpheme belongs to it by an arbitrary tradition.

There are two separate aspects of Bloomfield's claim. First, the "arbitrary tradition" linking each morpheme with its meaning; second, the relation of compound word-forms to their components. Morphologically and syntactically, this second idea can be heard to echo in later writings. Chomsky (1965, p. 87). proposes that "in general, all properties of a formative that are essentially idiosyncratic will be specified in the lexicon." Similarly, Chomsky and Halle (1968, p. 12) write, "Regular variations are not matters for the lexicon, which should contain only idiosyncratic items . . . not predictable by a general rule."

The first idea has received less attention, but clearly for a compound (i.e. polymorphemic) word to be used correctly either it must be linked to its meaning by an arbitrary tradition, or its meaning must be a predictable function of its components (cp. Aronoff, 1976). In the former case, the compound must necessarily be listed in the lexicon.

It may be a tautology to claim that anything not available via a rule must be separately listed, it is by no means a tautology to claim that everything available via a rule must be available only in that way. Following this line of reasoning, let us consider what would be involved if the FLH were rejected and only idiosyncracies were to be listed (leaving out of account aspects which this approach would share with a FLH approach).

(i)   A listing of base forms – e.g. *sing*
(ii) A set of lexical rules to permit the computation of all regular compounds – e.g.

(3rd singular present) V $\rightarrow$ V + *-s*
(agentive) V $\rightarrow$ V + *-er*

(iii) A listing of all irregular compounds (perhaps with tags on the base indicating where rules in (ii) should not be applied) – e.g.

(past participle) V $\rightarrow$ *sung*

(iv) A set of syntactic rules to permit the computation of (a) subcategorization frames for compounds, and (b) major categories of compounds – e.g. V + *ing* following part of the verb *to be*; agentive *-er* is a noun where the base was a verb.
(v)   A set of semantic rules which permit the computation of the meanings of the compounds of the base – e.g.

(Past Tense) V' $\rightarrow$ [Past] V'

(where V' indicates the meaning of the base V, and [past] V' indicates the meaning of the past tense of V. The exact interpretation of these terms is not relevant to our argument here, since the same issues appear in relation to the FLH as well. There will be some discussion of these issues further on).

(agentive) V' – Someone or something that Vs

By contrast, the FLH implies the following kind of arrangement: a form (e.g. *sings*) associated with a meaning (e.g. *sings'*, which is intended to denote the meaning of *sings*), a major category (V), and a list of suitable syntactic contexts, or subcategorization frames.

I should point out a quite general problem with rules, namely what is to count as "regular" and hence rule-governed. In English, as in other languages, there will be rules that apply to a large number of base forms, and rules that apply to smaller sets of base forms, and rules that apply to a singleton set (traditionally known as suppletive forms, e.g. *go* $\rightarrow$ *went; be* $\rightarrow$ *is*). So, in principle, any conjugation or declension CAN be generated by a rule, though rules which apply to only one LR do not seem to confer much usefulness or generality on this treatment. In any case, under a rule treatment, lexical entries would have to specify which rules are to apply in forming compounds, and it is possible to envisage a situation where the claimed advantages for this approach are lost by actually increasing the memory load to proportions comparable with the FLH model.

Notice also that rules can arise – be acquired – in two ways, and can also function in two ways. First, they can be learned *as* rules (as we learned to conjugate Latin verbs from a school grammar), or they can be induced from a corpus of exemplars. It seems quite likely that the pluralizing rule observed by Berko (1958) in children of three to four years of age, was learned by induction. However knowledge of a rule comes about, there is no logical guarantee that it is routinely employed to access compound forms. It is conceivable that LRs are routinely accessed from a full listing, but in certain circumstances – for new items, for items not accessible from the list for some other reason – the rules may serve as fall-back procedure. It may even be that, in these circumstances, the speaker does not retrieve an already learned rule but runs a quick induction over the relevant portions of the existing listing to come up with a rule suitable to the occasion.

An analogy from a related area may serve to illustrate the contrast between full-listing and rule-based procedure in a domain that is not wholly regular. Suppose a reader of English is confronted with a novel sequence of letters, e.g. YEAD, how might he read this sequence out loud? If he was using a rule-based procedure, he would have available six rules at least for pronouncing EA:

   (i)   EA $\rightarrow$ /iə/ as in *rear, beard*
   (ii)   EA $\rightarrow$ /i/ *bead*
   (iii) EA $\rightarrow$ /ɛ/ *head*
   (iv) EA $\rightarrow$ /ə/ *yearn*
   (v)   EA $\rightarrow$ /ɛə/ *bear*
   (vi) EA $\rightarrow$ /eɪ/ *break*

There would, in addition, have to be some system of cross-indexing to ensure that, say, (ii) applied just to BEAD, MEAD, LEAD etc and (iii) applied just to HEAD, DEAD, LEAD etc. (Cross-indexing will, of course, be needed even in a system which interprets EA according to the most frequently used rule, unless there is a specific indication to the contrary). When presented with YEAD, for which there is no cross-indexing, he may choose any of (i)–(vi), or prefer one that applies to more grapheme sequences (tokens *or* types) in the orthographic language.

With a full-listing procedure, each grapheme sequence standing for a word in English would be associated with its own pronunciation: HEAD – /hed/, BEAD – /bid/, LEAD – /led, li:d/ etc. Of course, there would be no listing for YEAD, and hence no way of pronouncing it. What can he do? He may know rules like (i) and (ii) from an induction over the many words he has experienced in his literature lifetime in which case, he would have a fall-back which would leave in the same position as if he were routinely using rules. Alternatively, he may construct rules for pronouncing YEAD by rapidly sampling other sequences containing the relevant subsequences for which he does know the pronunciation. That is, he will consult HEAD –/hɛd/, BEAD – /bid/ etc., until he derives a suitable rule. In an ingenious experiment, Kay and Marcel (1981) have shown that the pronunciation of YEAD depends on the samples consulted, and this in turn can be biased by presenting the reader with a relevant sample shortly before the target item. So, when the reader encounters the following list to read . . . GONE BEAD SHOE POUR YEAD . . . he will pronounce YEAD as /jid/; but when he encounters a list like . . . GONE HEAD SHOE POUR YEAD . . . he will pronounce it /jɛd/. This result also suggests that a sample size of one may be all that the reader uses; in which case, all that the speaker needs to assume is that the relation between graphemes and phonemes is not entirely random, even in English, and that a fair try at the pronunciation of a novel grapheme sequence may be based on a cursory examination of the pronunciation of similar sequences. That is, he does not need substantive rules at all associating graphemes with phonemes but only a kind of metarule which asserts in general some kind of relation between graphemes and their pronunciation. Notice also, to get the pronunciation correct of the -EA- words in a rule-based procedure virtually every word containing EA has to be cross-indexed to the appropriate rule, and the advantages of reduced memory load will not apply here.

An important condition for rejecting FLH is that compounds bear meanings that are predictable functions of their components. For inflexional compounds, for example conjugations, this seems straightforward, even though the morphology of the compounds may not be regular:

(1) bore,   bores,   boring,   bored
(2) sing,   sings,   singing,   sang
(3) be,   is,   being,   was

The semantic relation between *bore* and *bored* is the same as between *be* and *was* (under the infinitival interpretation of *bore*, and the third singular or first singular interpretation of *bored* – it would be clearer in languages where these morphological ambiguities did not exist). And it seems silly to deny that speakers have access to knowledge of this regularity. What they do with it is, of course, another matter.

Derivations, on the other hand, are another matter again. *-ion* can be applied in a fairly regular way to verbs to yield a noun, with predictable semantic results in many cases:

(4) digest   digestion – the act of digesting
(5) prohibit   prohibition – the act of prohibiting.

But *-ive* applied to the same bases to yield adjectives does not give such predictable results:

(6) digestive   – promoting digestion, pertaining to digestion
(7) prohibitive   – serving to prohibit, *pertaining to prohibiting (where *
                   indicates that this interpretation does not exist.

The compounds of *induce* are an interesting case. *Induce* has several meanings, but not all derivations can be used with all meanings nor do they have predictable results when they do (see Table 1). This sets the rule-based model some difficult problems. For instance, the application of the *-ment* addition rule seems to apply just under two readings of the verb. Extrapolating from this example would require derivational rules to be sensitive to meaning and not just to lexical identity. That is, the standard problem is that some rules apply just to some lexical items, so the rules must be stated in a

TABLE I

Five senses of *induce* and their derived senses

induce [induce] V V	*inducement* [[induce] ment] NV V N	*inductive* [[ind?] + ive] AV V A	*induction* [[ind?] + ion] NV V N	*inducible* [[induce] + ible] AV V
1. Persuade	Something that persuades	(Influences)†	*	*
2. Cause	Something that causes	*	*	(Causable)†
3. Produce current	*	Pertaining to producing current	Process of producing current Result of producing current	[current] is producible
4. Infer from cases	*	Pertaining to cases	Process of inference Result of inference	Inferrable
5. [Induct]	*	Introductory	Introduction Initiation of GIs Inauguration of President	*

† indicates that this derivation is marginal or doubtful.
* indicates that there is no derivation under this interpretation.

lexically-sensitive way; now we have an added complication. Of course, this is also a problem for a FLH model, but it may resolve into the usual problem of how to treat homonyms.

Certain other types of compound do appear more regular in their semantics. Comparatives being one such (Klein, 1980). Here major category is unaffected by derivation, though subcategorization is:

(8) The table is wider than the chair
(9) *The table is wide than the chair
(Where * indicates that the word sequence is ungrammatical)

Morphologically similar, but semantically quite distinct, is the -er used to form agentive and instrumental nouns from verbs: *walk–walker, cook–cooker*, respectively. Some forms may have both agentive and instrumental readings: *clean–cleaner* (one who cleans, something to clean with). It is not clear whether the verbs that take the instrumental reading form a well-defined, predictable type, though the class of verbs taking instruments as grammatical subjects seems to be a good candidate:

(10) The pot was cooking
(11) Ajax cleans well.

Nevertheless, and I shall return to this, derivational compounds where major category is changed by the derivational process, in general have unpredictable semantics and thus constitute a major problem for a model of LR which rejects to FLH.

A. FLH: Evidence from Speech Production

In this modality, the critical evidence comes from the analysis of certain classes of speech error in which words appear to break down into their component morphemes, and recombine in systematic ways. Garrett (1975, 1976, 1980) and myself in earlier papers (Butterworth, 1979, 1980) have argued that these analyses demonstrate that affixal morphemes – especially inflexions – are selected independently of lexical stems and are added to them at a relatively late stage in speech production. This position has been supported by studies of aphasia where affixal processes can be spared in patients where access to lexical stems has been severely impaired (Butterworth, 1979). I now think these conclusions were premature, and that the evidence against FLH is not particularly convincing.

It is well-established, and uncontroversial, that phonetic segments exchange positions to produce slips of the tongue. These exchanges occur for segments in the initial positions of words to produce classic "spoonerisms", like (12) from Fromkin (1971):

(12) *h*eft *l*emisphere   Target: *l*eft *h*emisphere

and for segments in other positions, including word-final positions (Fromkin, 1973):

(13)　to*tch* no*p*　　　　　　　　Target: to*p* no*tch*
　　　go*d* to see*n*　　　　　　　Target: go*ne* to see*d*

More than one segment or whole final syllables, also exchange, as in

(14)　the sing*est* bigg*le* problem　Target: sing*le* bigg*est* problem
(15)　pass*age* us*ive*　　　　　　Target: pass*ive* us*age*

(both from Garrett, 1980, p. 201). None of these errors involve the movement of identifiable morphemes.

　　Garrett (1975, 1976, 1980) has pointed out that final portions of words that
can be identified as morphemes also shift into erroneous locations:

(16)　I'd forgot about*en* that　　Target: I'd forgot*ten* about that
(17)　point out*ed*　　　　　　　Target: point*ed* out
(both from Garrett, 1980, p. 202)

And, more strikingly, morphemic stems can exchange "stranding" their
affixes in the intended locations, as in:

(18)　I want to get a cash check*ed*　Target: I want to get a check cash*ed*
(19)　It wait*s* to pay　　　　　　Target: It pay*s* to wait
(1980, p. 197)

From examples like these, Garrett infers that the source of bound
morphemes, and the processes for inserting them into the structure to be
output, are separable from the source of stems and the processes for inserting them. A sentence frame is constructed in which the bound morpheme is
located in the appropriate phrase marker slot, and then into these slots
lexical stems are inserted. In an earlier treatment (Garrett, 1975), Garrett
did not accord morphemes any special status, and treated stranding
exchanges and final position errors as simply involving word fragments –
segments or syllables. This earlier position can be seen to be consistent with
FLH, where these errors can be analysed in terms of elements in the string of
phonemes to be realized articulatorily. The current position, however,
keeps distinct stems and affixes, where the lexicon will list only stem forms,
inflexions being added later, on their insertion into the sentence frame. This
is how stranding exchanges add the wrong inflexion to the stem.

　　What are Garrett's grounds for this change in position? He offers two
pieces of distributional evidence.

(i)　Bound morphemes do not exchange, but other word final fragments
　　do (e.g. (13); (16) and (17) are shifts of one morpheme, not an
　　exchange). (1980: 201)
(ii)　Stems exchange stranding bound morphemes, but other word
　　"portions" – e.g. syllables not coextensive with a morpheme – do not
　　exchange stranding fragments. (1980: 197)

In both Garrett's corpus, and Fromkin's (esp. 1973, Appendix S) we can find
no examples which clearly contradict claim (i) but there are plenty of
examples which are inconsistent with claim (ii). In Fromkin's Appendix
AA, we find

(20) [dij sərd] of [θɛmbər]   Target: *th*ird of *Dec*ember

where a nonmorphemic syllable *Dec-* exchanges with an initial segment, and

(21) fran sanisko   Target: San Francisco

where *San* and *Fran* exchange leaving behind the nonmorphemic fragment *isko* (the medial /s/ has got lost somewhere along the way).

A second type of problematic exchange has been pointed out by Garrett himself, in which stems exchange stranding derivational morphemes, as in

(22) square it face*ly*   Target: face it square*ly*
(23) I've got a load of cook*en*   Target: I've got a load of chick*en*
     chick*ed*   cook*ed*

> In the MIT corpus, 64% of the stranding errors involve only inflectional morphemes, while 23% involve an inflexional morpheme and a derivational morph or a non-morph that is positionally and prosodically appropriate (and often phonetically identical) to an inflection. (1980, p. 198)

It is difficult to see how the involvement of derivational morphemes is reconcilable with Garrett's model. The explanation of stranding exchanges is that stems go into the wrong slots, and these slots are defined syntactically and marked with the appropriate syntactic device. Unless, Garrett wants to argue that *derivational* morphology is handled as a syntactic process rather than a lexical one, these examples surely constitute strong counterexamples to the separation of lexical selection and insertion from the processes of sentence frame construction. If he does want to handle derivational processes syntactically he will run into all the traditional problems of lexically-specified application of derivational rules (see above, p. 264). Thus one seems to be left with a case that rests solely on the nonexistence of bound morpheme exchanges.

If the process of selecting lexical bases is indeed distinct from other word-forming processes, like adding inflexional or derivational affixes, one would expect to find cases of language breakdown where just one of these processes is impaired while the others are intact. Perhaps the clearest evidence comes from the analysis of the speech of jargon aphasics. These patients appear to have unimpaired prosody, syntax and morphology, while they show fairly severe impairment in word-finding. What distinguishes them from other "anomic" aphasics is how they cope with this word-finding difficulty. Anomic patients resort to elaborate circumlocutions when they cannot find the appropriate word, or, on other occasions, they leave a gap in their output where the word should have been. Jargon cases, on the other hand, make up words to fill these gaps. These neologisms are generally phonotactically regular – i.e. they sound like English words (if the patient is an English speaker) – and frequently the neologisms seem to be constructed from a nonsense stem plus derivational and inflexional affixes (Butterworth, 1979) as in the following examples:

(24) I remember the other [dɒkjumən] and was [pleɪzd] to see the other
    ['dɒkjumən]
(25) he [mɪvz] in a love-beautiful home
(26) she ['wiksɨz] a [zɛn] from me
(27) but there are a few [zʌmrəz]
(28) the great ['ziːmləs] where I used to work
(29) It was about in [ɛd'zɪmərɪks] in ['ɛksʃiə] neares to ['ɛmtʃɜtʃ]

In (24)–(27) he produces appropriate inflexional affixes on nonsense stems.
[pleɪzd] has an appropriate past participle -d; [mɪvz] and ['wiksɨz] have the
appropriate allomorphs of the third person present singular, -z and -əz;
[zʌmrəz] has a plural ending in a plural context following a few . . . In (29) the
derivational affix, -less is added to the nonsense stem [ziːm]; and (30) shows
that the patient still has control of the arcana of English place-name
morphology with -shire and -church. (These examples are from
Butterworth, 1979.)

Examples like these are consistent with the Garrett–Butterworth (1980)
position that endings are added after stems have been selected, or, in this
case, made-up. However, this is not the only interpretation. A supporter of
FLH is not forced to deny that affixing rules are unknown to speakers (as
opposed to linguists), but only that they are not routinely used. Clearly, in
language breakdown, all kinds of language routines can be affected, and
knowledge of rules may then come into play in fall-back procedures. We
shall see below that normal speakers also use rules in the (erroneous)
construction or derived forms that they surely know, and in others which
they may not. You may never have come across the word undigitalizable, but
you would be able to understand it if you heard it, and you may even be able
to construct it if you needed a word with this meaning. (It was invented (or
reinvented) by David Howard (pers. commun.) to illustrate just this point.)
As Goldstein (1948) has remarked, aphasic patients have to call on many
different kinds of fall-back procedures to cope with their language-dis-
ability, and it would not be surprising if they called on knowledge of
morphological rules in their attempts to communicate with others.

Thus, the evidence from speech production in both normal and language-
impaired speakers is by no means decisive in rejecting FLH.

B. FLH: Evidence from Speech Perception

There is very little experimental evidence bearing directly on FLH in hearing, and theorists, bold on other modalities, are curiously reticent here. One
exception is an early paper by Morton (1968), in which he describes a
sophisticated model of word recognition and production within a broader
framework of language processing. Central to this model is the idea of a
"logogen". This is a unit which makes available a word as a response when
its threshold is exceeded. "All information relevant to a single word

response converges [on the logogen] regardless of the source of information" (1968, p. 501) and raises the level of activation in it towards the threshold. Logogens are thus modality-neutral, in my sense, so what he claims in general for them will apply, *mutatis mutandis*, to hearing, and he does make certain predictions about FLH which he says will be open to experimental test. "For reasons of economy, it is suggested that all inflected forms of a word affect the same logogen. Thus 'walk', 'walks', 'walked', 'walking', and possibly 'walker' will all give rise to M_{walk}" (1968, p. 516) where "M_{walk}" is the output from the *walk* logogen in a morphemic code which is analysed by a "surface structure analyser" and labelled with a syntactic category for later semantic interpretation by a "dictionary". "The bound morphemes -*s*, -*ed*, -*ing* would then be identified separately, and it would not be rational to call such identifying units 'logogens', for such morphemes are not normally produced as single responses". (1968, p. 516)

The model then rejects the FLH, preferring instead the independent listing and identification of stems and affixes. Morton's current position, however, differs from this in two important ways. First, he has offered evidence suggesting that instead of one modality-neutral representation for a word, separate modality-specific logogens are required (see Section IV below for further discussion of this evidence). Second, irregular compounds will have to have their own logogens. Thus [sɪŋ, sɪŋz, sɪŋgɪŋ] all affect the *sing* logogen, but [sæŋ] affects only the *sang* logogen.

Morton (1981) cites an unpublished experiment by himself and Kempley which supports this second point. Auditory recognition of a word in noise can be facilitated by a previous hearing of a related compound. Thus recognition of *looks* will be made easier by a previous hearing of *looking*, indeed the size of this effect is as great as with a previous hearing of the identical word. However, and this is the crucial point, prior exposure to *stink* has no facilitatory effect on *stank*. Morton is led to postulate an organization of logogens such that access to a regular compound activates all other regular compounds of that base; but irregular forms which have their own logogen units are not so linked. It is not clear whether this change implies abandoning the morphemic character of logogens, and the adoption of some form of the FLH (see especially Fig. 3, p. 393 of Morton, 1981).

One final point about the Kempley and Morton experiment. In the design, they rigidly separated regular and irregular verbs. That is, they did not test to see whether the regular compounds of *stink* (*stinks*, *stinking*) could facilitate each other, so it remains possible that it is not just irregular forms that behave differently, but any verb with at least one irregular compound.

C. FLH: Evidence from Reading

The evidence here is more extensive, and can be interpreted as consistent with FLH provided that a base and its compounds are grouped together in certain ways.

Murrell and Morton (1974) showed that recognition of a compound is facilitated by "pretraining" with its base. Using tachistoscopic presentation of words, they found that if the subject had previously been shown SEE, then the exposure needed for him to recognize SEEN was briefer than if he had previously been exposed to an unrelated word. Moreover, prior presentation of words which were merely phonetically similar – like SCENE – has no facilitatory effect, nor did words which were merely visually similar – like SEED. Murrell and Morton argue for a common morphemic representation of SEE, SEEN, SEES etc. to account for this effect, but alternative explanations are possible. Compounds share many semantic attributes and it is known that pretraining with a semantically related word facilitates subsequent recognition, thus recognition of DOCTOR is facilitated by recent prior experience of the word NURSE; and SEEN will be semantically related to SEE, but not to SCENE or SEED. Morton, more recently, has claimed that this kind of semantic facilitation effect decays very rapidly in just a few seconds and thus could not have operated the intervals used in the Murrell and Morton experiment, which were between 10 and 45 minutes (Morton, 1979, 1981). But the evidence for this distinction between long-term and short-term effects still awaits decisive experimental test.

Bobrow and Bell (1973) and Swinney and Cutler (1979) have reported results which strongly suggest that idioms behave more like lexical items than a function of their parts. Of course, the meaning of phrases like *kick the bucket* is not predictable from the component words and syntax. So one would expect a special listing. Swinney and Cutler found that readers could judge idioms as "sensible" more quickly than normal, matched control phrases. This, they argue, indicates that idioms are "lexicalized", though not held in a separate list (as claimed by Bobrow and Bell). They do not specify how reading processes are organized so that idiomatic interpretations are arrived at. Presumably, their data show that idiomatic phrases are processed literally and idiomatically in parallel. This implies that every time a word appears which could be the first item in an idiomatic phrase, this lexicalized phrase is accessed. One problem is that there seems to be no correlation between decision times and the "frozenness" of the phrase – i.e. the extent to which it can undergo syntactic variation (Fraser, 1970) *the bucket was kicked by John* is not possible variant of *John kicked the bucket*, but *the ice was broken by John* does seem to keep its idiomatic reading.

A study by Stachowiak et al. (1977) shows that German aphasics, who have relatively poor comprehension of individual words and texts, are nevertheless not specifically (differentially) impaired, as compared with normals, on the correct interpretation in context of idiomatic expressions. These subjects were presented with texts like (A) – translated from the German – and asked to match them to one of a set of five pictures.

(A) Mr. Bauer works in an office. He has volunteered to replace his colleagues during their holidays. But, after having been ill himself for a week, Mr. Bauer is unable to cope with the piles of files on his desk. He filled his soup with pieces of bread (= He got himself into a nice mess). That's what comes of his ambition. Which picture shows what situation he is in?

The critical pictures showed him (a) struggling through a mound of files and (b) filling a soup bowl with pieces of bread. Both normal and aphasic subjects readily rejected (b). For idioms where the "literal" meaning is closer to the idiomatic, both normals and aphasics made comparable numbers of mistakes on the critical pictures. For example, in a story about losing at poker, the critical sentence was "The others strip him right down to his shirt", and both types of subjects produced a substantial proportion of responses (15–25%) picking the picture showing the others stripping him right down to his shirt, but with the majority of responses, of course, being for the picture showing the others with large piles of money and him with none.

One might have thought, on Cutler and Swinney's thesis, that idioms would have been differentially affected, since they would be relatively infrequent lexical items, since every occurrence of *kick the bucket* will access *kick*, and in addition so will every occurrence of *kick* in literal contexts. And in general aphasics are worse on low frequency lexical items, than on high (Newcombe *et al.*, 1965; Howes, 1964) (on the other hand, given that aphasics are generally poorer than normals on syntactic and semantic processing, there might be a countervailing advantage for idiomatic units not needing these processes for comprehension).

Bradley (1978) proposes a version of FLH in which (at least some regular) compounds are listed together under a representation which she calls the "name" of the word. Thus *kick*, *kicking*, *kicker* will all be listed under "kick". She argues from this to the prediction that the word-frequency effect (which is extremely powerful in many reading tasks, Whaley, 1978) will be a function of the total frequency of all forms listed under one name, and not, as has been commonly supposed, the frequency of the tested form alone. So infrequent compounds which are part of a highly frequent "cluster" of forms should behave like frequent words not like infrequent ones. *Sharpness* and *briskness* have the same frequency of occurrence, but *sharp* and its compounds are much more frequent than *brisk* and its compounds. As predicted, in a task where subjects have to decide as quickly as possible whether a letter string is a word she finds that decision times are shorter for *sharpness* than for *briskness*. (In the complementary case, where the clusters are matched for overall frequency, but the test items contrast – *happiness* v. *heaviness* (low frequency), there is no effect of item frequency). Interestingly, this result is replicated for compounds using morphologically and semantically fairly regular affixes – *-er*, *-ment* as well as *-ness* – but the effect does not occur for irregular *-ion* compounds. Thus, she claims, these regular forms at least are clustered under their name, through which they are accessed. The irregular compounds, also fully-listed, may instead have their own names, and not form clusters of this sort.

III. Unit Type

The kind of unit or units that should be proposed for LRs is logically independent of the FLH. Of course, if FLH is accepted, there seems to be less reason for proposing some kind of morpheme-based LR. Nevertheless, it is possible in a full listing for all forms to have an internal structure marking morpheme boundaries. Bradley (1980), who seems to favour FLH, and Lyons (1981) who is presumably agnostic, propose two quite different kinds of unit: one kind is a unit that actually forms part of the speech chain; the second kind is more abstract and does not participate in this process. Bradley calls this second a "name" (see above), Lyons a "lexeme", where all forms of, say, *sing*, fall under the name "sing". It will be helpful to list some of the candidates for unit type.

A. Unit Type Candidates

(a) all forms, each with a separate listing, and with no internal morphemic structure (*sings*; *singing*; . . .).

(b) all forms, each with a separate listing, but with morphemic boundaries marked in (*sing + s*; *sing + ing*; . . .).

(c) all forms, grouped under a heading, where the heading may be any of the types (d)–(h) (*sing-sings-singing* . . .).

(d) base forms only which are directly realizable and enter into rule processes.

(e) citation forms, realizable, but do not enter into rule processes.

(f) names, or lexemes, not realizable, and do not enter rule processes.

(g) morphemes – proper parts of words, but not words themselves.

(h) underlying representations, in the style of "generative phonology", where this representation enters into rules, unlike lexemes, though may itself never be realized phonetically. The classic example is the underlying form of *divine* and *divinity* which Chomsky and Halle (1968) claim is /dɪviːn/. The vowel /iː/ is never found in any of the derived forms since the rules always change it into another vowel – e.g. /aɪ/ in *divine* and /ɪ/ in *divinity*.

Linguists are by no means agreed on the proper analysis of LRs. Lyons (1981) distinguishes the principal candidates, much as I have done. Two kinds of evidence are relevant to the psychological issue. First, can people recognize and work with the proposed type? That is, do people notice that *terror* and *horror* are related to *terrify* and *horrify*; and that *horrid* is the adjective associated with *horror* and that *terrid* would be the adjective related to *terror* by the same rule, but happens not to be? Second, even if they can reconstruct these relations, are they "computationally effective" in the normal processes of speech production and reception? Language users may have a full listing of all the words they can use which is employed in normal online processing, yet when they are off duty, not speaking or hearing, reading or writing, they may run inductions over this listing in order to find regularities which will be useful in certain circumstances. Off duty, do people behave like linguists?

In fact, this seems to be what children do. In the case of tensed forms, children start by using only present tense forms e.g. *go*, *goes* – perhaps because these are the most common in parents' talk to children. There is then a stage in which they appear to collect individual past tenses which are generally used in appropriate contexts to indicate past events – e.g. *went*. This is followed by a stage during which they seem to have discovered a past-tense forming rule, and they apply it indiscriminately to all verbs – e.g. *goed*. Finally, they are able to discriminate regular and irregular past tense forms – *went* again (Berko, 1958).

These data clearly demonstrate the computational effectiveness of rules in forming past tenses: the child will not have heard *goed*, so he will have had to apply the rule to construct it. Berko (1958) showed that children are able to apply this kind of morphological rule to new words. But the important question is this: once the child has constructed the past tense of *spank*, will he have to construct anew each time he needs it, or will he simply draw on the results of the first computation?

Unfortunately, there is little decisive psychological evidence on any of these questions.

B. Evidence from Speech Production

In the last section, we saw that the apparent involvement of inflectional and derivational affixes in stranding errors did not constitute decisive evidence for the separate representation of stems and affixes. Further relevant evidence comes from substitution errors in which an error form substitutes for the correct form. The examples in (30) come from Cutler (1980).

(30) (a) self-indúlgement   Target: self-indúlgence
     (b) deríval   Target: derivátion
     (c) dispútion   Target: disputátion
     (d) concédence   Target: concéssion
     (e) expéction   Target: expectátion
     (f) proféssoral   Target: professórial

It is hard to believe that the speakers did not know the correct forms of these words. Cutler points out that the targets in (b)–(f) change stress and vowel quality as compared to their roots. Thus *derivation* reduces the /aɪ/ in *derive* and moves the stress from /aɪ/ to /eɪ/; whereas the error forms are "transparent" with respect to their bases – that is, neither vowel quality nor stress location are altered. Out of 119 errors of this sort, Cutler found that 90 did not affect transparency – like (30)(a), 21 became more transparent – like examples (b)–(f), 8 became less transparent, like (31)

(31) inconsiderátion   Target: inconsíderateness

These errors are particularly interesting because they cannot all be explained as haplologies – contractions causing a fragment to be left out –*self-indulgement* and *inconsideration* are not contractions of their targets, nor is *concedence*, which looks exactly how one might expect it to look after the misapplication of a rule to the base verb *concede*. And, generally, the misapplication of a rule to a base seems to be the most plausible account. What can be said about these bases? First, they all seem to be real words; that is, rules seem to be applied to *indulge, derive, dispute, concede, expect, professor*, and not to forms like *derivate-, disputate-, concess-, expectate-*. This is consonant with Aronoff's linguistic treatment of word formation rules, in which he argues that the input to such rules is a real word, and not some nonrealizable morpheme base (1976). Even (31) can be interpreted as addition of *in* to the real word base *consideration*. Second, the forms which undergo these derivational processes seem to have the stressed syllable labelled as such, since this is generally preserved in the derivation.

Of course, the question arises, why do speakers produce these errors when they know what the correct word is? There are two possibilities. First, if the speaker has one set of lexical representations for hearing, and one for speaking (see below, Section IV), then the target may be in the hearing lexicon only, and thus only in that sense does he know it. It is not implausible to suggest that there are some words that a person has only heard (or seen) but never spoken. In this case, the speaker will have to construct an output representation. Normally, he will check this representation against his input representation, but occasionally, perhaps in less careful speech, he may omit to do this. The principles of new word construction will, perhaps, be, in the first instance, the most regular or transparent rules applied to some form – not necessarily the simplest base form, since in (31) the form *consideration*, rather than *consider* seems to have been used.

The second possibility is that, temporarily, the requisite form is not available, and therefore has to be constructed, with the same conditions as in the first.

There are some problems with the view that only real words are involved in these processes. Fromkin (1973, Appendix R) lists examples of derivational errors where the source seems to be a nonword morpheme:

(32) acoustal theory   Target: acoustic theory   (acoust-)
     counter índicant   Target: counter indicátor   (indic-)
     percéptic monitoring   Target: perceptual   (percépt-)
     is not ambígual   Target: ambiguous   (ambígu-)
     introdúcting   Target: introducing   (introduc-)

I have also noted examples like these:

(33) volúptitude   Target: voluptuous   (volupt-)
      fortúity   Target: fortuitousness   (fortuit-)

(Note: although *indicant* and *fortuity* are real, if very rare, words, the speakers seem to have regarded these forms as errors.)

C. Evidence from Reading

Under the FLH, recognizing a letter string as a word will involve matching (an analysis of) a letter string to one from a stored list of letter strings. Alternative hypotheses as to how this matching is done are possible. Manelis and Tharp (1977), tested models in which unsuffixed words – like FANCY – would be recognized in a different way from suffixed words – like DUSTY (= DUST + Y). In such models, a suffixed word would be "decomposed" into base plus ending prior to matching with items in the orthographic lexicon (i.e. the stored list of letter strings). They postulate three models: (1) and (2) involve decomposition and predict differential effects for words like FANCY and DUSTY in a lexical decision task, and (3) which does not involve decomposition, and which, other things being equal, predicts no differences in reading performance.

1. *Decomposition first*

Step 1. Decompose the whole item into base and ending

Step 2. Test whether base and ending are valid in combination as an affixed word
    If YES, give a positive response
    If NO, do step 3

Step 3. Search lexicon for the whole item
    If present, give positive response
    If absent, give negative response
Under this model, DUSTY should give a positive response before FANCY

2. *Decomposition second*

Step 1. Search lexicon for whole item
    If present, give positive response
    If absent, go on to Steps 2 and 3

Step 2. Decompose whole item into base and ending

Step 3. Test whether base and ending are valid in combination as an affixed word

If YES, give a positive response
If NO, give negative response
Under this model, FANCY should get a positive response before DUSTY, since only the base (and affix separately) will be listed in the lexicon, and the reader will have to go on to do Step 3.

3. *Single-unit hypothesis*

Step 1. Search lexicon for the whole item
    If present, give positive response
    If absent, give negative response
This predicts no difference in response time between words like FANCY and DUSTY (provided they have matched on other attributes that may affect response times – e.g. word frequency, length, bigram and trigram frequencies etc.)

In their experiment, Manelis and Tharp used words whose endings were among the most regular, morphologically and semantically, and whose bases therefore should best candidates for base-only listing: -Y, -ING, -EST, -EN, -ER. In fact, it was found that there were no differences in response times for affixed words as compared with nonaffixed controls.

One problem with the logic of this kind of test may have already occurred to the careful reader. How is the reader to test whether a base and ending are valid in combination except by reference to a full listing of forms, and if there is a full listing of forms, why then bother with decomposing the letter string into base and ending? Without full listing, the reader faces all the problems of cross-indexing irregularities that we have mentioned above. Notice that it is not sufficient for both base and ending to be recognized as valid, since there will be many combinations of real base and real affix which will not be a word – e.g. desk + er, un + re + fit + ing + ly etc, etc.

A number of studies have employed lexical decision tasks to investigate the role of affixes, with somewhat variable results. Taft and Forster (1975) have found that it takes longer for readers to decide that a nonword containing a real prefix is not a word then matched unprefixed controls. However, Rubin, Becker and Freeman (1979) showed that, although stripping prefixes may be a strategy readers can employ, it actually slows down decision time, and so is presumably useful under certain, rather uncommon circumstances. Their study used prefixed words – like PROPOSE, REMARK – and "pseudoprefixed" words – like PROBABLE, RECKON presented as items in one of two kinds of context – (a) where the other words were prefixed, and the filler nonwords were prefixed (DEVIEW, ENPOSE), or (b) where the other words and nonwords were unprefixed (DANGER, CUSTOM, DEMPLE, CURDEN). The idea was that in context (a), readers would be encouraged to employ a prefix-stripping strategy, whereas in (b) they would be less inclined to do so. Two main results emerged. First, readers were quicker in (b) contexts, even for pseudoprefixed words. Second, pseudoprefixed words were classified more slowly than prefixed words in (a) contexts. Thus readers can be encouraged to decompose words, but this slows them down, especially when such decomposition leads them astray, as in PRO-BABLE or RE-CKON.

Acquired reading disabilities are relevant here. Patients with brain damage affecting general language skills often show rather specific reading deficits. Patterson (1982) reports a patient, A.M., who is quite unable to read aloud nonwords, though his reading of real words is fairly good. However, he made many errors that Patterson describes as "derivational", though they include inflexions as well, in which endings are added to or subtracted from the target word (presented singly)

(34) books   Target: book
     thinking   Target: think
     situate   Target: situated
     diseased   Target: disease
     eradicate   Target: eradicable
     amputation   Target: amputate
     offense   Target: offend

Interestingly, A.M. had no trouble distinguishing invalid combinations of real stems and real affixes – FEAREST, PASSLY – from similar real words – NEAREST, COSTLY. A.M. is classified as a "phonological dyslexic". Another class of acquired dyslexia – "deep dyslexia" – produces in addition, "semantic errors, where words semantically-related to their targets – *king* for QUEEN – as well as derivational errors are found (Coltheart, Patterson and Marshall, 1980), and it may be argued in these cases, that the derivational errors are simply a special type of semantic error; but since A.M. did not produce semantically related errors, and so this explanation will not hold for him. Since he can tell which stem-affix combinations are real words, he presumably has full-listing, but is, for some reason, unable to distinguish reliably between forms grouped together in the list.

Patterson (1980) in an earlier study of deep dyslexia, cautiously concluded that the evidence from two patients, P.W. and D.E., were compatible with decomposition. These patients were more likely to make errors reading words containing a suffix, and more likely to say that a nonword containing a real suffix – e.g. FIRCHING – was a word than a letter string not containing a suffix – e.g. FIRCH. One patient, P.W., was still more likely to accept a letter string if it contained both a real stem and a real suffix – e.g. THICK-ING. Patterson notes that the decompositional view implies that if QUICKLY is accepted, then QUICK will be too, though the reverse need not be the case, since the reader must have QUICK to accept QUICKLY, but may not have -LY, or knowledge of the legitimacy of the combination. Broadly, these patients were more likely to accept bases than their derivations. However, some patients will have -LY but not QUICK. This may make them more likely to accept strings ending in -LY, since these have at least some characteristics of a real word. But this wouldn't in itself create the confusion among suffixed forms. As Patterson points out, derived forms and bases are usually visually and semantically similar. Under FLH, readers who can extract only partial information from the letter string, may well end up confusing visually or semantically similar forms; and in a lexical decision task where there is at least partial information compatible with one or more stored items, they will be more likely to accept the string as a word.

D. Evidence from Writing

Writing disabilities, "agraphias", show syndromes analogous to the dyslexias. Shallice (1981) reports a patient, P.R., who writes much as Patterson's patient A.M. reads. P.R. was quite unable to write nonsense words to dictation, and when asked to write content words to dictation produced many derivational errors (in this instance, they were genuinely derivational). Examples from Shallice's Appendix 2 are given in (35).

(35) ascent   Target: ascend
     defect   Target: defection
     lovely   Target: loveliness
     true   Target: truth
     injury   Target: injure

Two inflexional errors are also reported

(36) depressed   Target: depress
     spilt   Target: spill

and some errors of derivation occurred,

(37) derivement   Target: derivative
     profligaty   Target: profligacy
     misfortunate Target: misfortune

The errors in (35) and (36) are compatible with a FLH model which groups similar and related items together, and where small malfunctions of access will lead to the writing of a related form. The source of errors in (37) is more problematic, since the written forms are not words. However, these forms look as though they may be derived from real words: *derive* + *ment*, *profligate* + *y*, *mis/un* + *fortunate*. This explanation is not wholly convincing, since it is not clear what kind of mechanism would be responsible for these errors.

These data do not throw much light on what the nature of LRs in writing might be, but there seems little reason to reject word forms as the best candidate.

E. Conclusions on Unit Type

Very little evidence has emerged from studies of any of the modalities which

would point to units other than words. The most problematic data come
from speaking and writing, where subjects produce errors that are not real
words. How can such errors arise is subjects have only a listing of word-
forms? I have suggested that rules might be used as fall-back procedures.
The input to such rules generally appears to be words, as in the analyses of
(30), (31) and (37), but (32) and (33) constitute prima facie counterevidence
pointing to some kind of morphemic representation.

IV. Modality-specific Lexical Representations

Let me first outline the four main alternative positions, and the kinds of
evidence that can be adduced in support of them. I shall then take each kind
of evidence in turn and discuss to what extent it favours one or another of the
main positions.

(a) *Modality-neutral LRs.* For each word (or morpheme etc) there will be
one LR in a code neutral with respect to modality. In keeping with the
terminological conventions adopted in this essay, such a LR will look like
this: *cat*. Under this model, modality-specific information will have to be
translated into the neutral code before the LR can be accessed. For
example, the acoustic signal [kæt] would have to be translated by rule into *c*,
a, *t*, and this neutral representation would be matched against listed LRs.

(b) *Modality-specific LRs.* There will be separate lists of LRs for each
modality, and items in each list will be in a code appropriate to that modality
i.e. a word can have LRs specific to speech, to hearing, to reading and to
writing. No neutral code LR is postulated. It is not necessary that each word
a speaker knows will have a LR in every modality. For example, a person
may have the orthographic LR AWRY, which he well understands, but may
have no LR for speech. Thus when asked to read AWRY, he will fall back on
rules and (mis)pronounce it ['ɔːri]. Translation among LRs serving the
various modalities may be by rule, or it may be by direct LR-LR mapping.
So if the reader does have a speech LR for AWRY he will pronounce it
correctly as [ə'raɪ]. Interpretation of LRs will be by direct mapping from
LR to meanings.

(c) *Modality-specific LRs plus a modality-neutral common form.* In effect,
a combination of (a) and (b). Proposals concerning word "names" as well as
word forms (cp. Bradley, 1980) would fall under this heading. Mapping from
LR to meaning may be via the neutral name only; and all modality specific
LRs will have a mapping onto the neutral LR. Subtypes of this model will
differ in the extent to which there exist mappings among modality-specific
forms themselves. (See Forster, 1978, for a proposal along these lines.)

(d) *"Emic" LRs.* Under this scheme, differences between input and output
are factored out for a common channel – i.e. for the auditory channel,

phon*emes*; for the visual channel, graph*emes*. Thus there will be just one LR for *cat* – perhaps the phonemic form /kæt/ – serving both hearing and speech. This allows the lexicon to capture commonalities in this channel. Similarly, there will be an graphemic lexicon serving both reading and writing. I have proposed a subtype of this model in which there is a "phonological lexicon" serving hearing and speech, mapped into a "semantic lexicon" serving hearing and speech, and can be extended to include a graphemic lexicon mapped into the semantic lexicon and into the phonological lexicon. For a similar proposal see Allport and Funnell (1981).

Three kinds of evidence can be brought to bear in assessing the value of these alternatives: (1) a comparison of lexical representation in the various modalities – does the evidence point to the same kinds of LR in each modality? (2) the existence of cross-modal effects of the same kind as intra-modal effects – does the evidence point to a common form mediating these effects? (3) modality-specific breakdown in aphasia – does the evidence point to the impairment of LRs in one modality but not in others? †

A. Evidence from the Comparison of Modalities

If we could find evidence that, say, inflected forms were treated as base + suffix in reading, but as single items in hearing, this would suggest that LRs for reading were separate from LRs for hearing. On the other hand, if both modalities seemed to behave in the same way, we would have no grounds for proposing the separation; logically, it would still be possible that separate lists of LRs were built to the same specification – i.e. both treated inflected forms as base + suffix. As it happens, the evidence is somewhat more complicated, but it provides no basis for a separation.

(a) *Reading.* Stanners *et al.* (1979) found, in a lexical decision task, that prior presentation of a base facilitates subsequent decision for that base, and that regularly inflected forms facilitates decision for the base as much as the base itself; irregular forms produce some, though a lesser degree of, facilitation. Stanners *et al.* conclude (p. 410): that

---

† There is a fourth kind of potentially relevant data: the linguistic capacities of young children. Children below, say, the age of three or four) can hear distinctions between words they are unable to reproduce in speech. Thus they will be able to understand both *mouth* and *mouse*, but pronounce each as [maus]; even words that are regularly mispronounced – for example, *duck* as [gʌk], *fish* as [fɪs] – would be rejected if an adult offered the same pronunciation (Smith, 1973). I shall not attempt to recapitulate the main points of Dr Menn's review in Chapter 1, but I would like to draw the reader's attention to one of her conclusions. She argues that these phenomena are most elegantly captured by an account that includes both an input and an output lexicon along with a (changing) set of mapping rules an output constraints for transducing (generally correct) input LRs into output LRs. There can be thought of as stored motor programs for known words. She also notes that this view has been challenged by Smith (1978), who argues for a single level of lexical representation plus nonlexical "realisation rules" employed at the moment of speaking to convert a phonological LR into output instructions.

> the reading of inflections appears to involve partitioning of the base and suffix and the direct accessing of the base verb in memory . . . accessing the irregular past tense does not result in full activation of base verbs. Since the semantic relationship for the case of past tense was the same . . . but the amount of priming (facilitation) was different, the conclusion was drawn that direct access of the base verb took place for inflections but not for irregular past tense words.

In the case of derivations, there is a facilitatory effect of derived forms on subsequent base forms, but it is smaller than the effects of base on base. Both adjectival forms (SELECTIVE, DESCRIPTIVE from the bases SELECT, DESCRIBE) and nominals (APPEARANCE, DESTRUCTION from the bases APPEAR, DESTROY), produced facilitation of the base decision, and the less "transparent" (or more regular) derivations (SELECTIVE, APPEARANCE) produced more facilitation than the less transparent forms (DESCRIPTIVE, DESTRUCTION).

(b) *Hearing*. A rather similar experiment in the auditory modality was carried out by Kempley and Morton (reported in Morton, 1981), but instead of using a lexical decision task, they used word recognition – hearers had to say what the word was they had heard. They found equal facilitatory effects for prior presentation of base and regularly-inflected form on subsequent presentation of the base form. However, irregular forms produced no facilitation in recognition of the base. That is, there was no advantage for the prior presentation of STANK on STINK, but there was an advantage for the prior presentation of WALKING on WALK. Morton proposes a list in which WALK, WALKING, WALKED are connected entries, but STINK and STANK are separate entries. These LRs are relatively peripheral and modality-specific, but even irregular forms are brought into relation in some more central device.

Why there should be no facilitation at all from irregular forms in this task is unclear. Several methodological differences from Stanners et al.'s study may be implicated. First, the interval between prime and target was in the order of minutes in Kempley and Morton, but of seconds in Stanners et al.; the longer interval may have resulted in decay of the semantic effects proposed by Stanners et al., leaving only the residual effects of access to base. Secondly, Kempley and Morton used word recognition, and counted just morphemes reported correctly (i.e. "stink" would count as correct for STANK); this measure may be less sensitive to small effects than a reaction-time measure.

In any event, both modalities show a clear distinction between regularly inflected forms and irregular inflections and derivations.

(c) *Speech*. The evidence for the separation of inflections comes from "stranding" errors, and these, as I have argued above, may be interpreted in other ways. The separation of derivational affixes and their bases emerges fairly clearly from derivational errors resulting in nonwords (see (30)–(33) for examples).

As you can see, the evidence here is rather sparse. Broadly, it points to close connexions among regularly related forms in the input modalities. Whether this close connexion should be interpreted as base + affixes, or as grouping under, and access via, the base cannot be decided on these data. Speech points to some autonomy for base forms in derivations.

(d) *Cross-modal effects.* If a LR serves all modalities (via transcoding processes of course), then effects found between two LRs in the same modality should also be found in between two LRs in different modalities. Facilitation effects, like those discussed above, should occur independently of the modality of the priming word, for a target in a given modality.

A series of studies by Winnick and Daniel (1970) and by Morton and his co-workers have explored cross-modal priming in some detail.

Winnick and Daniel (1970) found that recognition thresholds for tachistoscopically presented words were *not* shortened by prior presentation of a picture named by that word, or by the word's definition. These results have been replicated by Clarke and Morton (in press). Moreover, prior auditory presentation of a word does not facilitate subsequent visual recognition. In recognition, as opposed to decision, tasks, the subject actually has to say the word – whether to an auditory stimulus, a picture or a definition – so the absence of a facilitation effect indicates that saying the word does not affect visual or auditory recognition. It also rules out response bias in favour of the target in the intramodal cases where there is facilitation. Clarke and Morton conclude that there are, at least, three modality-specific lists of LRs – auditory, orthographic and spoken (which they call "phonological"). (Incidentally, though these effects are modality-specific, they do not depend on the exact form of the stimulus items. Clarke and Morton found that a handwritten word was as good a prime as a typed word when a typed word was the target; and Jackson and Morton (in Morton, *op. cit.*) noted that, in auditory priming, facilitation occurred, when prime and target were in different voices).

B. Modality-specific Language Breakdown

The classical statement of modality-specific LRs can be found in the writings of two nineteenth century pioneers of aphasia studies, Wernicke (1874) and Lichtheim (1885). They maintained that there are separate stores for "auditory word images" and "motor word images", and that these stores are anatomically distinct, the former in an area of the cortex (now known as Wernicke's area) close to the area serving audition generally, the latter in an area (known as Broca's area) close to the area serving control of movement generally. On this account, when Wernicke's area is damaged, comprehension of words will be affected, but not the production of them; and when Broca's area is damaged, production of words will be affected, but not comprehension. Lichtheim, somewhat less confident about the relation of orthographic LRs to this scheme, suggests that there are also separate stores for writing and for reading. These too should be affectable without consequent effects on hearing or speaking words.

The evidence for modality-specific breakdown has been extensively reviewed by Allport and Funnell (1981) and elsewhere in this volume by Cooper and Zurif, and will not be dealt with in detail here. Broadly, there is no strict dissociation between hearing and speech as predicted by the model. Although damage to Broca's area makes speech dysfluent, and damage to Wernicke's area impairs auditory comprehension, there does not appear to be a specific deficit to motor word images in the first type of case, and in the Wernicke's case there does appear to be difficulty in finding motor word images and to producing them correctly (Butterworth, 1979). Cooper and Zurif (this volume), in fact, point to a common problem in hearing and speech for Broca's patients: they have trouble both in producing "function words" and in understanding the syntactic role of these words in auditory comprehension. As Cooper and Zurif put it "Just as they speak ungrammatically, so too they be characterized as agrammatic comprehenders" (p. 228). Failure to utilize function words to compute the syntactic structure of heard sentences, leads to very limited comprehension of complex sentences, especially those sentences where simple semantic strategies using word-order and the meanings of the content words alone cannot provide the correct reading.

Following Bradley, Garrett and Zurif (1980), they propose that the effective use of function words depends on a separate store, which is accessed in a different manner from access to the store of content words, and is used in both comprehension and production. (I will discuss the evidence for this position in Section V below on the organization of the lexicon.)

Correlation of symptoms in production and comprehension words is not always a sure guide to underlying lexical deficits. In a recent study by Butterworth, Howard and McLoughlin (1982), various aphasic types were tested on auditory comprehension of object names and on the naming of objects. It was found, in all aphasic categories, that patients poor on comprehension were also poor at naming. However, it was not the same word which typically gave trouble on the two tasks. Thus, a patient who could not pick out an orange from an array of pictures of fruit when he heard "orange", may well have been able to name the orange when presented with a picture of one. Interestingly, the kinds of error the poor performers made was analogous in the two tasks and seemed to invoke a kind of partial mapping from sound to meaning. Patients who were able to point to the orange in an array of miscellaneous objects, were unable, reliably, to point to the orange in an array of fruits, indicating that they were able to derive some meaning from the word but not sufficient to discriminate it from other words of similar meanings. In naming, the most common error was to produce a word related in meaning to the target (rather than some quite unrelated word, or some phonemic distortion of the target). So when presented with an orange, the patient might say "lemon", rather than "locomotive" or "organ".

It is not clear whether this pattern of results should be explained in terms of some problem with semantics, or whether it should be explained as a disorder in mapping from LRs to semantics, and from semantics to LRs.

The general problem of distinguishing between impaired access (or mapping) and impaired LRs is discussed by Allport and Funnell (1981). They cite an early study by Bramwell (1897), whose patient was unable to understand the words she heard, though she was able to repeat quite long sentences. Her talking and writing were fluent, and she could understand written words well; in fact, when she was allowed to write down what she had heard she was able to understand it. It seems clear in this patient, that LRs serving hearing, speaking, reading and writing are intact, but that somehow the mapping from LRs serving hearing, and these alone, have lost their mappings with semantics; alternatively, the mappings from the phonemic LRs to semantics have been impaired (but not from semantics to LRs). The preserved ability to write to dictation favours this latter alternative.

Words with irregular spellings are the crucial test here. Procedures for converting graphemes to phonemes, and from phonemes to graphemes, will work adequately when spelling is regular, but not otherwise. Correct reading and spelling of irregular forms thus depends crucially on being able to access LRs. Beauvois and Derouesné (1981) report a case, R.G., who strikingly illustrates this point. R.G. could read irregular words, but not nonwords, even when they were spelled "regularly". At the same time, he could not spell irregular words correctly, rather he gave a "phonetic" spelling of them, and he was able to write nonwords to dictation. Thus in reading, he could use a route via LRs, but could not use grapheme–phoneme procedures; while in writing, he could not use a route via LRs, but could use phoneme–grapheme procedures. One explanation, is that reading LRs are intact, but writing LRs are impaired, with grapheme–phoneme correspondences available only in one direction. Alternatively, following Allport and Funnell (1981), there exists only one set of (graphemic) LRs serving both reading and writing, and that access to these LRs from the visual stimulus is intact, but access from sounds is impaired; again with the postulation of only unidirectional phoneme–grapheme mappings. Bramwell's patient, who could spell irregular words, suggests the latter explanation is more generalizable, though this case was far less thoroughly tested than Beauvois and Derouesné's. Overall, there seems to be fairly good evidence for separating the visual channel from the auditory channel, but the only results which clearly distinguish input from output modalities are those reported by Morton. None of the data points to a modality-neutral LR, though some kind of procedure, or lexical mapping, needs to be postulated so that CAT and [kæt] can be seen to have the same meaning (cp. the semantic lexicon postulated by Butterworth (1980)).

V. Organization of Lexical Representations

Cooper and Zurif (this volume) have suggested that function words are to be found in a separate list from content words. The explanation of frequency effects has been explained in terms of a frequency-organization of LRs (Forster, 1976) and a recurrent motif of the previous sections has been the idea that morphologically-related words are grouped together under a heading (Bradley, 1980; Morton, 1981). These are organizational questions, and will be addressed in this section. It should be noted that under the hypothesis of modality-specific LRs, or of "emic" LRs, the organization of different lists may be different, and thus there may be no one answer to the organizational question.

A. Frequency Organization

The effects of word frequency is one of the most widely attested in the psychological literature, and can be found in a whole range of tasks: lexical decision (Rubenstein *et al.*, 1971; Whaley, 1978), tachistoscope word recognition (Howes and Solomon, 1951), object-naming (Oldfield and Wingfield, 1965), same-different discrimination (Chambers and Forster, 1975) etc. It applies to aphasics as well as normal subjects (Newcombe *et al.*, 1965; Bradley *et al.*, 1980; Howes, 1964).

The organizational implications of the word-frequency effect depend on particular assumptions as to how words are accessed in the lexicon. One assumption is that given a stimulus item – say, a letter string – the reader searches through the list of LRs until a match is found. Under this assumption, the effect occurs because the words are arranged in order of their frequency of occurrence (Forster, 1976; Oldfield, 1966; Glanzer and Ehrenreich, 1979). There are two main problems with this deduction. First, frequency effects can be explained in terms of a model where access does not depend on search (e.g. Morton, 1979b). Second, frequency effects are highly correlated with other variables and may be second-order effects of them. For example, frequent words are more likely to have been used recently (Scarborough *et al.*, 1977); frequent words tend to have more meanings (Jastrzembski, 1981); in context, frequent words are more predictable (Beattie and Butterworth, 1979).

Frequency effects can, however, be a useful diagnostic when deployed in a way which does not depend critically on assumptions of access through search. Differential frequency effects for different classes of words would be a result which any access model would need to explain.

Such differential effects have been observed in lexical decision experiments by Bradley (1978). Like other investigators, she found that decision time was a function word frequency, but only for content words. Function words, which also have a range of frequencies, as in (38) and (39)

(38) High frequency: *the, a, and*
(39) Low frequencies: *nor, seldom, thereby*

show no sensitivity in decision times to frequency. This effect does not depend on subjects knowing where in the lexicon the words are drawn from. In her third experiment, Bradley found that when all the stimulus words were animal names – a known sublist for the subjects – there was no diminution of the frequency effect, although there was some advantage for the animal name list over a mixed, matched control list. She argues for a special set of items, the function words, outside the lexicon, which serve syntactic processing. In Broca's aphasics which are held to have special difficulty with syntactic processing (see Cooper and Zurif, this volume), function words, like other words, *do* show a frequency effect. This suggests that function words have a double representation – in the special store and in the general lexicon – and that Broca's patients who do not have this special store have to access these words from their general lexicon.

One problem is that attempts to replicate this result have failed (Gordon and Caramazza, 1981). A second problem is that some high frequency content words have shorter decision times than function words. It is not clear why this should be so; nor indeed is it clear why function words should not show an effect of frequency, even if they have separate listing. Why is there not simply a frequency effect consistent with access from a short list?

A second problem is that frequency effects are less convincingly demonstrated in word production. Although Newcombe *et al.* (1965) found them in object-naming by aphasics. And it is by no means well-established that frequency is effective in spontaneous speech production: Beattie and Butterworth (1979) found that low frequency words tended to follow pauses in speech, indicating a delay due to lexical search, but frequency is confounded with predictability in context. Although they were able to show an effect of predictability independent of frequency, they were not able to show an effect of frequency independent of predictability.

B. Are Content Words and Function Words Listed Separately?

We turn now to some evidence that supports Bradley's general contention, but with special reference to speech.

The speech of aphasic patients falls into one of two rough categories – content words relatively well-preserved but function words largely absent or used incorrectly, or function word use relatively well-preserved, but content words restricted to some common items, or made-up words when the appropriate content word cannot be found.

The first syndrome is apparent even when the subject has only to repeat a sentence he has heard (Saffran *et al.*, 1980):

(40) Experimenter (E): No, I do not like fish.
      Patient (P): No . . . fish (where ". . ." indicates a long pause)
      E: One morning, the girl was pulled by the man.
      P: One morning, the . . . the girl is pull . . . pull the boy.
      E: The girl runs to the man.
      P: The girl running the . . . the girl is running on the man.

The second syndrome can be seen in the speech in (43) (Butterworth, 1979):

(41) E: What is that?
      P: Oo that, that, sir, I can show you then what is a ['zæprɪks] for the
      ['ɛlənkɒm], with the ['pɪdlənd] thing to the . . . and then each of the
      ['pɪdləmz] has an [aɪjɪn] – one, two, three and so on.

The close connexion between function words and syntactic processing has
already been noted. Whether function word difficulties are consequent upon
a more general syntactic deficit (see Cooper and Zurif, this volume) or
whether they should be regarded as a separate deficit (Saffran *et al.*, 1981) is
still a matter of some controversy. It is interesting to note that a characteristic sympton of 'deep dyslexia" – a reading disorder found typically in
Broca's patients but in some fluent aphasics too – is a special difficulty in
reading function words (Coltheart *et al.*, 1980, passim).

One general difficulty is, as Kean (1980) has pointed out, that function
words do not form a homogeneous category. They comprise pronouns,
prepositions, some adverbs, articles etc. The same word can be a locational
preposition or part of a phrasal verb – e.g. *up* in *look up his nose* and *look up
his address*; *to* can be a locational preposition or the mark of an infinitival
verb; and so on. Some function words can be heads of phrases, e.g. proper
prepositions, others not, e.g. articles, conjunctions. As a consequence, their
role in syntactic processing cannot be expected to be homogeneous. Studies
distinguishing more carefully the subtypes are urgently needed for definitive
statements to be justifiable.

C. Are Compound Forms Listed under their Bases?

I have argued that there are no decisive reasons for rejecting FLH. But even
if all words are listed, there may still be an organizational principle in the
lexicon which groups compound forms under their base. The studies I have
described in this essay have frequently demonstrated that morphologically
related words seem to have a special affinity for each other which shows up in
the appropriate experimental tasks.

Bradley (1978) has shown that it is the total frequency of all related
compounds, rather than the frequency of the target itself that is effective in
determining decision times in a visual lexical decision task. In a lexical
decision task, with a priming manipulation, Stanners *et al.* (1979) found that
morphological relatives act as effective primes, and that regular relatives are
as effective as the base itself when the base is the target. Similarly, Morton

(1981) reports studies of auditory word-recognition with a priming manipulation, in which regular relatives are as effective primes as the target word itself. Here however, irregular relatives had no priming effect.

Errors in reading aloud in dyslexic patients involve morphological relatives (Patterson, 1980, 1982), as do writing errors in dysgraphic patients (Shallice, 1981).

These results, though pointing to some kind of grouping on morphological principles, do not compel us to accept the idea of grouping under a base, or some other heading.

VI. Conclusions

In summary then, there is, disappointingly, little solid evidence to support the strongest theories of lexical representation, and considerable evidence in favour of some weaker alternatives.

1. The idea that only base forms are listed, with inflexional or derivational compounds being computed online by rule, is not well-supported in any of the modalities. We are therefore left with the weaker alternative that all forms – base and compound – have their own LR.

2. Models which propose that LR represent morphemes rather than words are also not well-supported. The critical cases concern morphemes not equivalent to words. Misderivations in slips of the tongue seem to apply to both word stems and nonword morphemic stems. This is the best evidence, but I think it can be explained away; see below.

3. There is no evidence for modality-neutral LRs, either as the only kind of LR, or in a "master file" accessed by modality – specific LRs (cp. Miller, 1978; Forster, 1976, 1978). There seems to be a clear separation of graphemic and phonemic LRs, but the evidence for further separation by input and output functions is provisional. It is hard, on the present data, to distinguish empirically effects attributable to input and output access, from effects which would be due to input and output LRs.

Perhaps studies of inter- and intramodal facilitation would be decisive. David Howard (pers. commun.) has observed that object naming in severely aphasic patients can be dramatically improved by providing the first phoneme of the target word. This makes sense only if there is a phonemic LR serving both speech and hearing.

4. The postulation of separate listing for function words gains some support, but this is to some extent vitiated by the vagueness of the function word category and its supposed relation to other LRs and to syntactic processing.

5. The organization of LRs by their frequency of use has been widely claimed, but alternative explanations of the word frequency effect exist (Morton, 1969, 1979b), and weaken this claim.

6. The grouping together of morphologically-related forms is well attested in a variety of tasks in several modalities, but there is no clear evidence that such a group has the base form, or some other more abstract LR, as a heading.

These conclusions run counter to two indisputable facts. First, that word-formation is productive in the sense that we can and do construct new words, and we can and do understand new words, when both conform to certain principles (Cutler, 1980b, 1981). Thus, I can construct *undigitalizable*, and you can understand it. Second, literate native speakers know that the orthographic form CAT and the sound [kæt] are the same word.

To account for this apparent discrepancy between full listing in separate lexicons of phonemic and graphemic LRs, some further processes must be invoked. As I said in Section II, the FLH is not incompatible with having "fall-back procedures" when confronted by a new word, or the need to make-up a word when access to the full list fails. These procedures may be substantive rules, analogous to those proposed by Chomsky and Halle (1968) or Aronoff (1976), which provide a recipe for constructing, say, *divinity* from *divine* (or /dɪviːn/). Alternatively, they may be in the form of "meta-rules" which say something rather general, like, "if you want to construct a new word, have a look for a word that's similar, and try a construction which looks like it." One empirical advantage of the meta-rule proposal, is that it is consistent with speakers' variable responses given a base from which to form a new word (Cutler, 1980a): how the construction turns out will depend on which existing word the speaker chooses as a model. In reading novel letter strings, like YEAD, readers' pronunciation will depend on recently presented letter strings. He will read it as /jiːd/ following BEAD, or as /jɛd/ following HEAD (Kay and Marcel, 1981). Perhaps something similar occurs when subjects in Cutler's task had to make up an abstract noun from *jejune*: some produce *jejunity*, *jejuneness*. The differences will depend on which model comes to mind. It remains an open question the extent to which this kind of analogical word-formation process makes use of morpheme structure, as opposed to a more haphazard reconstruction of the model to provide a basis for constructing the new word out of the old.

The second problem can be resolved by postulating a common semantic unit which maps onto both the phonemic unit /kæt/ and the graphemic unit CAT. In a similar way, inflexional compounds of a verb, regular and irregular, can be mapped onto a common semantic unit. The mappings will be bidirectional, and will enable access from the semantic unit to the phonemic unit in speech, and to the graphemic unit for writing. The semantic unit can be thought of as being accessible from general semantics, and containing the addresses of the graphemic and phonemic units onto which it can be mapped, thus providing the link, determined by "an arbitrary tradition" (Bloomfield, 1933), between form and meaning. Further grounds for postulating such a unit can be found in Butterworth (1980).

Acknowledgements

Jean Aitchison, Ruth Campbell, Anne Cutler, Lindsay Evett, Gerald Gazdar, David Green, David Howard, Colin MacCabe, George Mandler, Tony Marcel and John Morton have discussed with me many of the ideas contained herein, and many I have left out. I think I have benefitted from these discussions. They may take a different view when they have read the result.

References

Allport, D. A. and Funnell, E. (1981). Components of the mental lexicon. *In* "The Psychological Mechanisms of Language", (H. C. Longuet-Higgins, J. Lyons and D. E. Broadbent, eds). The Royal Society and The British Association, London.

Aronoff, M. (1976). "Word Formation in Generative Grammar". *Linguistic Inquiry Monogaph 1*. MIT Press, Cambridge, Massachusetts.

Beattie, G. W. and Butterworth, B. (1979). Contextual probability and word frequency as determinants of pauses in spontaneous speech. *Language and Speech*, **22**, 201–211.

Beauvois, M.-F. and Derouesne, J. (1981). Lexical or orthographic agraphia. *Brain*, **104**, 21–49.

Berko, J. (1958). The child's learning of English morphology. *Word*, **14**, 150–168.

Bloomfield, L. (1933). "Language". Holt, New York.

Bobrow, S. and Bell, S. (1973). On catching on to idiomatic expressions. *Memory and Cognition*, **1**, 343–346.

Bradley, D. (1978). Unpublished Ph.D. Dissertation. MIT , Massachusetts.

Bradley, D. (1980). Lexical representation of derivational relation. *In* "Juncture", (M. Aronoff and M.-L. Kean, eds). MIT Press, Cambridge, Massachusetts.

Bradley, D., Garrett, M. and Zurif, E. (1980). Syntactic deficits in Broca's aphasia. *In* "Biological Studies of Mental Processes", (D. Caplan, ed.) MIT Press, Cambridge, Massachusetts.

Butterworth, B. (1979). Hesitations and the production of verbal paraphasias and neologisms in jargon aphasia. *Brain and Language*, **8**, 131–161.

Butterworth, B. (1980). Some constraints on models of language production *In* "Language Production Vol. 1", (B. Butterworth, ed.) Academic Press, London and New York.

Butterworth, B., Howard, D. and McLoughlin, P. (1982). Semantic errors in comprehension and naming by aphasic subjects. Internal report. University College London.

Chambers, S. and Forster, K. (1975). Evidence for lexical access in a simultaneous matching task. *Memory and Cognition*, **3**, 549–59.

Clarke, R. and Morton, J. (in press). Cross modality facilitation in tachistoscopic word recognition. *Quarterly Journal of Experimental Psychology*.

Chomsky, N. (1965). "Aspects of the Theory of Syntax". MIT Press, Cambridge, Massachusetts.

Chomsky, N. and Halle, M. (1968). "The Sound Pattern of English". Academic Press, New York and London.

Coltheart, M., Patterson, K. and Marshall, J. C. (1980). "Deep Dyslexia". Routledge and Kegan Paul, London.

Cutler, A. (1980a). Errors of stress and intonation. In "Errors of Linguistic Performance: Slips of the Tongue, Ear, Pen and Hands", (V. Fromkin, ed.) Academic Press, New York and London.

Cutler, A. (1980b). Productivity in word formation. CLS 14.

Cutler, A. (1981). Degrees of transparency in word formation. Canadian Journal of Linguistics, 26, 73–77.

Forster, K. (1976). Accessing the mental lexicon. In "New Approaches to Language Mechanisms", (R. J. Wales and E. C. T. Walker, eds). North-Holland, Amsterdam.

Forster, K. (1978). Accessing the mental lexicon. In "Explorations in the Biology of Language", (E. C. T. Walker, ed). Bradford Books, Montgomery, Vermont.

Fraser, B. (1970). Idioms within transformational grammar. Foundations of Language, 6.

Fromkin, V. (1971). The nonanomalous nature of anomalous utterances. Language, 47, 27–52.

Fromkin, V. (1973). "Speech Errors as Linguistic Evidence". Mouton, The Hague.

Garrett, M. (1975). The analysis of sentence production. In "The Psychology of Learning and Motivation", (G. Bower, ed.) Vol. 9. Academic Press, New York and London.

Garrett, M. (1976). Syntactic processes in sentence production. In "New Approaches to Language Mechanisms", (R. J. Wales and E. C. T. Walker, eds).

Garrett, M. (1980). Levels of processing in sentence production. In "Language Production" Vol. 1, (B. Butterworth, ed.) Academic Press, London and New York.

Glanzer, M. and Ehrenreich, S. (1979). Structure and search of the internal lexicon. Journal of Verbal Learning and Verbal Behaviour, 18, 381–98.

Goldstein, K. (1948). "Language and Language Disturbance". Grune and Stratton, New York.

Gordon, B. and Caramazza, A. (1982). Lexical decision for open- and closed-class items: failure to replicate differential frequency sensitivity. Brain and Language, 15, 143–160.

Howes, D. (1964). Application of the word frequency concept to aphasia. In "Disorders of Language", (A. V. S. De Reuck and M. O'Connor, eds). Churchill, London.

Howes, D. and Solomon, R. L. (1951). Visual duration thresholds as a function of word probability. Journal of Experimental Psychology, 41, 401–410.

Jastrzembski, J. (1981). Multiple meanings, number of related meanings, frequency of occurence, and the lexicon. Cognitive Psychology, 13, 278–305.

Kay, J. and Marcel, A. (1981). One process, not two, in reading aloud: lexical analogies do the work of non-lexical rules. Quarterly Journal of Experimental psychology, 33A, 397–413.

Kean, M.-L. (1980). Grammatical representations and the description of language processing. In "Biological Studies of Mental Processes", (D. Caplan, ed.) MIT Press, Cambridge, Massachusetts.

Klein, E. (1980). A semantics for positive and comparative adjectives. Linguistics and Philosophy, 4, 1–45.

Lichtheim, L. (1885). On aphasia. Brain, VII, 433–484.

Lyons, J. (1981). "Language and Linguistics". Cambridge University Press.

Manelis, L. and Tharp, D. (1977). The processing of affixed words. *Memory and Cognition*, **5**, 690–95.

Miller, G. A. (1978). Semantic relations among words. *In* "Linguistic Theory and Psychological Reality", (M. Halle, J. Bresnan and G. A. Miller, eds). MIT Press, Cambridge, Massachusetts.

Morton, J. (1968). Consideration of grammar and computation in language behaviour. *In* "Studies in Language and Language behaviour", (J. C. Catford, ed.) Progress Report IV, US Office of Education.

Morton, J. (1969). The interaction of information in word recognition. *Psychological Review*, **16**, 165–78.

Morton, J. (1979a). Facilitation in word recognition: experiments causing change in the Logogen model. *In* "Processing Visible Language", (P. A. Kolers, M. E. Wrolstad and H. Bouma, eds). Plenum, New York.

Morton, J. (1979b). Word recognition. *In* "Psycholinguistics Series 2", (J. Morton and J. C. Marshall, eds). Elek, London.

Morton, J. (1981). The status of information processing models of language. *In* "The Psychological Mechanisms of Language", (H. C. Longuet-Higgins, J. Lyons and D. E. Broadbent, eds). The Royal Society and The British Association, London.

Murrell, G. A. and Morton, J. (1974). Word recognition and morphemic structure. *Journal of Experimental Psychology*, **102**, 963–68.

Newcombe, F., Oldfield, R. C. and Wingfield, A. (1965). Object-naming by dysphasic patients. *Nature*, **207**, 1217–18.

Oldfield, R. C. (1966). Things, words and the brain. *Quarterly Journal of Experimental Psychology*, **18**, 340–53.

Oldfield, R. C. and Wingfield, A. (1965). Response latencies in naming objects. *Quarterly Journal of Experimental Psychology*, **7**, 273–81.

Patterson, K. (1980). Derivational errors. *In* "Deep Oyslexia", (M. Coltheart, K. Patterson and J. C. Marshall, eds). Routledge & Kegan Paul, London.

Patterson, K. (1982). The relation between reading and phonological coding: further neuropsychological observations. *In* "Normality and Pathology in Cognitive Functioning", (A. W. Ellis, ed.) Academic Press, London and New York.

Rubenstein, H., Lewis, S. S. and Rubenstein, M. A. (1971). Evidence for phonemic recoding in visual word recognition. *Journal of Verbal Learning and Verbal Behavior*, **10**, 645–657.

Rubin, G. S., Becker, C. A. and Freeman, R. H. (1979). Morphological structure and its effect on visual word recognition. *Journal of Verbal Learning and Verbal Behavior*, **18**, 757–67.

Saffran, E. Schwartz, M. and Marin, O. (1980). Evidence from aphasia: isolating the components of a production model. *In* "Language Production", (B. Butterworth, ed.) Vol. 1. Academic Press, London and New York.

Scarborough, D. L., Cortese, C. and Scarborough, H. S. (1977). Frequency and repetition effects in lexical memory. *Journal of Experimental Psychology: Human Perception and Performance*, **3**, 1–17.

Shallice, T. (1981). Phological agraphia and the lexical route in writing. *Brain*, **104**, 413–429.

Smith, N. V. (1973). "The Acquisition of Phonology: A Case Study". Cambridge University Press, Cambridge.

Smith, N. V. (1978). Lexical Representation and the Acquisition of Phonology. *In* "Linguistics in the Seventies: Directions and Prospects", (B. J. Kachru, ed.) (Studies in the Linguistic Sciences, **8**, Part II).

Stachowiak, F.-J., Huber, W. Poeck, K. and Kerschensteiner, M. (1977). Text comprehension in aphasia. *Brain and Language*, **4**, 177–95.

Stanners, R. F., Neiser, J. J., Hernon, W. P. and Hall, R. (1979). Memory representations for morphologically related words. *Journal of Verbal Learning and Verbal Behavior*, **18**, 399–412.

Swinney, D. A. and Cutler, A. (1979). The access and processing of idiomatic expressions. *Journal of Verbal Learning and Verbal Behavior*, **18**, 523–534

Taft, M. and Forster, K. (1975). Lexical storage and retrieval of prefixed words. *Journal of Verbal Learning and Verbal Behavior*, **14**, 638–647.

Taft, M. and Forster, K. (1976). Lexical storage and retrieval of polymorphemic and polysyllabic words. *Journal of Verbal Learning and Verbal Behavior*, **15**, 607–620.

Wernicke, C. (1874). Der Aphasische Symptomen Complex. Breslau: Weigart.

Whaley, C. P. (1978). Nonword classification time. *Journal of Verbal Learning and Verbal Behavior*, **17**, 143–154.

Winnick, W. A. and Daniel, S. A. (1970). Two kinds of response priming in tachistoscopic recognition. *Journal of Experimental Psychology*, **84**, 74–81.

Zimmer, K. (1964). Affixal Negation in English and Other Languages: an investigation of restricted productivity. *Word: Monograph Supplement*, **5**

Author Index

Page numbers in italics refer to reference lists

A

Abbs, J. H. 209, *221*
Abramovitch, R., 63, *98*
Abramson, A. S., 214, 216, *221*
Aitchison, J. 148, 152, 153, *196*
Alden, D. G. 124, 127, *141*
Allport, D. A., 281, 284, 285, *291*
Amidon, A., 63, *93*
Anderson, S., 220, *223*
Anglin, J. M., 60, 61, 67, *93, 96*
Aronoff, M., 259, 261, 275, 290, *291*
Asatryan, D., 105, *141*
Atkinson, M., 72, *93*
Aurbach, J., 154, 171, *199*

B

Baars, B. J., 148, 171, 195, *196, 198*
Baddeley, A. D., 103, *146*, 148, 150, 185, *199*
Bader, L., 228, *255*
Bailey, P. J., 218, *221*
Baker, E., 234, 237, *251, 253*
Baker, W., 228, *255*
Baldwin, P., 63, 64, *96*
Balfour, G., 63, *95*
Barnard, P., 115, *141*
Barrett, M. D., 56, 57, 58, *93*
Barrie-Blackey, S., 63, *93*
Barton, D. P., 10, 11, 17, 37, *46, 47*
Basso, A., 165, *196*
Bawden, H. H., 103, *141*
Beattie, G. W., 158, *196*, 286, 287, *291*
Beauvois, M.-F., 285, *291*
Becker, C. A., 277, *293*
Beebe, B., 6, *49*
Beil, R. G., 206, *221*
Bell, A., 17, *46*
Bell, S., 271, *291*
Bellugi, U., 74, 88, *94*
Benedict, H., 58, *97*
Bennett, S. L., 6, *49*
Berko Gleason, J., 34, 41, *46, 48*, 262, 274, *291*

Berlin, B., 58, *93*
Berndt, R. S., 228, 233, 234, *252*
Bernstein, N., 110, 117, 129, *141*
Beuckelaer, R. de, 238, *253*
Bever, T. G., 136, 138, *141, 197*, 231, *251*
Biber, C., 231, 235, *252*
Bierwisch, M., 57, *93*
Binet, A., 107, *141*
Bisiach, E., 233, *251*
Bizzi, E., 106, *141*
Bjork, L., 206, *221*
Black, M., 54, *93*
Bloom, L., 53, 56, 59, 61, 72, 74, 75, 76, 77, 78, 86, 87, 92, *93*
Bloomfield, L., 261, 290, *291*
Blumstein, S. E., 212, *224*, 228, 231, 234, 235, 237, *251, 252, 255*
Bobrow, S., 271, *291*
Bolinger, D., 239, *252*
Bond, Z. S., 36, *47*
Bonvillian, J. D., 89, 90, *97*
Book, W. F., 103, 104, 127, 133, 135, *141*
Boomer, D. S., 157, 163, 164, *196*
Bowe, T., 61, *94*
Bowerman, M., 58, 59, 73, *93*
Boyes-Braem, P., 58, 68, *98*
Brabb, B., 120, *144*
Bradbury, R. J., 158, *196*
Bradley, D. C., 229, 230, 238, *252*, 259, 260, 272, 273, 280, 284, 286, 288, *291*
Brady, S. A. 214, *221*
Braine, M. D. S., 54, 73, 74, 76, 78, 79, 81, 84, 87, 91, *93*
Braitenberg, V., 115, *142*
Branigan, G., 6, *46*, 242, *252, 255*
Breckenridge, J., 241, *252*
Brewer, W. F., 63, *94*
Broen, P. A., 214, 221, *224*
Brown, J., 229, 234, *252, 254*
Brown, R., 67, 71, 73, 74, 76, 78, 82, 83, 84, 88, *94*
Brownell, H., 234, *252*
Bruner, J., 66, 72, *94, 97*

295

Bryan, W. L., 103, 104, 110, 127, 133, *142*
Buckingham, H. W. Jr., 247, 248, *252*
Bullowa, M., 51, *94*
Buren, P. van, 60, *95*
Butsch, R. L. C., 136, *142*
Butterworth, B., 136, *142*, 160, 170, *196*, 236, 238, 246, 247, 249, *252*, 266, 268, 269, 284, 285, 286, 287, 288, 290, *291*

C

Campbell, R. N., 61, 63, 64, 72, *94, 96*, *98*
Capatides, J. B., 77, *93*
Caplan, D., 231, 234, *252*
Caramazza, A., 216, 218, 220, *221*, 228, 230, 233, 234, 235, 237, *251, 252*, *255, 256*, 287, *292*
Carbone, E., 216, 218, 220, *221*
Carey, P., 63, *93*
Carey, S., 63, 64, 65, 68, 91, *94*
Carney, P. J., 209, *222*
Carskaddon, G., 89, 90, *97*
Cazden, C. B., 73, 83, 88, 89, *94*
Chafe, W., 71, 75, *94*
Chalkley, M. A., 84, 87, 91, *97*
Chambers, S., 286, *291*
Chapman, R. S., 59, 60, *98*
Chedru, F., 148, 165, 185, *196*
Chiat, S., 54, *93*
Chomsky, C., 62, *94*
Chomsky, N., 52, 53, 71, *94*, 147, *196*, 260, 261, 273, 290, *291*
Clark, E. V., 56, 57, 58, 62, 63, *94, 95*
Clark, R., 60, *95*
Clarke, R., 283, *291*
Clumeck, H., 7, *46*
Coekaerts, M.-J., 238, *253*
Cole, R. A., 171, *196*
Coltheart, M., 161, 181, *196*, 278, 288, *292*
Comrie, B., 62, *95*
Conway, E., 117, 119, *143*
Cooper, F. S., 208, 209, 210, 215, *222*
Cooper, W. E., 136, *142*, 232, 234, 237, 238, 239, 241, 242, 243, 244, 245, 246, 248, *251, 252, 253*
Coover, J. E., 120, *142*

Cortese, C., 286 *293*
Courtier, J., 107, *141*
Culicover, P. N., 71, *99*
Cutler, A., 170, 171, 178, 183, 185, *196*, *199*, 229, *255*, 271, 274, 290, *292*, *294*
Cutting, J. E., 213, *222*

D

Daniel, S. A., 283, *294*
Daniels, R. W., 124, 127, *141*
Daniloff, R. G., 207, 209, 216, *222*
Danks, J. H., 63, *95*
Danly, M., 232, 241, 242, 243, 244, 246, 248, *252, 253*
Darwin, C. J., 214, *221*
Dealy, W. L., 104, *142*
DeClerk, J. L., 203, 216, *222, 223*
Delattre, P. C., 208, 210, *222*
Delis, D., 236, 240, *253*
Dell, G. S., 172, *196*
Demeurisse, G., 238, *253*
Demol, O., 238, *253*
Denes, G., 228, *253*
Denier van der Gon, J. J., 104, 105, 106, 115, *142*
Derouck, M., 238, *253*
Derouesné, J., 165, *198*, 285, *291*
Deschamps, A., 238, *254*
Dev, P., 106, *141*
Dixon, R. M. W., 80, *95*
Dockrell, J., 61, 68, 69, *94, 95*
Donaldson, M., 63, *95*
Dooling, R. J., 214, *223*
Drachman, G., 43, *46*
Ducarne, B., 247, *254*
Duchan, J. F., 246, 247, *253*
Duncan, S. Jr., 157, *196*
Dvorak, A., 104, *142*

E

Easton, T. A., 216, *222*
Eden, M., 104, *142*
Ehrenreich, S., 286, *292*
Ehrlich, S. F., 245, *252*
Eichelman, W. H., 132, *142*
Eilers, R. E., 63, *95*

Eimas, P. D., 214, *222*
Ellington, J., 63, *95*
Ellis, A. W., 148, 163, 165, 173, 190, *196*
Erickson, D. M., 218, *222*
Escourolle, R., 247, *254*

F
Farwell, C. B., 12, 13, 14, *46*
Fay, D. A., 170, 171, 183, 185, *196*
Feldman, A. G., 105, 106, *141*, *142*
Ferguson, C. A., 4, 7, 12, 13, 18, *46*, *50*, 51, 52, *98*
Fey, M., 18, *46*
Fillimore, C., 71, 75, *95*
Fiske, D. W., 157, *196*
Fitch, H. L., 218, *222*
Fitts, P. M., 109, *142*
Flege, J. E., 17, *46*
Fodor, J. D., 242, 244, *253*
Fodor, J. A., 57, *96*, *197*, 234, *253*
Foldi, N. S., 236, 240, *253*
Folger, M. K., 13, *47*
Ford, G. C., 104, *142*
Forster, K. I. 173, 180, *197*, *199*, 259, 277, 280, 286, 289, *291*, *292*, *294*
Fourcin, A. J., 212, 215, 219, *222*, *223*
Fowler, C. A., 217, *222*, *224*
Fox, J. G., 125, 126, *142*
Fradis, A., 238, *254*
Francis, W. N., 161, *197*
Frank, J. S., 109, *144*
Fraser, B., 271, *292*
Fraser, C., 74, *94*
Frazier, L., 231, *253*
Freeman, F. N., 104, 105, 110, 111, 115, *142*
Freeman, R. H., 277, *293*
Friederici, A., 230, 237, *253*
Fries, C. C., 157, *197*
Frith, U., 165, *197*
Fromkin, V. A., 148, 157, 163, 164, 170, 171, 172, *197*, 216, *222*, 266, 267, 275, *292*
Fry, D. B., 148, *197*
Fujimura, O., 206, *222*
Funnell, E., 281, 284, 285, *291*

G
Galanter, E., 147, *198*
Galen, G. P. van, 104, *145*
Galvin, J., 234, *256*
Gandour, J., 18, *46*
Gardner, H., 228, 234, 236, 240, *253*
Garnica, O. K., 62, *95*
Garrett, M. F., 152, 164, 191, *197*, 229, 230, 234, *252*, *253*, 266, 267, 269, 284, 286, *291*, *292*
Gay, T., 205, 209, 212, *222*, *223*
Gelman, R., 60, 62, *95*
Genest, M., 131, 133, 138, *142*
Gentner, D. R., 61, 62, *95*, 117, 119, 120, 127, 134, *143*, 235, *253*
Geoffroy, A., 132, *143*
Geschwind, N., 148, 165, 185, *196*, 226, 227, *253*
Gibson, E. J., 173, *197*
Gigley, H., 231, *252*
Glanzer, M., 286, *292*
Gleason, J. B., 51, *95*, 236, *253*
Gleitman, H., 52, 89, 90, *97*
Gleitman, L. R., 52, 89, 90, *97*
Glucksberg, S., 63, *95*
Goldin-Meadow, S., 60, 62, *95*
Goldman-Eisler, F., 136, *142*, 160, *197*, 238, *253*
Goldstein, K., 269, *292*
Goldstein, U., 22, *46*
Golinkoff, R. M., 77, 78, *95*
Goodenough, C., 228, 230, *253*, *256*
Goodglass, H., 227, 231, 234, 235, 236, 237, 238, 242, 244, *251*, *252*, *253*, *255*
Gordon, B., 287, *292*
Gordon, N., 228, *255*
Gordon, P., 63, *95*
Gottlieb, J., *251*
Gray, W., 58, 68, *98*
Green, E., 228, 247, *253*, *256*
Greenberg, M. T., 62, *97*
Grieve, R., 63, 64, *96*
Grober, E., 234, *254*
Grosjean, F., 238, *254*
Grosjean, L., 238, *254*
Grossman, M., 234, *254*
Grudin, J. T., 117, 119, 126, 129, *143*
Gruendel, J., 58, *97*
Guinet, L., 173, *197*

H

Hafitz, J., 83, 86, 87, 92, *93*
Haggard, M. P., 214, *224*
Hall, R., 281, 288, *294*
Halle, M., 260, 261, 273, 290, *291*
Halliday, M. A. K., 7, *47*, 72, *96*
Halpin, G., 120, *143*
Halwes, T., 218, *222*
Hamby, S., 236, 240, 246, 248, *252*, *253*
Hammarberg, R. E., 207, 216, *222*
Hamp, E. H., 35, *47*
Hardwick, J., 104, 129, 131, 133, 136, *145*
Harris, Z. S., 30, *50*
Harrison, B., 56, *96*
Harter, N., 103, 104, 127, 133, *142*
Haselkorn, S., 7, *48*
Hattori, S., 206, *222*
Hawkins, B., 109, *144*
Hawkins, S., 9, 43, *47*
Hay, A., 63, *95*
Hayes, V., 120, *143*
Hebb, D. O., 110, *143*
Heeschen, C., 235, 237, *254*
Helm, N. A., 243, *254*
Henke, W. L., 216, *222*
Hernon, W. P., 281, 288, *294*
Hershman, R. L., 131, 136, *143*
Hier, D. B., 165, 166, *197*
Hill, A. A., 173, *197*
Hillix, W. A., 131, 136, *143*
Hirose, H., 209, *222*
Hockett, C. F., 148, 171, *197*
Hollerbach, J. M., 104, 106, *143*
Holt, K. G., 105, 109, *144*
Hood, L., 76, *93*
Hoogenraad, R., 63, 64, *96*
Hooper, P. J., 80, *96*
Hotopf, W. H. N., 148, 149, 150, 152, 155, 159, 160, 170, *197*
Howard, D., 284, *291*
Howe, C. J., 66, 77, *96*
Howell, P., 213, 218, *222*, *223*
Howes, D., 272, 286, *292*
Huber, W., 271, *294*
Hutcheson, S., 60, *95*
Huttenlocher, J., 59, 61, *96*
Hutton, A., *254*
Hyde, M., 236, *253*
Hymes, D., 72, *96*

I

Ingram, D., 9, 15, 17, 20, 23, 29, *47*
Itkonen, T., 11, *47*

J

Jaeger, J. J., *47*
Jaffe, T., 6, *49*
Jakimik, J., 171, *196*
Jakobson, R., 13, *47*
Jarvella, R. J., 173, *199*
Jastrzembski, J., 286, *292*
Johnson, C. N., 62, *96*, *98*
Johnson, D., 58, 68, *98*
Johnson-Laird, P. N., 55, 62, *97*
Jones, L. G., 6, *47*
Jones, R. G., 131, 133, *145*
Jordan, M. I., 117, *143*

K

Kanarick, A. F., 124, 127, *141*
Kaplan, E., 227, 236, 238, *253*
Karmiloff-Smith, A., 73, 83, *96*
Katz, J. J., 57, *96*
Kavanagh, J., 4, *50*
Kay, D. A., 60, 61, *96*
Kay, J., 263, 290, *292*
Kay, P., 58, *93*, *96*
Kean, M. L., 229, *254*, 288, *292*
Keating, P. A., 17, *50*
Kellar, L., 229, 234, *254*
Kelly, W. J., 214, *223*
Kent, R. D., 37, *47*, 135, *143*, 209, *222*
Kerschensteiner, M., 271, *294*
Kertesz, A., 236, *252*
Kinkead, R., 127, *143*
Kirk, R., 136, 138, *141*
Kisseberth, C. W., 17, *47*
Klatt, D. H., 136, *143*, 242, *254*
Klein, E., 266, *292*
Klemmer, E. T., 127, *143*
Klitzke, D., 131, *144*
Knoll, R. L., 104, 120, 126, *145*
Kolk, H. H. L., 228, *254*
Korte, S. S., 36, *47*
Koster, W. G., 104, *145*
Kreindler, A., 238, *254*
Kripke, S. A., 55, *96*

Kristofferson, A. B., 120, *146*
Kroemer, K. H. E., 127, *143*
Kucera, H., 161, *197*
Kuczaj, S. A., 63, 73, *96*
Kugler, P. N., 105, 109, *143, 144*
Kuhl, P. K., 214, *222*

L

Labov, W., 58, *96*
Lackner, L. R., 136, 138, *141*
Lacquaniti, F., 107, *145*
Ladefoged, P., 203, *222*
Lahy, J. M., 120, 124, *143*
Lane, H., 238, *254*
LaRochelle, S., 126, *143*
Lashley, K. S., 110, *143*, 148, *198*
Laver, J. D. M., 157, 163, 164, 171, 172, *196, 198*
Lea, W. A., 239, *254*
Lecours, A. R., 148, 185, *198*, 236, 246, 247, 249, *254*
Lehiste, I., *222*
Lehman, S., 110, *146*
Lenneberg, E. H., 159, *198*
Leonard, L. B., 13, *48*
Leopold, W. F., 5, 38, *47*, 56, *96*
Levine, D. N., 226, 227, *254*
Levy-Schoen, A., 136, *143*
Lewis, M. M., 56, *96*
Lewis, S. S., 286, *293*
Llermitte, F., 165, *198*, 247, *254*
Liberman, A. M., 203, 208, 210, 215, 218, *222*
Lichtheim, L., 283, *292*
Lieberman, P., 171, *198*, 238, 241, *254*
Lifter, K., 83, 86, 87, 92, *93*
Lightbown, P., 76, *93*
Lindau, M., 203, *222*
Lindblom, B. E. F., 136, *143*, 205, 209, 212, *223*
Linell, P. 42, *47*
Lisker, L., 214, 216, *221*
Lock, A., 51, *96*
Lubker, J. F., 205, 212, 216, *223*
Luria, A. R., 223, 234, 237, *254*
Lyberg, B., 242, *254*
Lyons, J., 54, 55, *96*, 257, 273, *292*

M

McAllister, R., *254*
McBride, K. E., 227, *255*
McCawley, J., 75, *96*
McClelland, J. L., 136, *143*
McCollum, G., 107, 110, 112, *145*
McDill, J. A., 110, *145*
McDonald, J. S., 106, *143*
Mace, W., 105, *145*, 216, *224*
Macken, M. A., 5, 9, 10, 11, 13, 17, 19, 20, *46, 47*
MacKay, D. G., 148, 163, 164, 171, 195, *196, 198*
Maclay, H., 157, 158, *198*
McLoughlin, P., 284, *291*
MacNeilage, P. F., 104, 136, *143*, 148, *198*, 216, *223*
McNeill, D., 53, 71, *97*, 157, *198*
McShane, J., 51, 53, 56, 59, 72, 83, *97*
MacWhinney, B., 5, 10, 42, *47, 48*
Maeda, S., 239, *254*
Malikouti-Drachman, A., 43, *46*
Manels, L., 276, 277, *293*
Maratsos, M. P., 63, 71, 84, 87, 91, *96, 97*
Marcel, A., 263, 290, *292*
Marie, P., 227, *255*
Marin, O. S. M., 225, 228, 232, *255*, 287, *293*
Marshall, J. C., 181, *196, 198*, 248, *255*, 278, 288, *292*
Martin, J. G., 136, *144*, 241, *255*
Marvin, R. S., 62, *97*
Massaro, D. W., 131, *144*
Massey, K. P., 17, *46*
Matthei, E., 231, *252*
Mayer, K., 148, 149, *198*
Maysner, M. S., 126, *144*
Menn, L., 5, 6, 7, 13, 15, 23, 25, 26, 28, 34, 39, 42, *47, 48, 50*
Menyuk, P., 11, 39, *48*, 220, *223*
Meringer, R., 148, 149, 184, *198*
Merrick, N. L., 104, *142*
Merton, P. A., 110, *144*
Mervis, C. B., 58, 68, *98*
Michel, F., 111, *144*
Michon, J. A., 120, *144*
Mihailescu, L., 238, *254*
Miller, G. A., 55, 62, 70, *97*, 147, *198*, 258, 289, *293*
Miller, J. D., 214, *222, 223*

Miller, J. L., 214, *222*
Minfie, F. D., 135, *143*
Miscione, J. L., 62, *97*
Mohr, J. P., 165, 166, *197*
Moll, K., 209, *222*
Monsell, S., 104, 120, 126, *145*
Morasso, P., 106, *141*
Morton, J., 173, 180, 192, *198*, 260, 269, 270, 271, 282, 283, 286, 288, 289, *291, 293*
Moskowitz, A., 5, 11, 29, 36, *48*
Motley, M. T., 148, 171, 195, *196, 198*
Murphy, C. M., 66, *97*
Murray, D., 63, 64, *96*
Murrell, G. A., 173, *198*, 271, *293*
Myerson, R., 42, *48*, 228, 230, 234, *256*

N

Naeser, M. A., 43, *48*, 234, *255*
Nakazima, S., 11, *48*
Nau, H., 154, 171, *199*
Nauclér, K., 148, 185, *198*
Neiser, J. J., 281, 288, *294*
Neisser, U., 212, *223*
Nelson, K. E., 58, 62, 89, 90, *97*
Newcombe, F., 181, *198*, 272, 286, 287, *293*
Newman, S. E., 159, *198*
Newport, E. L., 52, 89, 90, *97*
Nicholson, L. R., 159, *198*
Ninio, A., 66, *97*
Nooteboom, S. G., 163, 164, 184, *198*, *199*, 203, 215, *223*
Norman, D. A., 117, 120, 132, *143, 144*
North, E., 233, 234, *255*

O

Obler, L., 236, *253*
O'Brien, R. G., 62, *97*
Ohman, S. E. G., 135, *144*
Oldfield, R. C., 272, 286, 287, *293*
Oliva, J., 246, 247, *253*
Oller, D. K., 63, *95*
O'Regan, K., 136, *143*
Osgood, C. E., 157, 158, *198*
O'Shaughnessy, D., 239, *255*
Oshika, B. T., 154, 171, *199*
Ostry, D. J., 104, 126, *144*

P

Paccia-Cooper, J., 238, *253*
Paillard, J., 115, 117, *144*
Palermo, D. S., 63, *97, 99*
Papcun, G., 203, *222*
Parkes, C. H., 234, *253*
Pastore, R. E., 214, *223*
Patterson, K., 181, *196*, 278, 288, 289, *292, 293*
Peizer, D. B., 7, *46*
Perecman, E., 234, *254*
Perkell, J. S., 212, 216, *223, 224*
Perkell, K., 117, *144*
Peters, A. M., 6, 43, *48*
Pew, R. W., 115, *144*
Pick, A., 236, *255*
Pinker, S., 71, *97*
Pisoni, D. B., 214, *223*
Platt, C., 10, *48*
Poeck, K., 271, *294*
Polit, A. 106, *141*
Postal, P. M., 57, *97*
Potter, J. M., 148, *199*
Potter, R. K., 207, *223*
Pribram, K. H., 147, *198*
Priestly, T. M. S., 19, 20, *48*
Prins, R., 238, *255*
Putnam, H., 55, *97*

Q

Qualster, H., 120, *144*
Quinn, J. T., 109, *144*

R

Raffler-Engel, W. von, 6, *49*
Rapp, K., 136, *143*
Rayner, K., 192, *199*
Reich, P. A., 172, *196*
Remez, R. E., 217, *222*
Rescorla, L., 58, *97*
Richards, M. M., 62, 63, *98*
Riordan, C. J., 204, 212, *223*
Robaye, E., 238, *253*
Rochford, G., 236, *255*
Rosch, E., 58, 68, *98*
Rosen, S. M., 213, 214, *223*
Rosner, B. S., 213, *222*
Ross, J. R., 158, *199*

Rouillon, F., 236, 246, 249, *254*
Rubenstein, H., 286, *293*
Rubenstein, M. A., 286, *293*
Rubin, G. S., 277, *293*
Rubin, P., 217, *222*
Rubin, W., 231, *255*
Rumelhart, D. E., 117, 120, *144*, 158, *199*
Ryan, J., *199*

S

Saffran, E. M., 225, 228, 232, *255*, 287, *293*
Sander, E. K., 22, *48*
Scarborough, D. L., 286, *293*
Scarborough, H. S., 286, *293*
Schaffer, H. R., 51, *98*
Schieffelin, B. S., 80, *98*
Schlesinger, I. M., 75, 76, 78, *98*
Schmidt, R. A., 109, *144*
Schulhoff, C., 242, 244, *253*
Schwartz, M. F., 225, 228, 232, *255*, 287, *293*
Schwartz, R. G., 13, *47*, *48*
Schwartz, S. P., 55, *98*
Scott Kelso, J. A., 105, 109, *143*, *144*
Seligman, M., 60, 62, *95*
Severeid, L. R., 209, *222*
Shaffer, L. H., 104, 120, 127, 129, 131, 133, 135, 136, *144*, *145*, *199*
Shallice, T., 279, 289, *293*
Shankweiler, D. P., 215, 218, *222*, *223*
Shapiro, B. E., 232, 242, 243, 244, *253*
Shattuck, S. R., 162, 185, *199*
Shatz, M., 60, *98*
Shaw, R., 105, *145*, 216, *224*
Simon, C., 219, *223*
Simonini, R. C., 148, *199*
Skinner, B., 71, *98*
Slobin, D. I., 3, *48*, 71, 75, 76, 78, 80, 87, *98*
Smith, B. L., 17, *49*
Smith, N. V., 5, 9, 11, 17, 24, 27, *49*, 281, *293*
Snodgrass, J. G., 173, *199*
Snow, C., 6, *49*, 51, 62, *98*, 238, *255*
Solomon, R. L., 286, *292*
Sorensen, J. M., 232, 239, 242, 243, 248, *253*

Søvik, N., 104, *145*
Stachowiak, F. J., 271, *294*
Stampe, D., 23, *49*
Stanley, S., 63, *96*
Stanners, R. F., 281, 288, *294*
Stansfield, R. G., 125, 126, *142*
Stark, L., 110, *145*, *146*
Statlender, S., 231, 235, *251*, *252*
Steinberg, J. C., 207, *223*
Stelmach, G. E., 124, *145*
Stengel, M. L., 246, 247, *253*
Sternberg, S., 104, 120, 126, *145*
Sterne, D., 6, *49*
Stetson, R. H., 110, *145*
Stevens, K. N., 22, *49*, 212, *223*, *224*
Stockert, T. R. von, 228, *255*
Stokes, W., 242, *255*
Stone, J. B., 63, *94*
Strackee, J., 104, 106, *142*
Strange, W., 214, 218, 221, *223*, *224*
Studdert-Kennedy, M., 203, 215, *222*, *224*
Summerfield, A. Q., 214, 218, *221*, *224*
Sweet, E., 226, 227, *254*
Swinney, D. A., 178, *199*, 229, *255*, 271, *294*

T

Taborelli, A., 165, *196*
Tackeff, J., 77, *93*
Taft, M., 173, *199*, 277, *294*
Terzuolo, C. A., 107, 109, 113, 114, 115, 117, 118, 120, 121, 122, 123, 124, 125, 126, 127, 129, 130, 132, 134, 138, 139, *145*
Teulings, J. L. H. M., 106, *145*
Tharp, D., 276, 277, *293*
Thomas, E. A. C., 131, 133, *145*
Thomassen, A. J. W. M., 106, *145*
Thompson, S. A., 80, *96*
Thomson, J. R., 59, 60, *98*
Thuring, J. Ph., 104, 105, 106, 115, *142*
Todd, P., 148, 152, 153, *196*
Tonkonogy, J., 227, *255*
Townsend, D. J., 63, *98*
Trehub, S. E., 63, *98*
Tresselt, M. E., 126, *144*
Tuller, B., 217, *224*

Turvey, M. T., 105, 109, *143, 144, 145,* 216, 217, *222, 224*
Tweel, L. H. van der, 115, *145*

U

Ulatowski, H., 228, *255*
Ushijima, T., 209, *222*

V

Velten, H. V., 17, *49*
Verbrugge, R. R., 218, *223*
Vignolo, L. A., 165, *196*
Vihman, M. M., 15, 19, 25, *49*
Villiers, J. G., de, 72, 83, 86, *95,* 232, 241, 244, *253*
Villiers, P. A. de, 83, *95*
Viviani, P., 107, 109, 110, 112, 113, 114, 115, 117, 118, 120, 121, 122, 123, 124, 125, 126, 127, 129, 130, 132, 134, 138, 139, *145*
Vogel, I., 43, *49*
Vorster, J., 52, *98*
Vredenbregt, J., 104, *145*
Vygotsky, L., 59, *98*

W

Wagenaar, E., 238, *255*
Wales, R. J., 63, 72, *94, 95, 98*
Walker, E. C. T., 234, *253*
Warden, D., 62, *98*
Waters, R. S., 214, *224*
Waterson, N., 9, 29, 30, 31, 35, 37, *49*
Weeks, R. V., 154, 171, *199*
Weeks, T., 7, *46*
Weintraub, S., 51, *95,* 230, 236, *253*
Weir, R., 6, 38, *50*
Weisenberg, T. H., 227, *255*
Welford, A. T., 109, *146*
Wellman, H. M., 62, *96, 98*
Wellmers, W. E., 30, *50*

Wernicke, C., 283, *294*
Westbury, J. R., 17, *50*
Wexler, K., 71, *99*
Whaley, C. P., 272, 286, *294*
White, T. G., 67, *99*
Wells, R., 148, *199*
Whitehouse, P., 234, *255*
Wickelgren, W. A., *199,* 211, *224*
Wieman, L., 77, *99*
Wieneke, G. H., 115, *142*
Wier, C. C., 214, *223*
Wilbur, R. B., 9, 42, *50*
Wilcox, M. J., 13, *47*
Wilcox, S., 63, *99*
Wilson, W. A., 214, *224*
Wing, A. M., 103, 104, 105, 110, 115, 120, *146,* 148, 150, 185, *199*
Wingfield, A., 272, 286, 287, *293*
Winnick, W. A., 283, *294*
Wise, C. M., 206, *224*
Wright, C. E., 104, 120, 126, *145*
Wright, P., 115, *141*

Y

Yamamoto, K., 206, *222*
Yarbus, A. L., 110, *146*
Yasuhara, M., 104, *146*
Yeni-Komshian, G. H., 4, *50,* 216, 218, 220, *221*

Z

Zangemeister, W. H., 110, *146*
Zelaznik, H., 109, *144*
Zimmer, K., 259, *294*
Zue, V. W., 154, 171, *199*
Zurif, E. B., 216, 218, 220, *221,* 228, 229, 230, 234, 235, 236, 237, 240, *251, 252, 253, 255, 256,* 284, 286, *291*
Zwicky, A. M., 39, *50*

Subject Index

A

Action theory,
  of handwriting, 105–106, 108
  of speech processing, 216–219
Anagrammatic word formation, *see*
  Letter anticipation error
Angular velocity, in handwriting, 107
Anomic aphasia, 165, 227, 237–238, 268
  form-class effects in, 165, 238
Anticipation error, 151, 159, 164
  absolute frequency of, 154–157
  frequency of, 151, 155
  letter, 184–192
  phoneme, 162–163, 266
Aphasia, *see* names of specific
  syndromes
Articulation,
  developmental model of, 28–36
  models of, 211, 214–221
  rules, in children, 21–28
  strategies in children, 12–21
  variations in, 204–209
Articulatory program,
  metaphor in phonological acquisition,
  32–36
Assimilation strategy, 15, 16, 17
Attention,
  as source of letter level slips, 164–165,
  191–192
  as source of lexical errors, 161–162,
  176–178
  variable in imitation tasks, 39
Auditory features, 211–214
Avoidance strategy, 13, 17, 18

B

Babble, 5–7
  circular babble, 40
Biomechanical factors,
  in handwriting, 105–115
  in typing, 117–122
Blends, 156, 159
  absolute frequency of, 154–157
  frequency of, 153, 155

Broca's aphasia, 226–227, 283
  assignment of reference in, 230
  comprehension strategies in, 228–229,
  231–232
  comprehension of syntax in, 228–233,
  250
  production of prosody in, 230–233,
  240, 241–246
  production of syntax in, 228, 231, 232,
  233, 243–248, 250
  relation between comprehension and
  production in, 228–233, 250–251,
  284
  speech planning in, 232–233, 240,
  242–243, 244–246

C

Canonical forms,
  in phonological rule acquisition, 29–
  30, 33–36
Case grammar, 75–82
Categories, 58
Change,
  lexical, 66
  in syntactic rules, 72, 92–93
Co-articulation, 15–16, 43, 204, 207, 211
  anticipatory, 218
  explanation of, 208–209
Cognition hypothesis,
  exposition of, 71
  in grammatical development, 82–84
Colour adjectives,
  comprehension and production, 62–
  63
  input factors in acquisition, 68–69
Communicative intent, 7, 40–41, 75
Compensatory articulation, 205
Conspiracy rule, 17–19
Continuation rise, 239, 240, 244 *see also,*
  Fundamental frequency
Contrastive feature theory,
  exposition of, 57
  problems with, 57, 58–59

Control aspects,
　in handwriting, 105, 106, 115, 116, 140
　in typing, 120, 140
Covert slips, 173–178

D

Declination, *see also* Fundamental
　frequency, 239, 240, 242, 243, 248,
　249, 250
　resetting, 239, 240, 242
Denotation, 55, 56
Derivational morpheme, 264–266, 273
　in aphasic speech, 268–269
　decomposition into, in reading, 276–
　278
　error in agraphics, 279
　error in dyslexics, 278
　priming effects on, 281–282
　slips in, 267, 268, 274–276
Devoicing, 17–18, 26
Diary studies, 60
Digram, 124, 129
　frequency effects on typing speed,
　124–126, 127
　interval, 135
　variability, 134
Dimensional adjectives,
　acquisition of, 64–65, 68, 91
Disharmonic sequence, 17, 20
Dogs, brains of, 158–159
Dyslexia,
　deep, 161, 181, 278–279, 288
　phonological, 278

E

Embryonic theory,
　in phonological acquisition, 3, 38, 45
Environment *see* Input
Evolution of langauge, 212, 214 *see also*
　speech specific mechanisms
Exploitation strategy, 13–14
Extension, 55
External constraints, on handwriting,
　115–116

F

Favoured phonemes, 22
Feature models, of speech processing,
　211–214

Fluency, 227
　fluent v. non-fluent distinction, 226,
　238
Form classes, in early syntactic
　development, 84–87, 91–92
Form class errors,
　in children, 84–87
　closed-class, 171, 183, 184–188, 194–
　195
　frequency of, 153–157, 158
　open class, 151–152, 170–171, 183–
　184, 194–195
Formant,
　frequency, 204, 205, 206, 207
　transition, 210, 219
Fitts law, 109–110
Fundamental frequency (F_0), 238
　in Broca aphasic speech, 230–233,
　241–246
　in Wernicke aphasic speech, 236

G

General systems theory, 52–54
Grammatical rules,
　acquisition of, 41–43, 70–73, 78–82,
　84, 85, 88–90, 262–263, 274
　in aphasics, 228–238, 250–251, 268–
　269, 284
　in dyslexics, 278
　lexical representation of, 264, 270–
　271, 282
　in slips of the tongue, 266–267
Graphological lexicon, 181, 182

H

Haplography, 186, 192
Haplology, 275
Haplophony, 189
Hesitations, *see also* Pauses
　discourse function of, 158
　lexical access function of, 160
Homophone error, 152, 159, 179, 168,
　169, 185, 186
　absolute frequency of, 154–157
　explanation of, 179, 181
　frequency of, 153, 155
Homothetic behaviours, 104, 115
　space, 110, 113
　time, 110, 113, 114, 128, 129

I

Idioms, 271–272
Imitation, 36–40
Immediate repetition error,
  absolute frequency of, 154–157
  definition of, 151
  frequency of, 151, 155
Inertia effects, on articulation, 208, 215, 216
Inflectional morpheme, 264, 273
  acquisition of, 41–43, 82–87, 88–90
  errors in dyslexics, 278–279
  slips of the tongue in, 267, 268
  in Wernicke aphasics, 266, 268–269
Innateness,
  of cognitive capacities, 75, 76
  of grammatical categories, 53
  of phoneme perception, 212–214, 219–220
  of production rules, 71
Input lexicon, see Two lexicon models
Input – output relations,
  in language acquisition,
  in grammatical development, 71, 84, 88–90
  in lexical development 65–70
  impoverishment of input, 52
Intension, 55
Intervention studies, 89–90
Intonation contour, *see* Fundamental frequency
Invariance, 104
  in articulation, 216–219
  in handwriting, 105–117
  in typing, 117–124, 128*, 129, 140
Isochrony, 104, 111, 113
  interaction with Isogony, 110, 112
  in typing speed, 129
Isogony principle, 104,
  in handwriting, 106–109, 115
Item-by-item learning, 84

J

Jargon aphasia, *see* Wernicke's aphasia

L

Letter level errors,
  anticipatory, 184–192
  categories of, 163
  explanations of, 163–165

Lexicon,
  form class effects in, 229–230, 250, 260, 284, 286–288, 289
  frequency effects in, 229–230, 250, 260, 272, 286–288
  full-listing hypothesis in, 260, 261–272, 289
  irregular forms in, 259, 264
  modality-specificity, 259–260, 270, 280–285, 290
  parsimony of, 259, 264
  separation of hearing and speaking, in, 260, 285
  unit of organization, 260, 269–270, 271, 273–280, 288–290
  see also Two Lexicon Model
Lexical access,
  errors, in aphasics, 162–163, 164, 229–233, 238, 240, 248–249, 250, 268–269
  errors, in children, 59, 61
  frequency effects in, 229–230, 250, 260, 272
  selection time effects, on, 159–161, 174, 175, 194–195
  slips, in speech, 151–152, 154–162, 169–171, 175, 176, 181, 182–184, 194
  slips, in writing, 151–152, 154–162, 175, 177–178, 183, 184, 194–195
Lexical exceptions, 24, 25, 26
  theoretical implications, 28–29
Lexical rules, 259, 262–266, 269–270, 289–290
  context effects on, 263–264, 290
  derivational, 274–279
  fall-back rules, 262, 263, 269, 274, 280, 290
  irregular forms, 259, 263–264, 270
  overlearned rules, 262, 263, 274
Lexical smoothing, 25, 27, 28
Lexical stress, effects of,
  on Broca aphasic comprehension, 229
  on Broca aphasic speech, 242
  on retrieval errors, 274–275
Limited scope formula,
  for two word utterances, 73, 78–82, 87, 91
  for verb inflections, 87
Linear extent, in handwriting, 110, 111
Logogen theory, 269–270

M

Mean length of utterance (M.L.U.), 83
Malapropisms,
  access, 182–184
  storage, 183
Means–ends separation,
  in phonological development, 40–41
Medium of transmission effects,
  in articulation, 206, 215
Metalinguistic awareness,
  phonological, 13, 42
Misspellings, 159, 185, 186
  categories of, 178–181
  explanation of, 181–184
Modulated babble, 5–6
Morpheme, *see also,* Derivational
  morpheme, Inflectional morpheme
  priming effects, 271, 281–282
  stranding, 267–268, 269, 282–283
  as unit of lexical organization, 266–
  269, 273, 288–290
Morse code, 103, 127, 133
Motor equivalence, 104
  in handwriting, 110, 113, 140
Motor commands,
  in articulation, 208
    overlap of, 208–216
  in perception, 216
  in typing, 135–138
Motor theory,
  of speech processing, 215–216, 219
Mush-mouthed kids, 6, 43

N

Naming,
  input for, 66–69
Neologisms, 227, 236, 240
  location of, 247
  special generation device for, 246–
  249, 250–251, 268–269
Non-linguistic bias, 63–64
Non-natural rules,
  in early articulation, 23, 27

O

One-word omissions,
  absolute frequency of, 154–157
  in closed-class words, 161
  frequency of, 151, 155

Onomatopoeia, 5
Oscillatory system, *see* Spring–Mass
  model
Output constraints,
  articulation model, 16–19
  on consonant clusters, 17
  explanation of phonological
  acquisition, 28, 30–32
Output lexicon, *see* Two lexicon models
Overextensions, of names,
  as a communicative strategy, 59, 61
  in comprehension, 60–62
  input factors in, 67–68
  in production, 56–59
Overgeneralization,
  of phonological rules, 26–29
  of syntactic rules, 85, 262–263, 274
Overregularization, *see*
  overgeneralization

P

Paraphasias, 227, 240, 249, *see also*
  Neologisms
Patterns in typing
  higher order, 135–137
  subunits, 133–135
Pauses,
  in Broca aphasic speech, 242–243
  in Wernicke aphasic speech, 236, 246–
  249, 250–251, 268–269
Perception, of phonemes, 203, 210
  adult human, 212–214
  animal, 214, 219
  bilinguals, 216, 218–219, 220
  children, 37, 219, 220–221
Perception, of non-speech sounds,
  adult human, 213–214, 219, 220
Phoneme sequencing, 208–209, 214, 215
Phoneme variation in production, 204–
  209
Phonemic level slips, 162–163, 266–267
Phonetic spelling errors, *see* Misspellings
Phonological-graphological conversion,
  159–161, 172–173, 194
  breakdown of, 285
  in letter anticipation effects, 189–190
  in letter level errors, 163–164
  in misspellings, 181–182

Phonological idioms, 29
  misspellings as, 180–181
  role in early articulation, 31–32
Phonological rules, 171, 259–261
  allophonic, 41, 42–43
  allomorphic, 41–42, 43
  creation of, 21–27, 28
  generalisation of, 25–27
  productivity of, 41–42
  in slips of the pen, 183–184, 188–190
  in slips of the tongue, 163, 163–165, 188–190
  strategies of articulation, 4–16
Phonological similarity, 165
  explanation of structural slips, 159
  in speech errors, 163
  in writing errors, 163, 167–169
Polymorphemic words,
  irregular, 272
  lexical representation of, 261, 273–280
  slips of the tongue, and, 267–268
Pre-articulatory editing, see also Covert slips, suppressed slips, 171–172
Pre-phonemic speech, 11–12
Priming effects, 271, 281–282, 288–289
  cross modal, 283, 289
Problem-solving,
  theory of phonological acquisition, 3, 38–41, 45
  theory of syntactic development, 83
Productivity,
  of grammatical rules, 82–83
  of phonological rules, 41–42
Prototype,
  input strategy, 67–68
  theory in grammatical development, 72, 73, 86–87
  theory in lexical development, 58–59
Protowords, 5–7
Pseudowords, 126, 131, 132

Q

Quasi-homophone error, 159, 168, 169, 180

R

Radius of curvature, in handwriting, 107, 108, 112

Rate modulation, see also Timing of strokes, in typing, 140
Recidivism, see Overregularization
Reference,
  definition of, 54–55, 56
  input for, 66–69
Relative onset time, 214, 220
Repetition error, 158
  absolute frequency of, 154–157,
  frequency of, 151, 155
Resonant frequency, 204

S

Segmentation in typing, 131
Segmentation, in handwriting, 115,
  continuous model, 105–109, 110
  discontinuous effects, 106–115, 140
Self-monitoring,
  phonological 10–11, 37–39
Semantic categories,
  criteria for inference of, 77–82
  generality of, 78–82
  relation to cognition, 78
Semantic Feature Theory, 91
  exposition of, 57
  in non-lexical domains, 63–65
  problems with, 57, 58–59, 62
Semantic features, see also Semantic Feature Theory
  aphasic comprehension of, 234–235
  comprehension of, 234
  development of, 57–65
Sense, 55–56
Sensory feedback, see also Visual feedback
  in handwriting, 115, 118
  in typing, 124
Short term memory, 159, 175
  demands, in speech and writing, 159–162, 163–164
  explanation of speech errors, 176–177
  explanation of written errors, 177–178, 194
Silent period, 6, 40
Slips of the pen, see Letter level errors, Lexical access slips, Misspellings
Slips of the tongue, see Lexical access slips, Morpheme stranding, Phonemic level errors

Sound play, 6
Span ahead,
  of speech and writing, 159
Speech production models, 170–173, 266–268
  parallel v. sequential, 170
Speech prosody,
  in Broca aphasics, 240, 241–246, 250
  in normals, 238–239, 240–241
  in Wernicke aphasics, 240, 246–249, 250
Speech rate effects,
  on articulation, 208, 211, 215
  on perception, 214
Speech-specific mechanisms, 212, 219–220
Speech type,
  effects on errors, 156–157
Stem variants error, 169
  absolute frequency of, 154–157
  frequency of, 153–154, 155
Speed of execution, in handwriting, 110, 111
Spring-mass model, of handwriting,
  exposition of, 105, 106
  problems with, 106–115
State-output relations,
  in language acquisition, 53–54, 56, 71
Story grammar, 158
Strategy,
  phonological, in children, 12–21
Suppressed slips,
  verbal, 174
  written, 175–178, 186
Syllable stress,
  in lexical errors, 274–275
  in phoneme level errors, 163, 164
Symbols,
  development of, 7

T
Tangential velocity, in handwriting, 106, 107, 108, 110, 112, 114
Target invariance, see timing of strokes in typing
Task orientation,
  variable in imitation tasks, 39
Telegraphic speech,
  in aphasics, 226, 230, 232
  in children, 74

Template matching,
  model of speech processing, 211
  strategy in early articulation, 19–21
Terminal fall, 239, 240, 241, see also Fundamental frequency
Timing of strokes in typing
  pace keeping, 120, 122
  target invariance, 117–120
Trajectory, 105, 106, 107, 111
  Lissajou, 106
  segmentation of in handwriting, 105–109, 110, 106–115, 140
  in typing, 117, 119
Transformational grammar, 71–72
Transposition errors,
  reading, 192
  speech, 151, 154–157, 162–163, 164–165, 266–267
  suppressed, 175
  typing, 133, 136
  writing, 159–160, 163–165, 184–192
Trial-and-error learning,
  of phonological rules, 21, 24–25
Two lexicon models, for the production and comprehension of speech, 203–221, 280–281
  in aphasics, 228–237, 250–251, 283–285
  in phonological acquisition, 8–11, 32–36, 220–221
  in semantic acquisition, 60–62, 69, 92
Two-word combinations,
  pivot grammar, 74–75, 81
  semantic models of, 75–82
Typing speed,
  digram effects, 124–126
  higher-order effects, 137–138
  learning effects, 133, 140
  load compensation, 122–124
  random text effects, 132–133
  spacing effects, 131–133
  word effects, 127–131

U
Underextensions, of names, 61
  input factors in, 67–68

V
VOT see Voice Onset Time

Verbs,
  comprehension and production by Broca's aphasics, of, 231–232
  semantic development of, 62–63
  syntactic development of, 83
Visual feedback,
  in letter anticipation errors, 192–194
Vocal tract,
  size, effects of, 207, 211
  stable regions in, 212
  surgery on, 212, 215
Voice onset time, 11, 17, 212, 214, 216, 219, 220
Voicing, 17–18, 26

W

Wernicke's aphasia, 227, 228, 283
  comprehension, phonetic deficits in, 233–234, 237
  comprehension, semantic feature effects in, 234–235, 237
  comprehension, of syntax in, 235–236
  production, of syntax in, 236, 240
  production, failures of lexical access in, 236, 240, 268–269
  production, neologisms in, 236, 240, 268–269
  production, prosody in, 236, 248–249
  production, planning in, 240, 246–249
  relation between speech production and comprehension in, 233–237, 250–251, 284